Master the Dental Hygienist Exam

1st Edition

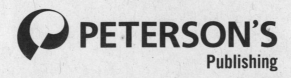

PETERSON'S

Publishing

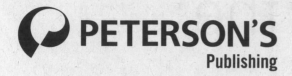

About Peterson's Publishing

To succeed on your lifelong educational journey, you will need accurate, dependable, and practical tools and resources. That is why Peterson's is everywhere education happens. Because whenever and however you need education content delivered, you can rely on Peterson's to provide the information, know-how, and guidance to help you reach your goals. Tools to match the right students with the right school. It's here. Personalized resources and expert guidance. It's here. Comprehensive and dependable education content—delivered whenever and however you need it. It's all here.

For more information, contact Peterson's Publishing, 2000 Lenox Drive, Lawrenceville, NJ 08648; 800-338-3282 Ext. 54229; or find us online at www.petersonspublishing.com.

© 2011 Peterson's, a Nelnet company

Facebook® and Facebook logos are registered trademarks of Facebook, Inc. Facebook, Inc. was not involved in the production of this book and makes no endorsement of this product.

Bernadette Webster, Director of Publishing; Mark D. Snider, Editor; Ray Golaszewski, Publishing Operations Manager; Linda M. Williams, Composition Manager

ISBN-13: 978-0-7689-3309-3
ISBN-10: 0-7689-3309-9

Printed in the United States of America

10 9 8 7 6 5 4 3 2 1   13 12 11

First Edition

By printing this book on recycled paper (40% post-consumer waste) 46 trees were saved.

Petersonspublishing.com/publishingupdates

Check out our Web site at www.petersonspublishing.com/publishingupdates to see if there is any new information regarding the test and any revisions or corrections to the content of this book. We've made sure the information in this book is accurate and up-to-date; however, the test format or content may have changed since the time of publication.

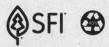

Certified Chain of Custody

60% Certified Fiber Sourcing and
40% Post-Consumer Recycled

www.sfiprogram.org

*This label applies to the text stock.

Sustainability—Its Importance to Peterson's Publishing

What does sustainability mean to Peterson's? As a leading publisher, we are aware that our business has a direct impact on vital resources—most especially the trees that are used to make our books. Peterson's Publishing is proud that its products are certified by the Sustainable Forestry Initiative (SFI) and that its books are printed on paper that is 40% post-consumer waste using vegetable-based ink.

Being a part of the Sustainable Forestry Initiative (SFI) means that all of our vendors—from paper suppliers to printers—have undergone rigorous audits to demonstrate that they are maintaining a sustainable environment.

Peterson's Publishing continuously strives to find new ways to incorporate sustainability throughout all aspects of its business.

Contents

PART I: A Career as a Dental Hygienist

Contents

PART II: Diagnosing Strengths and Weaknesses

PART III: NBDHE Component A Questions

PART IV: NBDHE Component B Questions

PART V: Two Practice Tests

APPENDIXES

SPECIAL ADVERTISING SECTION

f www.facebook.com/CareerResource

Before You Begin

OVERVIEW

- How this book is organized
- Special study features
- Special advertising section
- You are well on your way to success
- Find us on Facebook®

HOW THIS BOOK IS ORGANIZED

Dental hygienist is a good career choice for individuals who enjoy working with people and have an interest in proper dental care. Dental hygienists enjoy benefits such as job security, flexible schedules, and competitive salaries. The U.S. Bureau of Labor Statistics reports that the number of dental hygienist jobs is expected to grow 36 percent through 2018.

Those interested in becoming a dental hygienist must complete a 2-year associate degree or certificate program in dental hygiene accredited by the Commission on Dental Accreditation (CODA), pass the National Board Dental Hygiene Examination (NBDHE), pass a clinical exam, and apply for a license in their state. The American Dental Association's Joint Commission on National Dental Examinations (JCNDE) administers the NBDHE. State and regional testing agencies administer the clinical exam.

This book was carefully researched and written to help you prepare for the NBDHE. The chapters in this book explain what it is like to work as a dental hygienist and review important material that is likely to appear on the NBDHE. Completing the many practice exercises and practice tests in this book will help you pass this exam.

To get the most out of this book, take the time to read each section carefully and thoroughly.

- **Part I** provides an overview of a dental hygienist's job responsibilities and the places where dental hygienists work. It offers information about the education you need to become a dental hygienist and the subjects assessed on the NBDHE. Part I also outlines the steps you need to take to become a dental hygienist, including preparing and applying to take the NBDHE and how to become licensed.

- **Part II** is a preview of the written examination. This section introduces you to the kinds of questions you will see on the NBDHE, including questions about anatomy, histology and embryology, physiology, biochemistry and nutrition, microbiology and immunology, pathology and pharmacology, assessing patient characteristics, obtaining and interpreting radiographs, planning and managing dental hygiene care, performing periodontal procedures, using preventive agents, providing supportive treatment services, professional responsibility, promoting health and preventing disease within groups, participating in community programs, analyzing scientific literature, understanding statistical concepts, and applying research results.

- **Part III** is a comprehensive overview of the types of questions you will see on the NBHDE. A chapter is devoted to each subject area, or domain, on the test. Each chapter begins with a review of the subject matter to refresh your memory as to what you learned in school. At the end of each chapter are practice exercises. The multiple-choice questions in the practice exercises are just like those on the actual test. Complete the questions and study the answer explanations. You can learn a great deal from these explanations. Even if you answered the questions correctly, you may discover a new tip in the explanation that will help you answer other questions.

- When you feel that you are well prepared, move on to **Part IV**—the practice tests. These practice examinations contain new questions modeled after the samples provided in the *NBDHE Guide*, published by the Joint Commission on National Dental Examinations (JCNDE), the agency responsible for the development and administration of the National Board Dental Examinations. The questions on the practice tests in this book are not the *actual* questions that you will see on the exam. If possible, try to work through an entire exam in one sitting. On the actual test, you have 3.5 hours to complete the discipline-based items, and 4 hours to complete the patient-case items; there is a scheduled 1-hour break between the two sessions. Do not look at the correct answer until you have completed the exam. Remember, these tests are for practice and will not be scored. Take the time to learn from any mistakes you may make.

- The **Appendixes section** offers a list of abbreviations used on the NBDHE and a list of references recommended by the JCNDE. Study the abbreviations until you are sure that you know them. Consult the references if you are having trouble remembering information in a particular subject area.

SPECIAL STUDY FEATURES

Master the Dental Hygienist Exam is designed to be as user-friendly as it is complete. To this end, it includes several features to make your preparation more efficient.

Overview

Each chapter begins with a bulleted overview listing the topics covered in the chapter. This allows you to target the areas in which you are most interested.

Summing It Up

Each chapter ends with a point-by-point summary that reviews the most important items in the chapter. The summaries offer a convenient way to review key points.

Notes

Notes highlight need-to-know information about the NBDHE, whether it is details about scoring or the structure of a question type.

Tips

Tips provide valuable strategies and insider information to help you score your best on the NBDHE.

SPECIAL ADVERTISING SECTION

At the end of the book, don't miss the special section of ads placed by Peterson's preferred clients. Their financial support helps make it possible for Peterson's Publishing to continue to provide you with the highest-quality test-prep, educational exploration, and career-preparation resources you need to succeed on your educational journey.

YOU ARE WELL ON YOUR WAY TO SUCCESS

You have made the decision to become a dental hygienist and have taken a very important step in that direction. *Master the Dental Hygienist Exam* will help you score high and prepare you for everything you need to know on the day of the exam and beyond it. Good luck!

FIND US ON FACEBOOK®

Join the career conversation on Facebook® at www.facebook.com/CareerResource and receive additional test-prep tips and advice. Peterson's resources are available to help you do your best on these important exams—and others in your future.

GIVE US YOUR FEEDBACK

Peterson's publishes a full line of books—career preparation, test prep, education exploration, and financial aid. Peterson's publications can be found at high school guidance offices, college libraries and career centers, and your local bookstore and library. Peterson's books are now also available as eBooks.

We welcome any comments or suggestions you may have about this publication. Your feedback will help us make educational dreams possible for you—and others like you.

A Career as a Dental Hygienist

CHAPTER 1

What Is a Dental Hygienist?

OVERVIEW

- **Where dental hygienists work**
- **Educational requirements**
- **National Board Dental Hygiene Examination (NBDHE)**
- **Clinical examinations**
- **Salary and benefits**
- **Employment outlook**
- **Credentials**
- **The American Dental Hygienists' Association (ADHA)**
- **Advancement opportunities**
- **Summing it up**

Today's dental hygienists are performing tasks that were once performed by dentists. Dental hygienists have taken on these additional tasks because the population has grown, people now retain their teeth longer than they used to, and more emphasis is now placed on preventive dental care.

Dental hygienists of the twenty-first century clean teeth, educate patients on the best oral hygiene practices, and examine teeth for diseases or other abnormalities. They also take X-rays and sometimes make a diagnosis based on their findings.

WHERE DENTAL HYGIENISTS WORK

The vast majority of dental hygienists work in dentist offices. A very small number of hygienists work for employment services and in physician offices. The flexible schedule attracts many to the profession of dental hygiene. Hygienists are often hired to work 2 or 3 days a week, and therefore, may work part time if they choose to do so. Those who seek full-time employment may work for a single dentist or in multiple dentist offices. They are often able to work in the evening and during the weekend.

EDUCATIONAL REQUIREMENTS

To become a dental hygienist, you need a degree or certificate from a dental hygiene school that is accredited by the Commission on Dental Accreditation (CODA). Then you must take and pass the National Board Dental Hygiene

Examination (NBDHE), a regional or state clinical board examination and obtain a state license. Most programs offer a 2-year associate degree but some also offer a certificate, a bachelor's degree, or a master's degree. As of 2008, 301 dental hygiene programs were accredited by the Commission on Dental Accreditation (CODA). These schools offer laboratory, clinical, and classroom instruction. You can search for accredited colleges in your state on the American Dental Association's Web site (www.ada.org). It is recommended that high school students who want to pursue a career as a dental hygienist should take courses in biology, chemistry, and mathematics.

The course sequence for a dental hygienist program at an accredited college might look like this:

First Semester:
Head and Neck Anatomy
Microscopic Anatomy
Dental Hygiene Theory I
Oral Anatomy and Occlusion
Infection and Immunity
Dental Radiology
Periodontics I

Second Semester:
Dental Hygiene Theory II
Preventive Oral Health Education
Clinical Dental Hygiene I/Seminar
Nutrition
Dental Materials
Oral Pathology
Periodontics II

Third Semester:
Dental Hygiene Theory III
Community Dental Health
Clinical Dental Hygiene II/Seminar
Research Methods and Study Design
Management of Medicine Compromised/Medical
    Emergencies
Pharmacology and Pain Control

Fourth Semester:
Dental Hygiene Theory IV
Community Oral Dental Health Practicum
Current Issues, the Law and Ethics
Clinical Dental Hygiene III/Seminar

NATIONAL BOARD DENTAL HYGIENE EXAMINATION (NBDHE)

A dental hygiene student in an accredited dental hygiene program may take the National Board Dental Hygiene Examination (NBDHE) before graduation if the hygiene program director certifies that the student is prepared for the examination. A dental hygiene student might also wait until after graduation to take the exam. All graduates of dental hygiene programs from accredited colleges are eligible to take the examination once the Joint Commission of National Dental Examinations (JCNDE) has received evidence of graduation.

Graduates of non-accredited dental hygienist programs may also take the exam if the program they have taken is equivalent to an accredited program.

To register for the examination, go to the American Dental Association (ADA)'s Web site at www.ada.org and click the link for Education & Careers: Testing. Then choose the National Board Dental Hygiene Examination. You will then be directed to the JCNDE's registration page. Before registering, you should read the *NBDHE Guide* and obtain a DENTPIN (DENTal Personal Identifier Number), which is a unique number for applicants and students involved in the U.S. dental education system and standardized testing programs. Once you have a DENTPIN, you may register for the NBDHE electronically. When your NBDHE application has been processed, you will receive an e-mail confirming your eligibility for testing and giving you additional instructions from the American Dental Association (ADA).

Scheduling a Test Date

A company called Pearson VUE administers, or gives, the NBDHE at its nationwide testing centers. You need to register for the test 60 to 90 days prior to your desired testing date. You may register with Pearson VUE at www .pearsonvue.com once you have received your eligibility e-mail from the ADA. If you have a disability and need to make other arrangements for your exam, visit www.pearsonvue.com/faqs/state.asp to learn about what documents you should complete and submit.

Rescheduling and Withdrawing from the NBDHE

If you have to reschedule your test date, contact Pearson VUE through its Web site (www.pearsonvue.com) or by phone. There is a $25 transaction fee for every testing appointment rescheduled, whether via the Web site or call center. If you miss your test, you forfeit your application fee.

Special Accommodations

The JCNDE provides reasonable accommodations for individuals with documented disabilities. The Americans with Disabilities Act defines a disabled individual as one with a physical or mental impairment that limits one or more life activities. English as a second language, test anxiety, and slow reading without an identified underlying cognitive deficit are not considered disabilities.

If you have a documented disability, you should check the box indicating that you are requesting accommodations when you submit your application. You will have to submit a Testing Accommodation Request Form and a current evaluation report.

At the Testing Center

On the day of your scheduled exam, you should arrive at the Pearson VUE testing center at least 30 minutes before your exam begins. When you arrive at the testing site, you are required to show identification. The name and address on your identification must match the name and address on your registration.

Pearson VUE testing centers accept a government-issued passport, a driver's license, and a military ID as a form of identification. At the testing site, you will be given further instructions about where in the building you will take your exam.

The NBDHE is computer-based and given in two sessions, as shown here:

Optional tutorial	15 minutes
Session I: Discipline-based questions (200 multiple-choice questions)	3.5 hours
Optional scheduled break	1 hour
Session II: Patient-case questions (150 multiple-choice questions)	4 hours
Optional post-examination survey	15 minutes

The Structure of the NBDHE

Session I

The NBDHE is a comprehensive examination consisting of 350 multiple-choice items. The discipline-based section, Component A, includes 200 multiple-choice questions covering three topic areas, which are called domains. The percentage of each topic tested is also shown here:

1. Scientific Basis for Dental Hygiene Practice (30 percent)

2. Provision of Clinical Dental Hygiene Services (58 percent)

3. Community Health and Research Principles (12 percent)

The questions in these areas are mixed together throughout the first session of the examination.

Scientific Basis for Dental Hygiene Practice

Approximately 60 questions (30 percent) on the NBDHE are about the Scientific Basis for Dental Hygiene Practice. Questions in this domain assess your knowledge of the following areas:

- Histology and embryology

- Anatomic sciences, including anatomy of the head and neck, dental anatomy, general anatomy, and root anatomy

- Physiology

- Biochemistry and Nutrition

- Microbiology and Immunology

- General and oral pathology

- Pharmacology

Provision of Clinical Dental Hygiene Services

The NBDHE contains 116 questions (58 percent) about the Provision of Clinical and Dental Hygiene Services. Questions in this domain assess your skills in the following areas:

- **Assessing patient characteristics:** patient medical and dental histories, head and neck examinations, periodontal evaluations, oral evaluations, occlusal evaluations, and general characteristics

- **Obtaining and interpreting radiographs:** principles of radiophysics and radiobiology, principles of radiologic health, technique, recognition of normalities and abnormalities, and general interpretation

- **Planning and managing dental hygiene care:** the control of infection; recognition of emergency situations and provision of appropriate care; planning individualized patient education and instruction; provision of instruction for prevention and management of oral diseases such as dental caries, periodontal disease, and oral conditions; anxiety and pain control; recognition and management of compromised patients; dental hygiene treatment strategies such as diagnosis, treatment, and prevention; and general dental hygiene care

- **Performing periodontal procedures:** etiology and pathogenesis of periodontal diseases; prescribed therapy such as periodontal debridement, surgical support services, chemotherapeutic agents, and general therapy; reassessment and maintenance

- **Using preventive agents:** systemic and topical fluorides, mechanisms of action, toxicology, methods of administration, water fluoridation and self-administered fluoride, pit and fissure sealants, techniques for application, and other preventive agents

- **Providing supportive treatment services:** demonstrating properties and manipulation of materials, polishing natural and restored teeth, making impressions and preparing study casts, tooth desensitization, and other general supportive services

- **Professional responsibilities:** ethical principles such as informed consent, regulatory compliance, patient and professional communication, and other general professional responsibilities

Community Health and Research Principles

Twenty-four questions (12 percent) on the NBDHE are about Community Health and Research Principles. Questions in this domain assess your skills in the following areas:

- Promoting health and preventing disease within groups

- Participating in community programs; assessing populations and defining objectives; and designing, implementing, and evaluating programs

- Analyzing scientific literature, understanding statistical concepts, and applying research results

SESSION II

Session II, or Component B, of the NBDHE contains 150 case-based items that refer to 12 to 15 dental hygiene patient cases. The cases give information about adults and children by presenting their patient histories, dental charts, radiographs, and, at times, intra- and extra-oral photographs. Each examination includes at least one case with either geriatric, adult-periodontal, pediatric, special-needs, or medically-compromised patients. A compromised patient is one whose health status may require modification of standard treatment or special consideration.

To correctly answer these questions, you need to have knowledge and skills in the following areas:

- Assessing patient characteristics

- Obtaining and interpreting radiographs

- Planning and managing dental hygiene care

- Performing periodontal procedures

- Using preventive agents

- Providing supportive treatment services

- Professional responsibility

Scoring the NBDHE

Test results are mailed to you about a month after your test date. Due to JDNDE regulations, scores cannot be reported by phone, fax, e-mail, or even in person. Tests are scored by taking the number of correct answers and converting them into a standard score using the score-scale conversion formula for the examination. The minimum passing score is a standard score of 75. There is no penalty for guessing on the JCNDE.

Examination results are reported in standard scores of 49 to 99. Those receiving a standard score of 75 or better will receive an 8½" by 3½" National Board Certificate. In addition to the standard score, the JCNDE provides raw scores for each area of the examination. This includes the number of items in each section, the number of correct responses, and the national average. This information is useful because it allows you to determine your strengths and weaknesses. If you do not pass the NBDHE, you will know the areas in which you need to improve.

Both you and your dental hygiene program director will receive a copy of your score. Three dental licensing boards will also receive copies of your scores if you listed this information on your application. If you did not request that your scores be sent to three licensing boards on your application, you can pay to do this later. Score report requests can be obtained by visiting www.ada.org.

CLINICAL EXAMINATIONS

In addition to taking the NBDHE, you have to take and pass a clinical examination, which measures your hands-on skills in dental hygiene. You take this examination at a regional testing agency for one of the following organizations:

- Council of Interstate Testing Agencies, Inc. (CITA): www.citaexam.com

- Central Regional Dental Testing Service, Inc. (CRDTS): www.crdts.org

- North East Regional Board of Dental Examiners, Inc. (NERB): www.nerb.org

- Southern Regional Testing Agency, Inc. (SRTA): www.srta.org

- Western Regional Examining Board (WREB): www.wreb.org

For more information about exam schedules, fees, application requirements, patient treatment selection requirements, the radiographic component, any computer component, administration of local anesthesia requirements, and scoring information, visit the individual regional testing agencies' Web sites.

SALARY AND BENEFITS

Dental hygienists earn a salary that compares favorably to other health-care occupations requiring an associate degree. A dental hygienist's salary varies by geographical region. Dental hygienists are usually paid either hourly or with an annual salary. The Bureau of Labor Statistics reported in May of 2009 that dental hygienists earned between $44,900 and $92,860 annually or between $21.59 and $44.64 per hour.

The benefits that dental hygienists receive depend on the office in which they work. However, according to a 2009 survey conducted by the American Dental Hygienists' Association (ADHA), about half of all hygienists received some form of employment benefits such as paid vacation, paid sick time, and retirement benefits.

EMPLOYMENT OUTLOOK

The employment outlook for dental hygienists is extremely favorable. Dental hygienist is predicted to be among the fastest growing occupations. The U.S. Bureau of Labor Statistics expects the number of dental hygienist jobs to grow 36 percent through 2018. If you live in a geographic region with many accredited dental hygienist programs, you might face strong competition since dental hygienists must be licensed in the state in which they work. As older dentists who do not utilize dental hygienists retire, new dentists entering the profession will likely employ one or more dental hygienists.

CREDENTIALS

You need a license before you can work as a dental hygienist. Licensure is a way of protecting the public from unqualified people using unsafe practices. You must be licensed in the state in which you live. Each state has its own requirements for licensure. However, before you may be granted a license, you must

- graduate from an accredited dental hygiene program.

- pass the written National Board Dental Hygiene Examination (NBDHE).

- pass a regional or state clinical board examination.

Once these steps have been completed, you must contact the licensing authority in your state. Some states may also require

- successful completion of a jurisprudence exam, which is a legal exam, about the law as it applies to dental hygiene.

- proof of cardiopulmonary resuscitation (CPR) certification.

- letters of recommendation from dentists licensed in your state.

- official transcripts from the high school and college you have attended.

- official letters from the boards of dentistry where licensure is held.

THE AMERICAN DENTAL HYGIENISTS' ASSOCIATION (ADHA)

The American Dental Hygienists' Association (ADHA) is an organization formed to develop communication and mutual cooperation among dental hygienists. The ADHA is organized into three levels:

1. Component

2. Constituent

3. National

Component

The Component level of the ADHA implements community service programs, educational sessions, and offers ideas and gives information about state and national policies.

Constituent

The Constituent is the state dental hygiene association. Constituent organizations inform the components in their area of national policies and programs and new legislation.

National

The National level is comprised of twelve geographic districts. The administrative body at the National level is responsible for representing the interests of all dental hygienists.

Dental hygienists belonging to the ADHA may take advantage of benefits, such as exclusive access to products directly from Henry Schein Dental, a subscription to *Access* magazine, and access to the ADHA career resource center. You can learn more about the ADHA by visiting its Web site at www.adha.org.

ADVANCEMENT OPPORTUNITIES

Dental hygienists wishing to advance will most likely have to work outside of a typical dental practice as well as earn a bachelor's or master's degree in dental hygiene. Other advancement opportunities include teaching at a dental hygiene program, working in public health, or working in a corporate setting.

SUMMING IT UP

- Dental hygienists are licensed oral health professionals who focus on preventing and treating oral diseases and protecting patients' total health by educating them on the best oral hygiene practices.

- To become a dental hygienist, you must complete a dental hygiene program accredited by the Commission on Dental Accreditation (CODA). This program leads to a 2-year associate degree or certificate. Before becoming a dental hygienist, you must pass the National Board Dental Hygiene Examination (NBDHE), pass a regional or state clinical board examination, and apply for licensure with the state in which you live.

- Most dental hygienists work in dentist offices but a small number work for employment services and in physician offices.

- The National Board Dental Hygiene Examination (NBDHE) has two components. The discipline-based section includes 200 multiple-choice questions covering three topic areas: (1) Scientific Basis for Dental Hygiene Practice, (2) Provision of Clinical Dental Hygiene Services, and (3) Community Health and Research Principles. The second component includes 150 patient-case items that refer to 12 to 15 dental hygiene patient cases.

- In addition to passing the NBDHE, those wishing to work as a dental hygienist must pass a regional or state clinical examination.

- While a dental hygienist's salary varies by geographical location, in 2009 the U.S. Bureau of Labor Statistics reported that dental hygienists earn between $44,900 and $92,860 annually.

- The employment outlook for dental hygienists is very favorable. The number of dental hygienist jobs is expected to grow 36 percent by 2018. This is much higher than the national average.

CHAPTER 2

Becoming a Dental Hygienist

OVERVIEW

- **Step 1: Complete an accredited dental hygienist program**
- **Step 2: Register for the National Board Dental Hygiene Exam (NBDHE)**
- **Step 3: Prepare for the exam**
- **Step 4: Take the exam**
- **Step 5: Apply for your dental hygienist's license**
- **Step 6: Apply for jobs**
- **Step 7: Receive a job offer**
- **Step 8: Explore opportunities for advancement**
- **Summing it up**

STEP 1: COMPLETE AN ACCREDITED DENTAL HYGIENIST PROGRAM

To work as a dental hygienist, you must complete an accredited program in which you earn a certificate, an associate degree, or a bachelor's degree. Master's degree programs are also available. For a list of accredited programs, visit the American Dental Association (ADA) Web site (www.ada.org).

STEP 2: REGISTER FOR THE NATIONAL BOARD DENTAL HYGIENE EXAM (NBDHE)

To work as a dental hygienist, you must also take and pass the National Board Dental Hygiene Exam (NBDHE). It is possible to take this exam before graduating from an accredited program if the program director certifies that you are prepared. Otherwise, you may take this exam after graduation.

In some cases, students who have graduated from a program that is not accredited but equivalent to an accredited program may also take the NBDHE. The dean of an accredited dental school and the secretary of a board of dentistry of a U.S. licensing jurisdiction must write a letter stating that the non-accredited program met each requirement in terms of length of study, subjects studied, skills learned, and hours spent learning. Students who have graduated from a program that is not accredited must also contact Educational Credential Evaluators, Inc. (ECE) for an application form. They submit the completed application form to ECE along with official dental hygiene school

> **NOTE**
>
> The American Dental Hygienists' Association (ADHA) points out that both associate-degree and bachelor-degree programs are considered entry-level programs that prepare students to begin working as a dental hygienist in a private practice. Students enrolled in an associate-degree program complete 2,666 total clock hours of instruction while students enrolled in a bachelor-degree program complete 3,093 total clock hours of instruction.

transcripts. ECE will then send students a general evaluation report. ECE will send a copy of this report to the Joint Commission on National Dental Examinations (JCNDE). Once ECE deems the non-accredited program equivalent, a student may take the NBDHE.

> **NOTE**
>
> According to the American Dental Hygienists' Association (ADHA), students wishing to enroll in a dental hygienist program are usually required to have a high school diploma; completed high school courses in mathematics, chemistry, biology, and English; submitted college entrance test scores; and maintained at least a "C" average in high school. Individual programs may have additional requirements.

A dental student attending an accredited dental program is eligible to take the exam if the dean of the dental school certifies that the student has completed the equivalent of an accredited dental hygiene program. Dentists may take the NBDHE if they have met the eligibility requirements.

Registration

To register for the NBDHE, go to the American Dental Association (ADA) Web site (www.ada.org) and click the link for Education & Careers: Testing. Choose the National Board Dental Hygiene Examination (NBDHE). You will then be directed to the Joint Commission on National Dental Examination's (JCNDE) registration page. To register for the exam, you first need to read the *NBDHE Guide* and obtain a DENTPIN (DENTal Personal Identifier Number), which is a unique number for applicants and students involved with the U.S. dental education system and standardized testing programs. Once you have a DENTPIN, you may register for the NBDHE electronically. Once your NBDHE application has been processed, you receive an e-mail confirming your eligibility for testing and additional instructions from the ADA.

Test Date Selection

A company called Pearson VUE gives the test. You may register to take the test 60 to 90 days before your desired test date. You may register with Pearson VUE at www.pearsonvue.com once you have received your eligibility e-mail from the ADA. If you have a disability and need to make other arrangements for your exam, visit www.pearsonvue.com/faqs/state.asp to learn about what documents you should complete and submit.

STEP 3: PREPARE FOR THE EXAM

The NBDHE is a computer-based, multiple-choice test with two components. Component A consists of 200 questions addressing three major topic areas, which are called domains.

1. Scientific Basis for Dental Hygiene Practice

2. Provision of Clinical Dental Hygiene Services

3. Community Health and Research Principles

Component B of the exam contains 150 patient-case items. These items typically have a patient history and a chart showing the results of a clinical exam. The questions are based on the information in the history and on the chart. The case-based items assess your skills in these areas:

*   Assessing patient characteristics

- Obtaining and interpreting radiographs

- Planning and managing dental hygiene care

- Performing periodontal procedures

- Using preventive agents

- Providing supportive treatment service

- Professional responsibility

Study Tips

While each person must develop his or her own way of preparing for the NBDHE, you can use these tried-and-true methods to help you achieve a high score on the NBDHE:

- **Form a study group.** Group learning allows each member to benefit from the knowledge of others in the group. Your group may prefer to review a specific domain of the test each time you meet. Your group might also choose to assign a specific domain for each group member to research and develop questions to help the other group members retain the information. Study groups work well for students who learn best through speaking and conversation; however, make sure you are doing more studying than socializing. Otherwise, you are not really helping each other become dental hygienists.

- **Create note cards.** Some students find that studying with note cards helps them to remember information before a test. Creating note cards encourages you to separate large amounts of information into individual, concise thoughts that are easier to absorb and remember. For instance, you might create a note card for each individual disease or disorder that might appear on the NBDHE. Note cards are also an effective way to study on your own, without the support of a group. This method works well for students who remember facts by writing or typing them.

> **TIP**
> Only correct answers are scored on the National Board Dental Hygiene Examination (NBDHE). Therefore, it pays to guess. When you're unsure of an answer, eliminate answer choices that you know are incorrect, and then take your best guess.

- **Review all notes and textbooks.** Review the material in your course textbooks and read through your notes to refresh your memory of what you learned in your dental hygienist program. You might find that making outlines helps you organize the information so that it makes more sense to you and is easier to remember.

- **Use pictures and diagrams.** Drawing and labeling organ systems, radiographs, creating diagrams of dental tools, and color-coding material frequently helps learners store and recall information. This practice is most effective for visual learners, who often summon information that they have studied by picturing their study tools, such as diagrams or color-coded notes.

- **Practice, practice, practice.** Be sure to review the test questions in this book, which are very similar to those on the NBDHE. Review the chapters about specific subjects in this book and complete all practice questions. You will find a diagnostic test and two full-length practice tests in this book. When taking these tests, you should try to simulate the actual test-taking situation by eliminating distractions and tracking the amount of time it takes you to complete a full-length test. Practice taking Component A in 3.5 hours and Component B in 4 hours. If you find that you are exceeding the time limits you are allotted for the official test, brainstorm methods for improving your time, such as spending less time on questions you do not know and dedicating more study time to the difficult topics you encounter during the practice tests. The more you practice before taking the NBDHE, the less anxiety you will experience on test day.

- **Allow plenty of time to study.** The NBDHE is designed to test the knowledge a dental hygienist student has gained during a dental hygienist education program. You will need plenty of time to review all you have learned and to practice answering NBDHE-style questions. Start studying for the exam several months before you intend to take it. Keep in mind that engaging in frequent, short study sessions over a long period of time is generally more effective than cramming all the information into a few intense study sessions over a short period of time.

- **Take care of yourself.** Getting adequate sleep, staying hydrated, and eating are all great practices to help ensure that you are in the best frame of mind to take the NBDHE.

Test Day Tips

Taking a test can be a stressful experience. When the time comes to take the NBDHE, make sure you are prepared, focused, and feeling great. This section of the chapter provides you with suggestions to help you do your best on test day.

- **Get at least 8 hours of sleep the night before the test.** Sleep refreshes the body and allows you to think clearly. Do not take sleep-inducing medications the night before the test, as they may cause you to feel groggy instead of alert the next day.

- **Eat well.** Be sure to eat a healthy meal that will keep you full during the test so you are not distracted by hunger. However, avoid foods that are heavy or filled with sugar. Avoid carbohydrate-loaded foods such as pasta and potatoes, and instead opt for fresh fruits and veggies, eggs, and fish.

- **Avoid drinking caffeinated beverages or energy drinks that may overly excite you, making it difficult to concentrate.** Also stay away from alcohol the night before the test because alcohol causes dehydration. Staying hydrated with water or fruit juice will help you feel great on test day.

- **Stop studying.** Holding back from studying may seem counterproductive, but any information that you try to pack into your brain the night before the test will be quickly forgotten before it becomes a part of your long-term memory. Instead of cramming for the test the night before, try to find a relaxing activity such as reading a book or seeing a movie.

- **Gather the items that you will need for the test.** To avoid a chaotic rush the morning of the test, gather what you need ahead of time. Remember to bring two forms of identification (ID) to the testing center. One of the two IDs must contain a permanently affixed photo with your name and signature. The other should show your printed name and signature. Candidates will not be admitted to the test if the names on both forms of ID do not match the candidate's name as it is registered with Pearson VUE.

STEP 4: TAKE THE EXAM

You will not be allowed to bring any personal belongings into the room in which you will test. This includes items such as purses and handbags, hats, backpacks, books, notes, study materials, calculators, watches of any kind, electronic paging devices, recording or filming devices, radios, cellular phones, or food and beverages. You will be given a location in which to store personal items and may access them at scheduled breaks. During an unscheduled break, you may not access any personal items other than medication, food, or drink. To avoid any appearance of cheating, it is probably best not to take any study-related materials into the test center, and do not attempt to access any medically related Web sites or information while you are there.

Test Day

Note that you are not allowed to bring the following items with you into the test center:

- Electronic devices, including cell phones and iPods

- Purses, wallets, backpacks, or briefcases

- Books, notes, study materials, scratch paper, or tissues

- Highlighters, pens, erasers, and mechanical pencils

- Food and drinks

- Coats, jackets, gloves, or hats

- Watches or timing devices

- Good-luck charms or statues

- Dictionaries or translators

- Dental instruments, models, or materials

The Test-Taking Experience

Upon arrival at the Pearson VUE test center, the staff will teach you how to use the computer equipment and allow you to complete a short tutorial before taking the test.

You will have 3.5 hours to complete Session I (Component A) of the exam and 4 hours to complete Session II (Component B). The clock on your computer will help you track your time. During the test, you may take breaks, but the clock keeps running during your breaks so make sure you allow yourself enough time to complete the exam. There is a 1-hour scheduled break between Session I and Session II of the exam. Guessing on questions is not counted against you, so answer as many questions as you can on the NBDHE. You might also consider answering the questions you know first and then going back to answer the questions you are unsure of.

Test-Taking Tips

Test-taking can be a stressful experience. To reduce your test-taking anxiety and help yourself concentrate to achieve a better score, keep in mind the following tips:

- **Do not panic.** You have learned and studied the test material for 2 years and have most likely studied several weeks or months for the NBDHE. You are prepared to score high on the exam, so instead of worrying, focus on the content and feel confident about your chances for success.

- **Read each question carefully.** Be sure to understand exactly what each question is asking. Some questions will be more complicated than others. Regardless, make sure you fully comprehend each question before you answer.

- **Anticipate the answer.** Before answering the question, analyze the clues and decide what the answer may be. Then look at the choices to see if your preliminary answer is listed.

- **Read all the answer choices and think before answering the question.** If one of the choices matches your anticipated answer, mark it. If you are unsure of the answer, eliminate possible choices using logic and general knowledge. Then choose an answer from the remaining possibilities.

- **Visualize the answer.** When confronted with a situational question, visualize the patient in the situation. Thinking about the patient in a real-life scenario may make the test question seem more real and the correct answer to it more logical.

- **Do not get confused.** Test writers sometimes include distracting answers or answers containing bias. Analyze each answer choice individually, looking for distracters or bias that might mask the correct answer.

- **Anticipate the intent of the question.** When in doubt, think about what the question is intended to gauge. Which skill is being tested? Is the question trying to determine the best course of action to take with a patient, or is it asking you a specific definition?

- **Block out any previous negative test-taking experiences.** If you have ever had a tough time with a standardized test in the past, try not to bring that negative experience into the testing room with you. Remember, the NBDHE is not designed to torment and trick the test-taker. The aim of the NBDHE is to ensure the skill level and knowledge of dental hygienists.

Once you have mastered the NBDHE, you are ready to take the clinical exam in the state in which you wish to work.

STEP 5: APPLY FOR YOUR DENTAL HYGIENIST'S LICENSE

Licensure is granted by each individual state. To obtain your license you must

- graduate from an accredited dental hygiene program.

- obtain a passing score on the National Board Dental Hygiene Exam (NBDHE).

- pass a regional or state clinical board examination.

Once these steps have been completed, it is necessary to contact the licensing authority in your state because each state has different licensing requirements. You may be required to produce further information or complete additional requirements.

STEP 6: APPLY FOR JOBS

Before applying for professional jobs, assemble a file documenting your education and professional experiences. Gather and maintain the following documents in both paper and electronic format, if possible:

- Educational transcripts

- Any type of verifications of applicable experiences such as internships, jobs, or volunteer work in the dental field

- Letters of recommendation from people who have supervised you in school or at work

- A list of references and their contact information (phone numbers, physical addresses, and e-mail addresses)

- State licenses and other important medical training documents (i.e., CPR certification)

- Cover letter

- Resume

Bring these documents to interviews, or mail copies to prospective employers. The more prepared you are, the more you will impress a prospective employer, which will increase your chances of getting the job.

Write a Resume

Your resume should contain the following sections:

- **Contact information:** Your contact information includes your name, address, phone number, and e-mail address. If your e-mail address is not professional, get a new one to use during your job search. Many business-people simply use their first initial and their last name as their e-mail address, as in TSmith@youremailprovider.com.

- **Objective:** Your objective is your goal. The objective of your resume may be as simple as "To obtain a job as a dental hygienist."

- **Education:** List your education on your resume beginning with the most recent. If your resume is short, include a few bulleted points about your course of study. Be sure to include your school's name and address, the dates during which you attended, and the degree you obtained. (See the Sample Dental Hygienist Resume below.) If your work experience is stronger than your education, list your work experience first. The goal is to make your resume look as impressive as possible.

- **Work experience:** Begin with the most recent work experience, and keep in mind that it is not necessary to include every job that you have ever held. Include relevant experience, such as holding a job working with people or as a receptionist. If you held an unrelated job for several years, include this job because it shows that you are reliable.

- **License/certification/memberships:** Depending on the state in which you live, indicate that you are licensed. For example, you might add "New Jersey Licensed Dental Hygienist." Also indicate if you belong to any associations or organizations such as the American Dental Hygienists' Association (ADHA).

OPTIONAL SECTIONS

You might also want to include some of these sections on your resume:

- **References:** Some resumes include two or three references. If you have a reference from a dentist or someone who works in a dentist office, you might want to include this information. Past instructors are also good references. Be sure to ask each individual if it is okay to include him or her as a reference before doing so. It is also fine to list "Available upon Request" after the heading References on your resume.

- **Skills:** Some resumes include a list of skills or special qualifications that look impressive. For example, under the heading "Skills," you might include "Take radiographs" and "Excellent verbal and written communication skills."

- **Honors & awards:** If you have achieved a special honor or award, such as being a member of the National Honor Society in high school, you might want to list this on your resume.

Sample Dental Hygienist Resume

James Martinez
234 High Street
Seaside, New Jersey 08772
cell: 908-456-0087
JMartinez@youremailprovider.com

OBJECTIVE:
To work in a private dental practice as a dental hygienist

SKILLS:
- Perform oral assessments
- Use models of teeth to explain oral hygiene
- Record patients' health histories
- Clean and polish teeth
- Use X-ray machines and develop film
- Apply fluorides
- Apply sealants
- Perform dental cancer screenings

EDUCATION:
09–07 to 05–11: Bachelor's Degree in Dental Hygiene
Seaside College
Seaside, New Jersey 08772

EXPERIENCE:
2010–2011: Dental Hygiene Student
Duties included working under the supervision of a dental hygienist and dentist to provide patients with oral health care; clean and polish teeth; remove tartar, stains, and plaque; use X-ray machines; maintain patients' records and health histories; apply fluorides and sealants; and perform cancer screenings.
Seaside College Dental Clinic
Seaside, New Jersey 08772

2007–2011: Library Clerk
Assisted patrons by checking out books, shelving books, maintaining databases, answering telephones, supervising special events such as Story Hour.
Highland Public Library
Seaside, New Jersey 08772

LICENSURE:
National Board State Licensure, New Jersey

AWARDS & HONORS:
Graduated with honors

PROFESSIONAL AFFILIATIONS:
American Dental Hygienists' Association
New Jersey Dental Hygienists' Association

REFERENCES:
Available upon request

Prepare a Cover Letter

You should include a cover letter when you send your resume to dental offices. State your purpose in your cover letter, summarize your qualifications, mention any important or interesting information that is not on your resume, and express your interest in working at a particular facility. Your cover letter gives a prospective employer a glimpse of your personality, education, and experience, as well as your writing skills. It is not necessary to prepare a different cover letter every time you apply to a dental practice; save the body of your letter on a computer and add the date, dentist's or office manager's name, and the address of the practice before you send it.

Follow these guidelines when writing a cover letter:

- Your name and contact information should be centered at the top of page. Your contact information includes your address, home phone number, and e-mail address.

- Always include the date flush left.

- Include the name and address of the dentist and the practice (flush left) under the date. You can find the names of dentists in your area online or in the phone book. However, if the dentist office is very large or if you are applying to a practice with multiple dentists, finding the right name might not be so easy. In this case, call ahead and ask who should receive your resume. A large facility might have an office manager or a senior dentist who is in charge of hiring. When sending a cover letter to a dentist, always precede his or her name with "Dr."

> **TIP**
>
> Always spell check and carefully proofread your cover letter and resume. Read each of these documents word for word. Put your finger on each word and say it aloud. This will help you spot words that you inadvertently omitted. Have someone else proofread your cover letter and resume as well. Sometimes others will easily spot mistakes that you did not see. A cover letter and resume containing misspelled words and incorrect grammar will not make a good impression on a dentist.

- The salutation, or greeting, of your cover letter should simply say, Dear Dr. [surname] followed by a colon.

- Take time when drafting the body of your cover letter. Remember that a dentist or office manager will form a first impression of you based on your letter. The content of your message may vary, but in general you should

  o state your name and express your interest in working as a dental hygienist at that particular dental practice.

  o summarize your education and experience. If you do not have relevant experience, include the skills that you acquired at school or during an externship.

  o request an interview.

  o close your letter with "Sincerely" followed by a comma. Skip a few spaces and type your name. Sign your name in this space after you print your cover letter.

Your cover letter should be grammatically correct and informative and convey a warm and friendly tone. See the Sample Dental Hygienist Cover Letter below.

Sample Dental Hygienist Cover Letter

James Martinez
234 High Street
Seaside, New Jersey 08772
cell: 908-456-0087
JMartinez@youremailprovider.com

January 18, 20—

Dr. Cynthia Larson
Family Dental Practice
590 Main Street
Seaside, NJ 08772

Dear Dr. Larson:

As a recent graduate of Seaside College with a bachelor's degree in dental hygiene, I am very interested in joining your practice as a dental hygienist. While I am seeking full-time work, I would gladly work part time to gain experience. I also do not mind working evenings and weekends.

My education includes courses in oral pathology; radiography; periodontology; tooth morphology; head, neck, and oral anatomy; oral embryology and histology; dental materials; and pain management. In addition, I have completed course work in biomedical science and dental hygiene science as well as course work in general education such as oral and written communication, psychology, science, and sociology.

My clinical experience includes working as a dental hygiene student under the supervision of Suzette Mason, a registered dental hygienist (RDR), and Frederick Santos, a licensed dentist (DDS), at Seaside College Dental Clinic. As a dental student at the clinic, I provided oral health care and educational services to patients. I assisted in cleaning teeth and taking radiographs.

My other experience includes working the front desk at Highland Public Library, where I interacted with library patrons to check out books and conduct research using the library's facilities.

I hope you will contact me soon for an interview, even if you do not currently have an opening available. Friends and family have told me that you provide patients with excellent dental services, and I would really like to tour your facilities.

Sincerely,

James Martinez

James Martinez

eer as a Dental Hygienist

Online Job Listings

a click of a mouse, you can find dozens of dental hygienist jobs online. Many search engines allow you to ...arch for these jobs by state. Simply type "Dental Hygienist Jobs in PA" and you will access a listing. If you live in a large city, try searching for jobs within this city. Even your local newspaper most likely posts job ads online. A great resource for dental hygienist jobs is www.Dentalworkers.com.

Also, check the Web sites of national societies or associations such as ADHA. Individual states have their own associations, which you can easily access online.

Contact Dentists in Your Area

While online listings are helpful in locating a job, some dentists do not advertise jobs because they have many resumes on file. This is why it is important to be proactive in your job search. Send your resume and cover letter to dentists in your area. You can also drop off your resume and cover letter in person. However, if you do this, make sure you are dressed professionally. (See Dress for Success sidebar later in the chapter.) Also be prepared to fill out a job application, even if the dentist does not have any openings. You will learn what you need to bring with you to fill out a job application in the next section.

To find a list of dentists in your area, access Yellow Pages online or look in the Yellow Pages of your phone book. Make a list of the dental practices in your area. Some of them may have Web sites. If they do, spend a few minutes online to learn about their facilities. You might see something worth mentioning in your cover letter. Once you have a list, send a cover letter and a resume to each dental practice.

Applying for Jobs Online

Should you e-mail your resume to prospective employers? If you are responding to a job advertisement that says to apply via e-mail, then you should absolutely e-mail your cover letter and resume. However, when you are contacting dentists who are not advertising for a dental hygienist, snail mail is best. Imagine the number of e-mails dentists receive in one day. Do you think they reply to—or even read—every e-mail message they receive? Probably not. On the other hand, if you snail mail your resume, the person at the front desk may open it. He or she may be impressed by your qualifications and pass along your resume to the dentist or office manager. Furthermore, hardcopy cover letters and resumes are often kept on file while e-mails may be deleted.

Complete a Job Application

Some dental practices will ask you to complete a job application even if you have submitted a cover letter and a resume. A job application requires you to give specific details about yourself, your education, and your work history. If you are asked to come in for a job interview, expect to complete a job application. You might also be asked to fill out a job application if you are dropping off your cover letter and resume or if you are touring the dentist's facilities.

Gather these items ahead of time to help you accurately complete a job application:

- Your Social Security card

- Your driver's license

- The name and address of the college you attended and the dates you attended

- A copy of your occupational license

- The names, addresses, and phone numbers of your past employers and the dates when you worked there

- The names, phone numbers, and e-mail addresses of three references

While job applications vary, most ask for basically the same information. See the Sample Dental Hygienist Job Application as an example.

Sample Dental Hygienist Job Application

Application for Employment

Personal Employment

Last Name	First	Middle	Date
Street Address			**Home Phone** ( ) -
City, State, Zip			
Business Phone ( ) -			**E-mail Address:**
Are you over 18 years of age? ☐ Yes ☐ No If not, employment is subject to verification of minimum legal age.			
Have you ever applied for employment with us? ☐ Yes ☐ No If Yes: Month and Year _____ Location _____			**Social Security No.** - -
How did you learn of our organization?			
Are you legally eligible for employment in the United States? If no, when will you be able to work?			
Are you employed now? If so, may we inquire of your present employer?			
Have you ever been convicted of a crime in the past ten years, excluding misdemeanors and summary offenses, which has not been annulled, expunged, or sealed by the court? ☐ Yes ☐ No If yes, describe in full.			
Are there any reasons for which you might not be able to perform the job duties (with a reasonable accommodation)? ☐ Yes ☐ No If yes, please explain.			
Driver's License #	**State**	**Any Violations?** ☐ Yes ☐ No	

- 1 -

www.facebook.com/CareerResource

Education

School	Name and location of school	Course of study	No. of years completed	Did you graduate?	Degree or diploma
College				☐ Yes ☐ No	
High				☐ Yes ☐ No	
Trade				☐ Yes ☐ No	
Other				☐ Yes ☐ No	

Military

Complete this section if you served in the U.S. Armed Forces	Branch of Service
Describe your duties and any special training:	Period of Active Duty (Mo. & Yr.) From To
	Rank at Discharge
	Date of Final Discharge

Employment History

Please give accurate, complete full-time and part-time employment record. Start with the present or most recent employer.

	Company Name	Telephone ( ) -
1.	Address	Employed (Start Mo. & Yr.) From To
	Name of Supervisor	Hourly Rate Start Last
	Starting Job Title and Describe Your Work	Reason for Leaving

	Company Name	Telephone ( ) -
2.	Address	Employed (Start Mo. & Yr.) From To
	Name of Supervisor	Hourly Rate Start Last
	Starting Job Title and Describe Your Work	Reason for Leaving
	Company Name	Telephone ( ) -
3.	Address	Employed (Start Mo. & Yr.) From To
	Name of Supervisor	Hourly Rate Start Last
	Starting Job Title and Describe Your Work	Reason for Leaving
We may contact the employers listed above unless you indicate those you do not want us to contact.		Do not contact Employer number(s)_____ Reason_____

References: Below, list the names of three persons not related to you, whom you have known at least one year.

Name	Address	Business	Years Acquainted
1.			
2.			
3.			

The information provided in this Application for Employment is true, correct, and complete. If employed, any misstatements or omissions of fact on this application may result in my dismissal. I understand that acceptance of an offer of employment does not create a contractual obligation upon the employer to continue to employ me in the future.

_____   _____
            Date   Signature

- 3 -

Interviewing

If a dentist has a job opening or anticipates having one in the future, you may be asked to come in for a job interview. A job interview is a chance for a prospective employer to get to know you and determine whether you are a good fit for an organization. It is also the time for you to determine if a practice will be right for you. Preparation is the key to acing an interview. Keep these tips in mind:

- Research the practice or dental office where you are interviewing. Know enough about it to ask specific questions. This shows the interviewer that you care about the organization.

- Practice potential questions and answers. Anticipate what interviewers will ask and craft possible answers ahead of time. You can start by researching interview questions online and composing possible answers to these questions. Then ask a friend or colleague to conduct a mock interview. Remember that the best interviews become conversations between the interviewer and job candidate rather than an awkward series of questions and answers. Also, keep in mind that initial interviews are not the time to ask about benefits or salary; these topics should only be approached by the interviewer, if at all.

- Print several copies of your resume. Take at least two copies to the interview.

- Prepare a professional outfit to wear to job interviews.

- Practice relaxation techniques. The more relaxed you are, the better you will be able to sell yourself to a potential employer. Staying relaxed also allows you to pay attention to what an interviewer is telling you about the job, so that you can decide if it is the right fit for you.

If you find that you are not getting so many interviews as you had hoped, it might be wise to request a working interview. This allows you and the team to get a better picture of whether or not the job and the practice suit you. In addition, simply requesting a working interview will set you apart from the rest of the candidates and show that you are a confident individual.

Dress for Success

You should dress professionally for a job interview at a dentist's office. Regardless of whether you are male or female, you should wear a suit. Women can wear either a nice pant suit or a skirt and jacket. Make sure your hair is neat and away from your face. Remove any facial piercings. Men should shave all facial hair, although a neatly trimmed beard is often acceptable. Women should wear only light makeup.

STEP 7: RECEIVE A JOB OFFER

Compensation plans for dental hygienists vary with each dental practice and setting. You will probably learn the details of a potential employer's compensation plans once you receive a job offer. While many job offers are delivered orally, either in person or over the phone, it is a good idea to get the details of the offer in writing as well. This not only protects you legally by spelling out the terms of the agreement, but it also allows you to review the specific details several times before accepting or declining the offer.

Before accepting a job offer, be sure to come to an agreement and understand each of the following aspects of the employment package:

- The start date of employment

- Details about training or introductory programs for new employees

- Termination provisions and legitimate reasons for dismissal

- Frequency of formal job performance reviews (and what criteria will be used to evaluate dental hygienists)

- Payment of bonuses and the guidelines for receiving them

- Vacation time and sick days

- Working times, location of work, and specific duties within the practice

- How compensation will be determined (i.e., salary or hourly)

- Coverage of miscellaneous fees such as professional fees, licensure, and books and professional journals

- Specifics regarding health insurance, sick leave, disability, life insurance, and retirement plan

- Non-compete clause, if applicable

STEP 8: EXPLORE OPPORTUNITIES FOR ADVANCEMENT

One of your goals as a dental hygienist should be to keep up with trends in the dental industry, technology and legislation, and update your skills through continuing education. Write down where you want to be a year, five years, even ten years from now. Then, decide how you will get there and map out your career plan.

There are five professional roles in dental hygiene, with a public health component in each.

1. Clinician

2. Research

3. Teaching

4. Administration

5. Oral health advocate

A master's degree program will prepare you for a career as an educator, an administrator, or a researcher. For a list of schools that offer a master's degree in dental hygiene, visit www.adha.org. In addition, each state has different requirements for continuing education. These requirements, as well as course offerings, can also be found at www.adha.org.

> **NOTE**
>
> When you interview for a job as a dental hygienist, some of the questions you will be asked will be easy to answer. A dentist will likely ask about your education and your experience with adults and children. Other questions, however, may be more difficult to answer. Some interviewers ask questions such as, "What is your greatest strength and your greatest weakness?" Now, you are probably thinking, the strength part is easy, but what do I say is my greatest weakness? Choose a weakness that is true, but not serious—and always explain what you have done to overcome this weakness. For example, you might say that your greatest weakness is taking on too much at one time, and you have since learned to ask for help when you need it.

SUMMING IT UP

- The first step in becoming a dental hygienist is to complete an accredited dental hygienist program.

- To take the National Board Dental Hygiene Exam (NBDHE) you must first meet the eligibility requirements. In addition, you must obtain a DENTPIN to register for the exam.

- After you have successfully completed the NBDHE, you must take a clinical exam in the state in which you wish to work.

- Contact the licensing authority in your state to apply for a dental hygienist license. Some states may require additional information or credentials before a license can be issued.

- Create a professional portfolio containing educational transcripts, verification of any job experience, letters of recommendation, reference contact information, your dental hygienist state license, resume, and cover letter.

- Browsing job openings online is one way to search for a job as a dental hygienist. You should also make a list of local dentists and mail your resume and cover letter to each of them.

- When you are interviewing for a job, you may be asked to complete a job application. A job application asks for specific information that is usually not included on your resume, such as your Social Security number and the contact information of your former supervisors.

- Preparation is the key to easing your nerves during a job interview. Practice responding to questions that are commonly asked during job interviews. Suggest a working interview if you are not receiving as many interview requests as you had planned. Do not discuss salary or benefits during the initial interview unless these topics are approached by the interviewer.

- Get the details of any job offers in writing so that you clearly understand the employment package before accepting or declining the job.

- Enjoy your career as a dental hygienist! Write down your goals for the next few years and a plan for how you intend to achieve them. Keep abreast of the newest trends in the dental industry and investigate continuing education requirements for your state.

CHAPTER 3

The Types of Questions on the NBDHE

OVERVIEW

- **Question formats in Component A of the NBDHE**
- **Question formats in Component B of the NBDHE**
- **Summing it up**

The 350 items on the National Board Dental Hygiene Exam (NBDHE) are multiple-choice questions, but some of them may be in a format that is new to you. This chapter will acquaint you with the types of multiple-choice questions you will see on the NBDHE. You will answer these questions more easily and accurately if you are familiar with their format, or the way in which they are written.

The NBDHE is given in two parts called Component A and Component B. The multiple-choice questions in Component A test your knowledge of these three subject areas: (1) Scientific Basis for Dental Hygiene Practice, (2) Provision of Clinical Dental Hygiene Services, and (3) Community Health and Research Principles. Component B includes multiple-choice questions about patient cases. You will see examples of both Component A and Component B questions in this chapter.

QUESTION FORMATS IN COMPONENT A OF THE NBDHE

Multiple-choice questions, such as those on the NBDHE, consist of a stem and answer options. The *stem* is the part of a multiple-choice question that asks a question or gives a statement that you must complete. The *answer options* are the choices you are given. On the NBDHE, only one answer option is the correct answer. The NBDHE includes three to five answer options for each multiple-choice question. In this book, we include five answer options for the items in Component A to give you the most practice analyzing answer choices. The following types of items are on the NBDHE:

- Completion-type items
- Question-type items
- Negative items
- Paired true-and-false items

- Cause-and-effect items
- Testlets

Completion-Type Items

Completion-type items have an incomplete statement as the stem. You have to choose the answer option that correctly completes the statement. The following examples are completion-type items similar to those you might see on the actual NBDHE:

Example 1

Developmental cavities in the pit and fissures of teeth are
(A) Class I.
(B) Class II.
(C) Class III.
(D) Class IV.
(E) Class V.

Notice that all the answer options appear to correctly complete the sentence, but only one answer option, Choice (A), is correct.

Example 2

The place on a tooth where the fissures cross or the grooves come together is called the
(A) lobe.
(B) supplemental groove.
(C) furcation.
(D) pit.
(E) ridge.

The answer option that correctly completes this statement is choice (D), pit.

Question-Type Items

Question-type items are perhaps the most common type of multiple-choice item. These items contain a question followed by answer options. A question-type item on the NBDHE exam might look like this:

Example 1

Which of these is the tooth structure that is directly beneath the enamel?
(A) Cementum
(B) Dentin
(C) Pulp
(D) Roots
(E) Gingiva

Note that the answer options for this question are single words. Answer choice (B) is correct. Other question-type items may include complete sentences or long phrases as answer options, as in this question:

Example 2

A 41-year-old male suffering from diabetes mellitus (DM) shows signs of hypoglycemia while in the dental chair. Which of these medical treatments should be administered FIRST?
(A) Medicate the patient with oral antibiotics.
(B) Give the patient food or a drink with sugar.
(C) Give the patient an ammonia capsule.
(D) Test the patient's blood sugar.
(E) Help the patient administer insulin.

It is especially important to carefully read each answer option in questions that give scenarios and contain longer answer choices. If you read this question very quickly, you might choose (D). However, hypoglycemia is low blood sugar. To prevent the patient from going into insulin shock, you should first give the patient food or a drink containing sugar. Thus, choice (B) is correct. After this, a physician or an EMT may test the patient's blood sugar.

Negative Items

Some items on the NBDHE are negative items, or items that use the words **NOT**, **EXCEPT**, **EXCEPTION**, **NEITHER**, or **NOR**, which are usually capitalized and bolded. To answer these questions, you have to choose the answer option that is incorrect. A negative item on the NBDHE using the word **NOT** might look like this:

Example 1

Which of the following is **NOT** part of the oral cavity?
(A) Incisive papilla
(B) Lingual frenum
(C) Buccal mucosa
(D) Philtrum
(E) Uvula

To answer this question, you need to choose the answer option naming an organ that is *not* part of the oral cavity. The philtrum is not part of the oral cavity. It is the V-shaped depression between the bottom of the nose and the upper lip. Therefore, answer choice (D) is correct.

Example 2

Each of the following is a surface of the anterior teeth **EXCEPT** one. Which one is the **EXCEPTION**?
(A) Labial
(B) Mesial
(C) Lingual
(D) Incisal edge
(E) Buccal

Once again, look for the answer option that is incorrect according to the information in the stem. In this case, the answer is choice (E). Buccal is the outside surface of the posterior teeth.

Paired True-and-False Items

The true-and-false items on the NBDHE are probably different from the true-and-false items you have seen in the past. On the NBDHE, this type of item contains two statements that make up the stem. The answer options ask you if both statements are true, if both statements are false, if only the first statement is true, or if only the second statement is true. A true-and-false item on the NBDHE looks like this:

Example

The primary dentition begins to erupt in a child's mouth when the child is about 6 months old.

The teeth that eventually replace the primary teeth are called succedaneous teeth.
(A) Both statements are true.
(B) Both statements are false.
(C) The first statement is true, the second is false.
(D) The first statement is false, the second is true.

The answer options for paired true-and-false items on the NBDHE are always the same and look just like those above. In this example, both statements are true, so answer choice (A) is correct.

Cause-and-Effect Items

Like paired true-and-false items, cause-and-effect items on the NBDHE always have the same answer options. A cause-and-effect item contains a statement (the effect) and a reason (the cause). The statement and reason are written as a single sentence connected by the subordinate conjunction **BECAUSE**, which is usually capitalized and bolded. A cause-and-effect item on the NBDHE might look like the following:

Example

Dental hygienists must learn to efficiently transfer instruments **BECAUSE** they need to keep their eyes focused on the oral cavity.
(A) Both the statement and reason are correct and related.
(B) Both the statement and reason are correct but NOT related.
(C) The statement is correct, but the reason is NOT.
(D) The statement is NOT correct, but the reason is correct.
(E) NEITHER the statement NOR the reason is correct.

In this cause-and-effect statement, both the statement and reason are correct and related, so answer choice (A) is correct.

Testlets

On the NBDHE, a testlet consists of a scenario and a set of items. Testlets are used in Component A in the Community Health/Research Principles domain and in Component B. The following is an example of the type of testlet you might see in Component A:

> **NOTE**
>
> The scenarios in the testlets in Component A of the NBDHE are most often based on situations in which dental hygienists work. The scenarios in the testlets in Component B are patient-based case studies.

Use the following scenario to answer questions 1–3.

Teenagers in a developing country have eight times the number of decayed teeth as teenagers in other parts of the world. This makes them ten times more likely to develop periodontal disease, which may lead to cardiovascular disease, kidney disease, and diabetes. In an effort to reduce chronic disease in this country in the future, periodontists, dentists, and dental hygienists have established free oral health clinics in the country. Teenagers who visit the oral health clinics receive oral screenings, oral hygiene instruction, oral prophylaxes, and radiographs. Those at risk for serious diseases later in life are referred to a dentist or periodontist.

Example 1

Based on the above scenario, the free oral health clinics were designed to provide oral health-care services to teenagers **BECAUSE** the need for dental services in this developing country is lower than the available dental services.
(A) Both the statement and the reason are correct and related.
(B) Both the statement and the reason are correct but NOT related.
(C) The statement is correct, but the reason is NOT.
(D) The statement is NOT correct, but the reason is correct.
(E) NEITHER the statement NOR the reason is correct.

This is a cause-and-effect item that is part of a testlet. The second part of this—the words after the word *because*—is the effect. However, the second part of this statement is incorrect. The need for dental services in this country is higher than the available services. Therefore, answer choice (D) is correct.

Example 2

The primary focus of the dental clinics in this developing country is to
(A) reduce the number of dental carries in teens.
(B) reduce the risk of serious diseases later in life.
(C) increase the need for dental services.
(D) inform the public about dental services.
(E) treat dental carries in children and teens.

The primary focus of the free oral health dental clinic—the reason it was established—is to prevent serious diseases in teens related to dental decay. Answer choice (A) is correct.

Example 3

An initial professional responsibility of dental hygienists at the free oral health clinics is to determine the oral health status of teenagers. Which of the following represents the best approach?

(A) Meet with a consulting dentist.
(B) Meet with a teenager's parents.
(C) Review patient records.
(D) Conduct an oral screening.
(E) Give the patient a questionnaire.

This question asks you to identify the best approach, which is choice (D). The best way for dental hygienists at these clinics to determine the oral health status of teenagers is to conduct oral screenings.

QUESTION FORMATS IN COMPONENT B OF THE NBDHE

You learned earlier that all items in Component B are multiple-choice questions and patient-based scenarios. Component B of the NBDHE tests your knowledge of the following:

- Assessing patient characteristics

- Obtaining and interpreting radiographs

- Planning and managing dental hygiene care

- Performing periodontal procedures

- Using preventive agents

- Providing supporting treatment service

- Professional responsibility

All 150 items in Component B are part of testlets, or groups of questions about a scenario. Component B will include at least one case regarding one of the following patient types: geriatric, adult-periodontal, pediatric, special-needs, or medically compromised.

Testlets include patient histories and dental charts. Radiographs and/or clinical photographs are also included on the NBDHE.

The question formats in Component B are generally the same as in Component A. You might find completion-type items, question-type items, negative items, and cause-and-effect items. Read the following example case study and answer the questions based on it.

SYNOPSIS OF PATIENT HISTORY   CASE ___B___

Age ___72___

Sex ___Male___

Height __5'10"__

Weight __170_ lbs

__77.3_ kgs

Vital Signs

Blood pressure ___130/81___

Pulse rate ___100___

Respiration rate ___18___

---

1. Under Care of Physician
   Yes ☑ No ☐
   Condition: _____

2. Hospitalized within the last 5 years
   Yes ☐ No ☑
   Reason: _____
   _____

3. Has or had the following conditions:
   Emphysema _____
   _____

4. Current medications:
   MD is trying to find the right bronchodilator
   for him. _____
   _____

5. Smokes or uses tobacco products
   Yes ☐ No ☑

6. Is pregnant
   Yes ☐ No ☐ N/A ☑

MEDICAL HISTORY:
The patient smoked for 30 years and was diagnosed with emphysema 5 years ago, and then quit smoking. He uses a portable oxygen tank.

DENTAL HISTORY:
He comes in regularly for dental check-ups and cleanings. His last office visit was 6 months ago.

SOCIAL HISTORY:
He is divorced and retired from the military. He lives alone with his dog.

CHIEF COMPLAINT:
During a routine cleaning, he said his gums are a little sore on the lower right area.

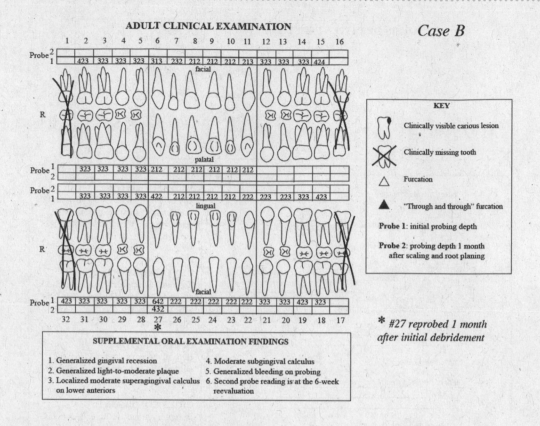

ADULT CLINICAL EXAMINATION

Case B

KEY

Clinically visible carious lesion

Clinically missing tooth

Furcation

"Through and through" furcation

Probe 1: initial probing depth

Probe 2: probing depth 1 month after scaling and root planing

* *#27 reprobed 1 month after initial debridement*

SUPPLEMENTAL ORAL EXAMINATION FINDINGS

1. Generalized gingival recession
2. Generalized light-to-moderate plaque
3. Localized moderate superagingival calculus on lower anteriors
4. Moderate subgingival calculus
5. Generalized bleeding on probing
6. Second probe reading is at the 6-week reevaluation

SUPPLEMENTAL ORAL EXAMINATION FINDINGS

- Good oral hygiene.

- Light calculus and stain.

- Pocket depths 1–4 mm with no bleeding upon probing, except for #27d facial, which measures 6 mm and has a small localized swelling. (Patient is unaware of this finding.) #27 is almost edge to edge with the opposing tooth. #27 is now extruding and has a mobility of one.

- Periapical of this area reveals bone loss on #27.

- Slight exudate present in the area of #27.

Examples 1–5 refer to Case B.

Example 1

Which of the following best describes this patient's condition?
(A) Gingivitis
(B) Early periodontitis
(C) Moderate periodontitis
(D) Severe periodontitis

The American Dental Association (ADA) classifies moderate periodontitis as pocket depths or attachment loss of 4 to 6 mm. The pocket depths in this diagnosis are 1 to 4 mm. This patient also has bleeding upon probing, which is another characteristic of moderate periodontitis. Choice (C) is correct.

Example 2

In the area of #27, the patient most likely has a(n)
(A) gingival abscess.
(B) periapical abscess.
(C) endodontic abscess.
(D) periodontal abscess.

The clinical appearance, as well as the localized pocketing and bone loss, indicates that the patient has a periodontal abscess. Therefore, choice (D) is correct.

Example 3

Which of the following is the treatment protocol for the abscessed area?
(A) Root canal
(B) Thorough debridement
(C) Vigorous polishing
(D) Immediate referral to the periodontist

A thorough debridement, which is a surgical excision of the contaminated tissue, is the best way to treat an abscess. Choice (B) is the correct answer.

Example 4

Each of the following is an additional treatment for this area **EXCEPT** one. Which one is this **EXCEPTION**?
(A) Possible antibiotic therapy
(B) Warm saline rinses
(C) Adjust occlusion
(D) Make the patient a night guard

Answer choices (A), (B), and (C) indicate additional treatment for a periodontal abscess and moderate periodontitis. Making the patient a night guard is not standard treatment for these conditions, however, so choice (D) is the answer.

Example 5

Which of the following is the best way to position the patient?
(A) Supine
(B) Semisupine or upright
(C) Supine, legs raised
(D) Prone

Because the patient has emphysema, the best way to position him is semisupine or upright. This positioning facilitates breathing. Choice (B) is correct.

SUMMING IT UP

- The questions on the National Board Dental Hygiene Examination (NBDHE) are divided into two components, each of which is taken in sessions. Component A contains questions about Scientific Basis for Dental Hygiene Practice, Provision of Clinical Dental Hygiene Services, and Community Health and Research Principles. The questions in Component B are based on patient case studies. All questions on the NBDHE are multiple choice.

- The multiple-choice items in Component A are not all in the same format. Expect to see completion-type items, question-type items, negative items, paired true-and-false items, cause-and-effect items, and testlets (or groups of questions about a scenario).

- The multiple-choice items in Component B are all about patient case studies. These items contain patient histories and dental charts. The format of the items in Component B is generally the same as for those in Component A.

PART II

Diagnosing Strengths and Weaknesses

ANSWER SHEET PRACTICE TEST 1: DIAGNOSTIC

Component A

1. Ⓐ Ⓑ Ⓒ Ⓓ Ⓔ	41. Ⓐ Ⓑ Ⓒ Ⓓ Ⓔ	81. Ⓐ Ⓑ Ⓒ Ⓓ Ⓔ	121. Ⓐ Ⓑ Ⓒ Ⓓ Ⓔ	161. Ⓐ Ⓑ Ⓒ Ⓓ Ⓔ
2. Ⓐ Ⓑ Ⓒ Ⓓ Ⓔ	42. Ⓐ Ⓑ Ⓒ Ⓓ Ⓔ	82. Ⓐ Ⓑ Ⓒ Ⓓ Ⓔ	122. Ⓐ Ⓑ Ⓒ Ⓓ Ⓔ	162. Ⓐ Ⓑ Ⓒ Ⓓ Ⓔ
3. Ⓐ Ⓑ Ⓒ Ⓓ Ⓔ	43. Ⓐ Ⓑ Ⓒ Ⓓ Ⓔ	83. Ⓐ Ⓑ Ⓒ Ⓓ Ⓔ	123. Ⓐ Ⓑ Ⓒ Ⓓ Ⓔ	163. Ⓐ Ⓑ Ⓒ Ⓓ Ⓔ
4. Ⓐ Ⓑ Ⓒ Ⓓ Ⓔ	44. Ⓐ Ⓑ Ⓒ Ⓓ Ⓔ	84. Ⓐ Ⓑ Ⓒ Ⓓ Ⓔ	124. Ⓐ Ⓑ Ⓒ Ⓓ Ⓔ	164. Ⓐ Ⓑ Ⓒ Ⓓ Ⓔ
5. Ⓐ Ⓑ Ⓒ Ⓓ Ⓔ	45. Ⓐ Ⓑ Ⓒ Ⓓ Ⓔ	85. Ⓐ Ⓑ Ⓒ Ⓓ Ⓔ	125. Ⓐ Ⓑ Ⓒ Ⓓ Ⓔ	165. Ⓐ Ⓑ Ⓒ Ⓓ Ⓔ
6. Ⓐ Ⓑ Ⓒ Ⓓ Ⓔ	46. Ⓐ Ⓑ Ⓒ Ⓓ Ⓔ	86. Ⓐ Ⓑ Ⓒ Ⓓ Ⓔ	126. Ⓐ Ⓑ Ⓒ Ⓓ Ⓔ	166. Ⓐ Ⓑ Ⓒ Ⓓ Ⓔ
7. Ⓐ Ⓑ Ⓒ Ⓓ Ⓔ	47. Ⓐ Ⓑ Ⓒ Ⓓ Ⓔ	87. Ⓐ Ⓑ Ⓒ Ⓓ Ⓔ	127. Ⓐ Ⓑ Ⓒ Ⓓ Ⓔ	167. Ⓐ Ⓑ Ⓒ Ⓓ Ⓔ
8. Ⓐ Ⓑ Ⓒ Ⓓ Ⓔ	48. Ⓐ Ⓑ Ⓒ Ⓓ Ⓔ	88. Ⓐ Ⓑ Ⓒ Ⓓ Ⓔ	128. Ⓐ Ⓑ Ⓒ Ⓓ Ⓔ	168. Ⓐ Ⓑ Ⓒ Ⓓ Ⓔ
9. Ⓐ Ⓑ Ⓒ Ⓓ Ⓔ	49. Ⓐ Ⓑ Ⓒ Ⓓ Ⓔ	89. Ⓐ Ⓑ Ⓒ Ⓓ Ⓔ	129. Ⓐ Ⓑ Ⓒ Ⓓ Ⓔ	169. Ⓐ Ⓑ Ⓒ Ⓓ Ⓔ
10. Ⓐ Ⓑ Ⓒ Ⓓ Ⓔ	50. Ⓐ Ⓑ Ⓒ Ⓓ Ⓔ	90. Ⓐ Ⓑ Ⓒ Ⓓ Ⓔ	130. Ⓐ Ⓑ Ⓒ Ⓓ Ⓔ	170. Ⓐ Ⓑ Ⓒ Ⓓ Ⓔ
11. Ⓐ Ⓑ Ⓒ Ⓓ Ⓔ	51. Ⓐ Ⓑ Ⓒ Ⓓ Ⓔ	91. Ⓐ Ⓑ Ⓒ Ⓓ Ⓔ	131. Ⓐ Ⓑ Ⓒ Ⓓ Ⓔ	171. Ⓐ Ⓑ Ⓒ Ⓓ Ⓔ
12. Ⓐ Ⓑ Ⓒ Ⓓ Ⓔ	52. Ⓐ Ⓑ Ⓒ Ⓓ Ⓔ	92. Ⓐ Ⓑ Ⓒ Ⓓ Ⓔ	132. Ⓐ Ⓑ Ⓒ Ⓓ Ⓔ	172. Ⓐ Ⓑ Ⓒ Ⓓ Ⓔ
13. Ⓐ Ⓑ Ⓒ Ⓓ Ⓔ	53. Ⓐ Ⓑ Ⓒ Ⓓ Ⓔ	93. Ⓐ Ⓑ Ⓒ Ⓓ Ⓔ	133. Ⓐ Ⓑ Ⓒ Ⓓ Ⓔ	173. Ⓐ Ⓑ Ⓒ Ⓓ Ⓔ
14. Ⓐ Ⓑ Ⓒ Ⓓ Ⓔ	54. Ⓐ Ⓑ Ⓒ Ⓓ Ⓔ	94. Ⓐ Ⓑ Ⓒ Ⓓ Ⓔ	134. Ⓐ Ⓑ Ⓒ Ⓓ Ⓔ	174. Ⓐ Ⓑ Ⓒ Ⓓ Ⓔ
15. Ⓐ Ⓑ Ⓒ Ⓓ Ⓔ	55. Ⓐ Ⓑ Ⓒ Ⓓ Ⓔ	95. Ⓐ Ⓑ Ⓒ Ⓓ Ⓔ	135. Ⓐ Ⓑ Ⓒ Ⓓ Ⓔ	175. Ⓐ Ⓑ Ⓒ Ⓓ Ⓔ
16. Ⓐ Ⓑ Ⓒ Ⓓ Ⓔ	56. Ⓐ Ⓑ Ⓒ Ⓓ Ⓔ	96. Ⓐ Ⓑ Ⓒ Ⓓ Ⓔ	136. Ⓐ Ⓑ Ⓒ Ⓓ Ⓔ	176. Ⓐ Ⓑ Ⓒ Ⓓ Ⓔ
17. Ⓐ Ⓑ Ⓒ Ⓓ Ⓔ	57. Ⓐ Ⓑ Ⓒ Ⓓ Ⓔ	97. Ⓐ Ⓑ Ⓒ Ⓓ Ⓔ	137. Ⓐ Ⓑ Ⓒ Ⓓ Ⓔ	177. Ⓐ Ⓑ Ⓒ Ⓓ Ⓔ
18. Ⓐ Ⓑ Ⓒ Ⓓ Ⓔ	58. Ⓐ Ⓑ Ⓒ Ⓓ Ⓔ	98. Ⓐ Ⓑ Ⓒ Ⓓ Ⓔ	138. Ⓐ Ⓑ Ⓒ Ⓓ Ⓔ	178. Ⓐ Ⓑ Ⓒ Ⓓ Ⓔ
19. Ⓐ Ⓑ Ⓒ Ⓓ Ⓔ	59. Ⓐ Ⓑ Ⓒ Ⓓ Ⓔ	99. Ⓐ Ⓑ Ⓒ Ⓓ Ⓔ	139. Ⓐ Ⓑ Ⓒ Ⓓ Ⓔ	179. Ⓐ Ⓑ Ⓒ Ⓓ Ⓔ
20. Ⓐ Ⓑ Ⓒ Ⓓ Ⓔ	60. Ⓐ Ⓑ Ⓒ Ⓓ Ⓔ	100. Ⓐ Ⓑ Ⓒ Ⓓ Ⓔ	140. Ⓐ Ⓑ Ⓒ Ⓓ Ⓔ	180. Ⓐ Ⓑ Ⓒ Ⓓ Ⓔ
21. Ⓐ Ⓑ Ⓒ Ⓓ Ⓔ	61. Ⓐ Ⓑ Ⓒ Ⓓ Ⓔ	101. Ⓐ Ⓑ Ⓒ Ⓓ Ⓔ	141. Ⓐ Ⓑ Ⓒ Ⓓ Ⓔ	181. Ⓐ Ⓑ Ⓒ Ⓓ Ⓔ
22. Ⓐ Ⓑ Ⓒ Ⓓ Ⓔ	62. Ⓐ Ⓑ Ⓒ Ⓓ Ⓔ	102. Ⓐ Ⓑ Ⓒ Ⓓ Ⓔ	142. Ⓐ Ⓑ Ⓒ Ⓓ Ⓔ	182. Ⓐ Ⓑ Ⓒ Ⓓ Ⓔ
23. Ⓐ Ⓑ Ⓒ Ⓓ Ⓔ	63. Ⓐ Ⓑ Ⓒ Ⓓ Ⓔ	103. Ⓐ Ⓑ Ⓒ Ⓓ Ⓔ	143. Ⓐ Ⓑ Ⓒ Ⓓ Ⓔ	183. Ⓐ Ⓑ Ⓒ Ⓓ Ⓔ
24. Ⓐ Ⓑ Ⓒ Ⓓ Ⓔ	64. Ⓐ Ⓑ Ⓒ Ⓓ Ⓔ	104. Ⓐ Ⓑ Ⓒ Ⓓ Ⓔ	144. Ⓐ Ⓑ Ⓒ Ⓓ Ⓔ	184. Ⓐ Ⓑ Ⓒ Ⓓ Ⓔ
25. Ⓐ Ⓑ Ⓒ Ⓓ Ⓔ	65. Ⓐ Ⓑ Ⓒ Ⓓ Ⓔ	105. Ⓐ Ⓑ Ⓒ Ⓓ Ⓔ	145. Ⓐ Ⓑ Ⓒ Ⓓ Ⓔ	185. Ⓐ Ⓑ Ⓒ Ⓓ Ⓔ
26. Ⓐ Ⓑ Ⓒ Ⓓ Ⓔ	66. Ⓐ Ⓑ Ⓒ Ⓓ Ⓔ	106. Ⓐ Ⓑ Ⓒ Ⓓ Ⓔ	146. Ⓐ Ⓑ Ⓒ Ⓓ Ⓔ	186. Ⓐ Ⓑ Ⓒ Ⓓ Ⓔ
27. Ⓐ Ⓑ Ⓒ Ⓓ Ⓔ	67. Ⓐ Ⓑ Ⓒ Ⓓ Ⓔ	107. Ⓐ Ⓑ Ⓒ Ⓓ Ⓔ	147. Ⓐ Ⓑ Ⓒ Ⓓ Ⓔ	187. Ⓐ Ⓑ Ⓒ Ⓓ Ⓔ
28. Ⓐ Ⓑ Ⓒ Ⓓ Ⓔ	68. Ⓐ Ⓑ Ⓒ Ⓓ Ⓔ	108. Ⓐ Ⓑ Ⓒ Ⓓ Ⓔ	148. Ⓐ Ⓑ Ⓒ Ⓓ Ⓔ	188. Ⓐ Ⓑ Ⓒ Ⓓ Ⓔ
29. Ⓐ Ⓑ Ⓒ Ⓓ Ⓔ	69. Ⓐ Ⓑ Ⓒ Ⓓ Ⓔ	109. Ⓐ Ⓑ Ⓒ Ⓓ Ⓔ	149. Ⓐ Ⓑ Ⓒ Ⓓ Ⓔ	189. Ⓐ Ⓑ Ⓒ Ⓓ Ⓔ
30. Ⓐ Ⓑ Ⓒ Ⓓ Ⓔ	70. Ⓐ Ⓑ Ⓒ Ⓓ Ⓔ	110. Ⓐ Ⓑ Ⓒ Ⓓ Ⓔ	150. Ⓐ Ⓑ Ⓒ Ⓓ Ⓔ	190. Ⓐ Ⓑ Ⓒ Ⓓ Ⓔ
31. Ⓐ Ⓑ Ⓒ Ⓓ Ⓔ	71. Ⓐ Ⓑ Ⓒ Ⓓ Ⓔ	111. Ⓐ Ⓑ Ⓒ Ⓓ Ⓔ	151. Ⓐ Ⓑ Ⓒ Ⓓ Ⓔ	191. Ⓐ Ⓑ Ⓒ Ⓓ Ⓔ
32. Ⓐ Ⓑ Ⓒ Ⓓ Ⓔ	72. Ⓐ Ⓑ Ⓒ Ⓓ Ⓔ	112. Ⓐ Ⓑ Ⓒ Ⓓ Ⓔ	152. Ⓐ Ⓑ Ⓒ Ⓓ Ⓔ	192. Ⓐ Ⓑ Ⓒ Ⓓ Ⓔ
33. Ⓐ Ⓑ Ⓒ Ⓓ Ⓔ	73. Ⓐ Ⓑ Ⓒ Ⓓ Ⓔ	113. Ⓐ Ⓑ Ⓒ Ⓓ Ⓔ	153. Ⓐ Ⓑ Ⓒ Ⓓ Ⓔ	193. Ⓐ Ⓑ Ⓒ Ⓓ Ⓔ
34. Ⓐ Ⓑ Ⓒ Ⓓ Ⓔ	74. Ⓐ Ⓑ Ⓒ Ⓓ Ⓔ	114. Ⓐ Ⓑ Ⓒ Ⓓ Ⓔ	154. Ⓐ Ⓑ Ⓒ Ⓓ Ⓔ	194. Ⓐ Ⓑ Ⓒ Ⓓ Ⓔ
35. Ⓐ Ⓑ Ⓒ Ⓓ Ⓔ	75. Ⓐ Ⓑ Ⓒ Ⓓ Ⓔ	115. Ⓐ Ⓑ Ⓒ Ⓓ Ⓔ	155. Ⓐ Ⓑ Ⓒ Ⓓ Ⓔ	195. Ⓐ Ⓑ Ⓒ Ⓓ Ⓔ
36. Ⓐ Ⓑ Ⓒ Ⓓ Ⓔ	76. Ⓐ Ⓑ Ⓒ Ⓓ Ⓔ	116. Ⓐ Ⓑ Ⓒ Ⓓ Ⓔ	156. Ⓐ Ⓑ Ⓒ Ⓓ Ⓔ	196. Ⓐ Ⓑ Ⓒ Ⓓ Ⓔ
37. Ⓐ Ⓑ Ⓒ Ⓓ Ⓔ	77. Ⓐ Ⓑ Ⓒ Ⓓ Ⓔ	117. Ⓐ Ⓑ Ⓒ Ⓓ Ⓔ	157. Ⓐ Ⓑ Ⓒ Ⓓ Ⓔ	197. Ⓐ Ⓑ Ⓒ Ⓓ Ⓔ
38. Ⓐ Ⓑ Ⓒ Ⓓ Ⓔ	78. Ⓐ Ⓑ Ⓒ Ⓓ Ⓔ	118. Ⓐ Ⓑ Ⓒ Ⓓ Ⓔ	158. Ⓐ Ⓑ Ⓒ Ⓓ Ⓔ	198. Ⓐ Ⓑ Ⓒ Ⓓ Ⓔ
39. Ⓐ Ⓑ Ⓒ Ⓓ Ⓔ	79. Ⓐ Ⓑ Ⓒ Ⓓ Ⓔ	119. Ⓐ Ⓑ Ⓒ Ⓓ Ⓔ	159. Ⓐ Ⓑ Ⓒ Ⓓ Ⓔ	199. Ⓐ Ⓑ Ⓒ Ⓓ Ⓔ
40. Ⓐ Ⓑ Ⓒ Ⓓ Ⓔ	80. Ⓐ Ⓑ Ⓒ Ⓓ Ⓔ	120. Ⓐ Ⓑ Ⓒ Ⓓ Ⓔ	160. Ⓐ Ⓑ Ⓒ Ⓓ Ⓔ	200. Ⓐ Ⓑ Ⓒ Ⓓ Ⓔ

Component B

1. Ⓐ Ⓑ Ⓒ Ⓓ	31. Ⓐ Ⓑ Ⓒ Ⓓ	61. Ⓐ Ⓑ Ⓒ Ⓓ	91. Ⓐ Ⓑ Ⓒ Ⓓ	121. Ⓐ Ⓑ Ⓒ Ⓓ
2. Ⓐ Ⓑ Ⓒ Ⓓ	32. Ⓐ Ⓑ Ⓒ Ⓓ	62. Ⓐ Ⓑ Ⓒ Ⓓ	92. Ⓐ Ⓑ Ⓒ Ⓓ	122. Ⓐ Ⓑ Ⓒ Ⓓ
3. Ⓐ Ⓑ Ⓒ Ⓓ	33. Ⓐ Ⓑ Ⓒ Ⓓ	63. Ⓐ Ⓑ Ⓒ Ⓓ	93. Ⓐ Ⓑ Ⓒ Ⓓ	123. Ⓐ Ⓑ Ⓒ Ⓓ
4. Ⓐ Ⓑ Ⓒ Ⓓ	34. Ⓐ Ⓑ Ⓒ Ⓓ	64. Ⓐ Ⓑ Ⓒ Ⓓ	94. Ⓐ Ⓑ Ⓒ Ⓓ	124. Ⓐ Ⓑ Ⓒ Ⓓ
5. Ⓐ Ⓑ Ⓒ Ⓓ	35. Ⓐ Ⓑ Ⓒ Ⓓ	65. Ⓐ Ⓑ Ⓒ Ⓓ	95. Ⓐ Ⓑ Ⓒ Ⓓ	125. Ⓐ Ⓑ Ⓒ Ⓓ
6. Ⓐ Ⓑ Ⓒ Ⓓ	36. Ⓐ Ⓑ Ⓒ Ⓓ	66. Ⓐ Ⓑ Ⓒ Ⓓ	96. Ⓐ Ⓑ Ⓒ Ⓓ	126. Ⓐ Ⓑ Ⓒ Ⓓ
7. Ⓐ Ⓑ Ⓒ Ⓓ	37. Ⓐ Ⓑ Ⓒ Ⓓ	67. Ⓐ Ⓑ Ⓒ Ⓓ	97. Ⓐ Ⓑ Ⓒ Ⓓ	127. Ⓐ Ⓑ Ⓒ Ⓓ
8. Ⓐ Ⓑ Ⓒ Ⓓ	38. Ⓐ Ⓑ Ⓒ Ⓓ	68. Ⓐ Ⓑ Ⓒ Ⓓ	98. Ⓐ Ⓑ Ⓒ Ⓓ	128. Ⓐ Ⓑ Ⓒ Ⓓ
9. Ⓐ Ⓑ Ⓒ Ⓓ	39. Ⓐ Ⓑ Ⓒ Ⓓ	69. Ⓐ Ⓑ Ⓒ Ⓓ	99. Ⓐ Ⓑ Ⓒ Ⓓ	129. Ⓐ Ⓑ Ⓒ Ⓓ
10. Ⓐ Ⓑ Ⓒ Ⓓ	40. Ⓐ Ⓑ Ⓒ Ⓓ	70. Ⓐ Ⓑ Ⓒ Ⓓ	100. Ⓐ Ⓑ Ⓒ Ⓓ	130. Ⓐ Ⓑ Ⓒ Ⓓ
11. Ⓐ Ⓑ Ⓒ Ⓓ	41. Ⓐ Ⓑ Ⓒ Ⓓ	71. Ⓐ Ⓑ Ⓒ Ⓓ	101. Ⓐ Ⓑ Ⓒ Ⓓ	131. Ⓐ Ⓑ Ⓒ Ⓓ
12. Ⓐ Ⓑ Ⓒ Ⓓ	42. Ⓐ Ⓑ Ⓒ Ⓓ	72. Ⓐ Ⓑ Ⓒ Ⓓ	102. Ⓐ Ⓑ Ⓒ Ⓓ	132. Ⓐ Ⓑ Ⓒ Ⓓ
13. Ⓐ Ⓑ Ⓒ Ⓓ	43. Ⓐ Ⓑ Ⓒ Ⓓ	73. Ⓐ Ⓑ Ⓒ Ⓓ	103. Ⓐ Ⓑ Ⓒ Ⓓ	133. Ⓐ Ⓑ Ⓒ Ⓓ
14. Ⓐ Ⓑ Ⓒ Ⓓ	44. Ⓐ Ⓑ Ⓒ Ⓓ	74. Ⓐ Ⓑ Ⓒ Ⓓ	104. Ⓐ Ⓑ Ⓒ Ⓓ	134. Ⓐ Ⓑ Ⓒ Ⓓ
15. Ⓐ Ⓑ Ⓒ Ⓓ	45. Ⓐ Ⓑ Ⓒ Ⓓ	75. Ⓐ Ⓑ Ⓒ Ⓓ	105. Ⓐ Ⓑ Ⓒ Ⓓ	135. Ⓐ Ⓑ Ⓒ Ⓓ
16. Ⓐ Ⓑ Ⓒ Ⓓ	46. Ⓐ Ⓑ Ⓒ Ⓓ	76. Ⓐ Ⓑ Ⓒ Ⓓ	106. Ⓐ Ⓑ Ⓒ Ⓓ	136. Ⓐ Ⓑ Ⓒ Ⓓ
17. Ⓐ Ⓑ Ⓒ Ⓓ	47. Ⓐ Ⓑ Ⓒ Ⓓ	77. Ⓐ Ⓑ Ⓒ Ⓓ	107. Ⓐ Ⓑ Ⓒ Ⓓ	137. Ⓐ Ⓑ Ⓒ Ⓓ
18. Ⓐ Ⓑ Ⓒ Ⓓ	48. Ⓐ Ⓑ Ⓒ Ⓓ	78. Ⓐ Ⓑ Ⓒ Ⓓ	108. Ⓐ Ⓑ Ⓒ Ⓓ	138. Ⓐ Ⓑ Ⓒ Ⓓ
19. Ⓐ Ⓑ Ⓒ Ⓓ	49. Ⓐ Ⓑ Ⓒ Ⓓ	79. Ⓐ Ⓑ Ⓒ Ⓓ	109. Ⓐ Ⓑ Ⓒ Ⓓ	139. Ⓐ Ⓑ Ⓒ Ⓓ
20. Ⓐ Ⓑ Ⓒ Ⓓ	50. Ⓐ Ⓑ Ⓒ Ⓓ	80. Ⓐ Ⓑ Ⓒ Ⓓ	110. Ⓐ Ⓑ Ⓒ Ⓓ	140. Ⓐ Ⓑ Ⓒ Ⓓ
21. Ⓐ Ⓑ Ⓒ Ⓓ	51. Ⓐ Ⓑ Ⓒ Ⓓ	81. Ⓐ Ⓑ Ⓒ Ⓓ	111. Ⓐ Ⓑ Ⓒ Ⓓ	141. Ⓐ Ⓑ Ⓒ Ⓓ
22. Ⓐ Ⓑ Ⓒ Ⓓ	52. Ⓐ Ⓑ Ⓒ Ⓓ	82. Ⓐ Ⓑ Ⓒ Ⓓ	112. Ⓐ Ⓑ Ⓒ Ⓓ	142. Ⓐ Ⓑ Ⓒ Ⓓ
23. Ⓐ Ⓑ Ⓒ Ⓓ	53. Ⓐ Ⓑ Ⓒ Ⓓ	83. Ⓐ Ⓑ Ⓒ Ⓓ	113. Ⓐ Ⓑ Ⓒ Ⓓ	143. Ⓐ Ⓑ Ⓒ Ⓓ
24. Ⓐ Ⓑ Ⓒ Ⓓ	54. Ⓐ Ⓑ Ⓒ Ⓓ	84. Ⓐ Ⓑ Ⓒ Ⓓ	114. Ⓐ Ⓑ Ⓒ Ⓓ	144. Ⓐ Ⓑ Ⓒ Ⓓ
25. Ⓐ Ⓑ Ⓒ Ⓓ	55. Ⓐ Ⓑ Ⓒ Ⓓ	85. Ⓐ Ⓑ Ⓒ Ⓓ	115. Ⓐ Ⓑ Ⓒ Ⓓ	145. Ⓐ Ⓑ Ⓒ Ⓓ
26. Ⓐ Ⓑ Ⓒ Ⓓ	56. Ⓐ Ⓑ Ⓒ Ⓓ	86. Ⓐ Ⓑ Ⓒ Ⓓ	116. Ⓐ Ⓑ Ⓒ Ⓓ	146. Ⓐ Ⓑ Ⓒ Ⓓ
27. Ⓐ Ⓑ Ⓒ Ⓓ	57. Ⓐ Ⓑ Ⓒ Ⓓ	87. Ⓐ Ⓑ Ⓒ Ⓓ	117. Ⓐ Ⓑ Ⓒ Ⓓ	147. Ⓐ Ⓑ Ⓒ Ⓓ
28. Ⓐ Ⓑ Ⓒ Ⓓ	58. Ⓐ Ⓑ Ⓒ Ⓓ	88. Ⓐ Ⓑ Ⓒ Ⓓ	118. Ⓐ Ⓑ Ⓒ Ⓓ	148. Ⓐ Ⓑ Ⓒ Ⓓ
29. Ⓐ Ⓑ Ⓒ Ⓓ	59. Ⓐ Ⓑ Ⓒ Ⓓ	89. Ⓐ Ⓑ Ⓒ Ⓓ	119. Ⓐ Ⓑ Ⓒ Ⓓ	149. Ⓐ Ⓑ Ⓒ Ⓓ
30. Ⓐ Ⓑ Ⓒ Ⓓ	60. Ⓐ Ⓑ Ⓒ Ⓓ	90. Ⓐ Ⓑ Ⓒ Ⓓ	120. Ⓐ Ⓑ Ⓒ Ⓓ	150. Ⓐ Ⓑ Ⓒ Ⓓ

CHAPTER 4

Practice Test 1: Diagnostic

COMPONENT A

Directions: Choose the option that best answers the questions.

1. Which of the following is also referred to as a reactive airway disease?
   (A) Asthma
   (B) Apnea
   (C) Hypoxia
   (D) COPD
   (E) Emphysema

2. Fat from foods can coat the teeth and prevent food particles from sticking to the teeth.

   Periodontal disease is unrelated to consuming a high-fat diet.
   (A) Both statements are true.
   (B) Both statements are false.
   (C) The first statement is true, the second is false.
   (D) The first statement is false, the second is true.

3. The white areas on a radiograph are
   (A) radiolucent.
   (B) radiopaque.
   (C) radioactive.
   (D) radiographic.
   (E) radiosensitive.

4. A patient who is overweight and uses a wheelchair comes in the dental office. Which of these actions will be most beneficial for the patient?
   (A) The workers should use the sliding board method to get the patient into the chair.
   (B) The workers should use the single-provider wheelchair transfer method.
   (C) The patient should be transferred to a dental office that has specialized mobilization equipment.
   (D) The workers should use the two-provider wheelchair transfer method.
   (E) The patient should be examined in his or her wheelchair.

5. What does the mean represent in population studies?
   (A) The middle numbers
   (B) The average number
   (C) The total number of participants
   (D) The number of participants in the control group
   (E) The number of times the same number appears

6. Ceramic, Arkansas, India, and Composition are all types of
   (A) probes.
   (B) explorers.
   (C) sharpening stones.
   (D) ultrasonic devices.
   (E) curettes.

7. Each of the following conditions presents with red lesions **EXCEPT** one. Which one is the **EXCEPTION**?
   (A) Erythroplakia
   (B) Pyogenic granuloma
   (C) Candidiasis
   (D) Hemangioma
   (E) Leiomyoma

8. During the first ten days of employment, the Occupational Safety and Health Administration (OSHA) requires that employers offer which immunization to new dental personnel?
   (A) Hepatitis A
   (B) Hepatitis B
   (C) Hepatitis C
   (D) Hepatitis D
   (E) Hepatitis E

9. After performing a Gram stain procedure, bacteria may change to a violet color **BECAUSE** the bacteria have tested as Gram-negative.
   (A) Both the statement and reason are correct and related.
   (B) Both the statement and the reason are correct but NOT related.
   (C) The statement is correct, but the reason is NOT.
   (D) The statement is NOT correct, but the reason is correct.
   (E) NEITHER the statement NOR the reason is correct.

10. Which gingival fiber group anchors teeth?
    (A) Dentogingival
    (B) Alveologingival
    (C) Dentoperiosteal
    (D) Circular
    (E) Transeptal

11. What is the primary difference between hyperglycemia and hypoglycemia?
    (A) The amount of oxygen present in one's blood
    (B) The amount of blood pumped through one's heart
    (C) The amount of beta cells present in one's body
    (D) The amount of sugar present in one's blood
    (E) The amount of oxygen reaching one's brain

12. Which of the following is the largest and strongest muscle of mastication?
    (A) Lateral pterygoid
    (B) Medial pterygoid
    (C) Temporalis
    (D) Masseter
    (E) Procerus

13. Which of the following best describes the cap stage of tooth development?
    (A) Epithelial cells become the ectomesenchyme of the jaw.
    (B) The epithelial tissue thickens and produces dental lamina.
    (C) The enamel organ is created and enamel is produced.
    (D) Tissues start to morphodifferentiate into ectoderm and mesenchyme tissue.
    (E) Epithelial tissue becomes the enamel organ, ameloblasts, and enamel matrix.

14. Written and verbal mandatory consent must be given in each of the following situations **EXCEPT** one. Which one is the **EXCEPTION**?
    (A) Medication administration
    (B) Use of a patient's photograph
    (C) Lengthy treatments
    (D) Emergency treatment
    (E) Treatment of a minor

15. Each of the following is a characteristic of a grand mal seizure **EXCEPT** one. Which one is the **EXCEPTION**?
    (A) Loss of consciousness
    (B) Temporary confusion
    (C) Muscle stiffening
    (D) Extreme fatigue
    (E) Prolonged coma

16. Periodontal diseases are reversible **BECAUSE** the gingival tissues are easy to repair.
    (A) Both the statement and reason are correct and related.
    (B) Both the statement and reason are correct but NOT related.
    (C) The statement is correct, but the reason is NOT.
    (D) The statement is NOT correct, but the reason is correct.
    (E) NEITHER the statement NOR the reason is correct.

17. What is the standard prophylactic regimen for dental, oral, respiratory tract, or esophageal procedures for adults?
    (A) 2.0 grams of ampicillin
    (B) 600 milligrams of clotrimazole
    (C) 2.0 grams of amoxicillin
    (D) 1.0 grams of cefazolin
    (E) 600 grams of oseltamivir

18. You are performing an examination on a patient. You would be most likely to notice enamel pearls
    (A) in the mandibular second molar.
    (B) on the root surfaces near CEJ.
    (C) on the velum, or soft fleshy palate.
    (D) on the hard palatal surfaces.
    (E) in the maxillary lateral incisors.

19. How do chemotherapeutic agents help treat periodontal diseases?
    (A) They break up plaque between teeth.
    (B) They eliminate potentially pathogenic organisms.
    (C) They flush away debris from the gum line.
    (D) They help speed up the healing of gingiva.
    (E) They stop bleeding of inflamed gums.

20. Each of the following is an enteral route of administering medications **EXCEPT** one. Which one is the **EXCEPTION**?
    (A) Oral
    (B) Intradermal
    (C) Sublingual
    (D) Rectal
    (E) Gastrointestinal

21. What are the three parameters of sterilization of reusable dental instruments?
    (A) Time, temperature, steam pressure
    (B) Cleaning agent, time, consistency
    (C) Method, time, temperature
    (D) Packaging, method, pressure
    (E) Consistency, time, temperature

22. A client expresses her concerns about having a root canal. You listen to her concerns and understand the emotions she's feeling. What is this called?
    (A) Empathy
    (B) Paraphrasing
    (C) Genuineness
    (D) Responsiveness
    (E) Respect

23. Which of the following is added to dentifrices to deter bacterial growth?
    (A) Flavoring agents
    (B) Coloring agents
    (C) Detergents
    (D) Preservatives
    (E) Nutrients

24. Dental office bleaching kits typically contain
    (A) 3.9–6.0 percent hydrogen peroxide.
    (B) 6.5–14.0 percent hydrogen peroxide.
    (C) 15.0–21.9 percent hydrogen peroxide.
    (D) 22.0–25.0 percent hydrogen peroxide.
    (E) 30.0–35.0 percent hydrogen peroxide.

25. The mesiobuccal surface and distolingual surface converge at a(an)
    (A) anatomical crown.
    (B) line angle.
    (C) point angle.
    (D) attrition.
    (E) abrasion.

26. Each of the following is considered a supply employers are required to give dental hygienists **EXCEPT** for one. Which one is the **EXCEPTION**?
    (A) Eyewear
    (B) Protective clothing
    (C) Face masks
    (D) Antibacterial soap
    (E) Gloves

27. If the CEJ to the mucogingival junction measured 5 mm, and the CEJ to the base of the pocket measured 2 mm, what would the attached gingiva (AG) be?
    (A) 2 mm
    (B) 3 mm
    (C) 7 mm
    (D) 9 mm
    (E) 10 mm

28. Which of the following will **NOT** scratch the titanium surface of dental implants?
    (A) Air abrasive powders
    (B) Plastic curettes
    (C) Ultrasonic tips
    (D) Metal instruments
    (E) Coarse prophylaxis pastes

29. The mandibular tori is a radiological landmark that can be identified by a(an)
    (A) radiopaque area that is a flattened attachment of the sphenoid bone.
    (B) radiopaque area that joins the ramus to the body of the mandible.
    (C) horizontal radiolucent area where the inferior alveolar nerve and vessels exit the mandible.
    (D) radiopaque area on the lingual surfaces of the mandible where additional bone growth happened.
    (E) inferior radiopaque area of the mandible with thick cortical bone.

30. Each of the following is true of cements **EXCEPT** one. Which one is the **EXCEPTION**?
    (A) They attach a prosthesis to the tooth structure.
    (B) They adhere orthodontic bands to teeth.
    (C) They attach pins and posts to teeth.
    (D) They provide protective covering to the pulp.
    (E) They are poor thermal conductors.

31. To assess the seriousness of a medical emergency, one should use the acronym AVPU. What does the acronym AVPU stand for?
    (A) Assess, vitals, pain, and under duress
    (B) Aware, voice, patient, and unresponsive
    (C) Alert, verbal, pain, and unresponsive
    (D) Assess, vitals, position, and unresponsive
    (E) Alert, voice, pain, and under duress

32. A patient has been told that he needs a root canal. The patient says that he cannot afford to pay for the procedure. The dentist informs the patient of the risks of refusing treatment, and the patient still refuses to consent to the procedure. Which action has the patient taken?
    (A) Informed consent
    (B) Implied consent
    (C) Implied contract
    (D) Express contract
    (E) Informed refusal

33. Which of the following actions builds trust between the dental hygienist and client?
    (A) Gestures
    (B) Self-disclosure
    (C) Hesitation
    (D) Paraphrasing
    (E) Body orientation

34. Each of the following should be kept in a Basic Life Support (BLS) kit **EXCEPT** one. Which one is the **EXCEPTION**?
    (A) Oxygen
    (B) Aspirin
    (C) Epinephrine
    (D) Nitroglycerine
    (E) Albuterol

35. The main difference between herpes simplex virus type 1 and herpes simplex virus type 2 is
    (A) only herpes simplex virus type 1 can be brought on by stress.
    (B) only herpes simplex virus type 2 can occur due to sun exposure.
    (C) only herpes simplex virus type 2 is extremely contagious.
    (D) herpes simplex virus type 1 and type 2 present in different locations.
    (E) herpes simplex virus type 1 and type 2 have different modes of transmission.

36. Which of these best describes what analgesic drugs do?
    (A) They reduce anxiety.
    (B) They treat pain.
    (C) They kill bacteria.
    (D) They aid in digestion.
    (E) They ease heartburn.

37. The acronym CAB helps people remember what to do when they are administering CPR. The acronym CAB stands for
    (A) compression, assessment, blow.
    (B) circulation, airway, breathing.
    (C) compress, administer, blow.
    (D) circulation, adjustment, bleeding.
    (E) compressing, alleviating, breathing.

38. A high flow rate of saliva increases the pH level of the oral cavity.

The oral cavity becomes less acidic with a high flow rate of saliva.
(A) Both statements are true.
(B) Both statements are false.
(C) The first statement is true, the second is false.
(D) The first statement is false, the second is true.

39. Neutral sodium fluoride (NaF), stannous fluoride (SnF_2), and acidulated phosphate fluoride (APF) are
(A) added to town water supplies to achieve optimal fluoride levels.
(B) safe to use on porcelain veneers, crowns, bridges, or composite restorations.
(C) effective types of fluorides to prevent caries in pits and fissures.
(D) in-office fluorides that are applied topically to a patient's teeth.
(E) types of dentifrices that are used to deter bacterial growth.

40. A patient complains of sensitive teeth during his office visit. You recommend using desensitizing toothpaste. On his next visit, he again complains of sensitive teeth despite using desensitizing toothpaste for 6 months. What should you suggest?
(A) Putting sealants on his teeth to reduce the sensitivity
(B) Switching to another brand of desensitizing toothpaste
(C) Using germicidal mouthwash twice a day for the next 6 months
(D) Switching from a manual toothbrush to an electric toothbrush
(E) Switching to the Leonard method of tooth brushing

41. Lesions that began but remineralized before more deterioration of the tooth could occur are called
(A) cavitation.
(B) pits and fissures.
(C) arrested caries.
(D) deep carious lesions.
(E) aphthous ulcers.

42. The chi-square test compares the observed measurement of a given characteristic with the expected measurement for a sample.

The chi-square test computes the positive square root of variation.
(A) Both statements are true.
(B) Both statements are false.
(C) The first statement is true, the second is false.
(D) The first statement is false, the second is true.

43. Which of these is another name for calciferol?
(A) Vitamin A
(B) Vitamin C
(C) Vitamin D
(D) Vitamin E
(E) Vitamin K

44. Custom mouth guards are preferable over a stock mouth guard **BECAUSE** custom guards make breathing easier.
(A) Both the statement and reason are correct and related.
(B) Both the statement and reason are correct but NOT related.
(C) The statement is correct, but the reason is NOT.
(D) The statement is NOT correct, but the reason is correct.
(E) NEITHER the statement NOR the reason is correct.

45. Each of the following is recommended to assist in caring for dental implants **EXCEPT** one. Which one is the **EXCEPTION**?
(A) Acidulated fluorides
(B) Air polishers
(C) Neutral sodium
(D) Tufted floss
(E) Germicidal mouthwash

46. Which of these types of drugs can cause gingival hyperplasia?
(A) Vasodilators
(B) Antihypertensive drugs
(C) Beta-adrenergic blocking agents
(D) Cardiac glycosides
(E) Antihyperlipidemic drugs

47. Meckel's cartilage contributes to both the formation of the middle ear and the
    (A) tongue.
    (B) eye cavity.
    (C) foramen cecum.
    (D) trigeminal nerve.
    (E) bone of the mandible.

48. Individuals who need supervision and assistance with some activities of daily living; may use gestures, demonstration, or adaptive equipment to help them communicate; and are not able to give informed consent are considered
    (A) high functioning.
    (B) moderate functioning.
    (C) low functioning.
    (D) minimal functioning.
    (E) nonfunctioning.

49. You are caring for a young female patient. The patient's mother asks you to apply sealants to the child's teeth. Her daughter is in her final year of preschool. What is the first thing you should do?
    (A) Give the patient the requested treatment.
    (B) Request that the mother sign a consent form for the treatment.
    (C) Check to see if the child has 6-year molars.
    (D) Explain that the treatment is inappropriate for a preschooler.
    (E) Determine whether the child will need braces.

50. What is one problem associated with panoramic radiographs?
    (A) They are large and often make a patient gag.
    (B) They lack definition and detail.
    (C) They are not helpful when checking form pathology.
    (D) They are not useful for an edentulous patient.
    (E) They require more radiation than normal radiographs do.

51. Self-curing sealants should be allowed to set for
    (A) 1–2 minutes.
    (B) 1–3 minutes.
    (C) 3–4 minutes.
    (D) 4–5 minutes.
    (E) 5–6 minutes.

52. During what week of embryonic development does the tongue start to form?
    (A) Week four
    (B) Week five
    (C) Week six
    (D) Week seven
    (E) Week eight

53. Each of the following is true about over-the-counter teeth whitening products **EXCEPT** one. Which one is the **EXCEPTION**?
    (A) They have the ability to reduce deep stains.
    (B) They are available in many forms.
    (C) They are a temporary solution.
    (D) They may cause enamel damage.
    (E) They do not work on tooth-colored fillings.

Use the following scenario to answer questions 54–57.

A new patient comes into your practice for a routine checkup. She has not had a checkup in 6 months. The patient is a young woman of about 25. The patient notes that she is allergic to shellfish and has asthma. She regularly takes medication for her asthma and allergies. She also takes birth-control pills. After performing the periodontal evaluation, you note that the patient has a periodontal reporting and screening (PRS) score of 0.

54. Which of the following would be a normal heart rate for this patient?
    (A) 25
    (B) 70
    (C) 110
    (D) 130
    (E) 160

55. Which piece of information in the patient's medical history indicates that the patient may be at risk for a latex allergy?
    (A) The fact that she has not had a checkup for 6 months.
    (B) The fact that the patient is allergic to shellfish.
    (C) The fact that the patient takes birth-control pills.
    (D) The fact that the patient has asthma.
    (E) The fact that the patient has a PRS score of 0.

56. Why is it important for the dental hygienist to know that the patient is on birth-control pills?
    (A) Birth-control pills can put women at risk for gingivitis.
    (B) Birth-control pills can increase the amount of calculus on a patient's teeth.
    (C) Birth-control pills can become less effective if antibiotics are prescribed for certain periodontal diseases.
    (D) Birth-control pills can raise a patient's blood pressure during periodontal procedures.
    (E) Birth-control pills can put women at risk for endocarditis.

57. What does a PRS score of 0 indicate about the patient?
    (A) No deposits
    (B) Plaque
    (C) Calculus
    (D) Supragingival calculus
    (E) Subgingival calculus

58. Each of the following is an appropriate treatment to offer to a patient suffering from periodontal disease **EXCEPT** one. Which one is the **EXCEPTION**?
    (A) Root planing
    (B) Gingival curettage
    (C) Fissure sealants
    (D) Bone grafting
    (E) Implants

59. Adrenergic drugs block the actions of the parasympathetic nervous system.

    Adrenergic drugs stimulate the adrenergic receptors and produce effects similar to those of the sympathetic nervous system.
    (A) Both statements are true.
    (B) Both statements are false.
    (C) The first statement is true, the second is false.
    (D) The first statement is false, the second is true.

60. Each of the following is a sign of acute fluoride toxicity **EXCEPT** one. Which one is the **EXCEPTION**?
    (A) Excessive salivation
    (B) Abdominal pain
    (C) Severe bleeding
    (D) Cardiac arrest
    (E) Vomiting

61. All of the following are responsibilities of the state board of dental examiners **EXCEPT** one. Which one is the **EXCEPTION**?
    (A) Regulate dental licenses.
    (B) Grant dental licenses.
    (C) Institute continuing education standards.
    (D) Inspect dental practices.
    (E) Revoke dental licenses.

62. Each of the following is an advantage to using a power-driven ultrasonic scaler for debridement purposes **EXCEPT** one. Which one is the **EXCEPTION**?
    (A) It makes it easier to establish a fulcrum.
    (B) It helps alleviate clinical fatigue.
    (C) It uses water to control heat.
    (D) It does not require the use of proper angulation.
    (E) It operates 20,000–50,000 cycles per second.

63. Each of the following is a step in the planning process for educating patients **EXCEPT** one. Which one is the **EXCEPTION**?
    (A) Reviewing a patient's current oral health
    (B) Coordinating with other dental professionals
    (C) Identifying proper treatments
    (D) Explaining the benefits of treatment
    (E) Implementing the plan with the patient

64. When should a patient's medical record be updated?
    (A) Every five years
    (B) Every two years
    (C) Once a year
    (D) Every office visit
    (E) Every two office visits

65. Which material is 70 percent inorganic, 18 percent organic, and 12 percent water?
    (A) Pulp
    (B) Bone
    (C) Dentin
    (D) Enamel
    (E) Cementum

66. Which of the following is true about nitrous oxide?
    (A) It allows the patient to stay awake and be consciously sedated.
    (B) The patient can control the flow of nitrous oxide as needed.
    (C) Patients cannot eat for 24 hours before receiving it.
    (D) Only anesthesiologists can administer it to patients.
    (E) It is usually considered to be a local anesthetic.

67. How long does it take for an alginate hydrocolloid impression to set?
    (A) 30–45 seconds
    (B) 1–2 minutes
    (C) 2–5 minutes
    (D) 5–8 minutes
    (E) 8–12 minutes

68. Which tissue comes from oral ectoderm?
    (A) Bone
    (B) Enamel
    (C) Cardiac muscle
    (D) Smooth muscle
    (E) Connective

69. When should children begin ingesting optimally fluoridated water to receive maximum benefits?
    (A) When their 6-year-old molars erupt
    (B) When they start school
    (C) Before 6 months of age
    (D) At the onset of tooth development
    (E) After they turn 16

70. The peripheral nervous system consists of twelve pairs of cranial nerves and thirty-one pairs of spinal nerves. The afferent nerve that controls the function of the ear and epiglottis is the
    (A) vagus.
    (B) abducens.
    (C) accessory.
    (D) hypoglossal.
    (E) vestibulocochlear.

71. Nitrous oxide and oxygen are both stored in colored tanks. In what color tank is nitrous oxide stored?
    (A) Blue
    (B) Green
    (C) Red
    (D) Yellow
    (E) Orange

72. What is the most important aspect of a good community dental program?
    (A) A lesson plan with defined goals and objectives
    (B) A summary of the material covered
    (C) Information that patients can easily relate to
    (D) Audience participation and use of humor
    (E) Quizzes and discussion material

73. Which of the following intraoral techniques directs the primary X-ray beam perpendicular to the film and the long axis of the tooth?
    (A) Bisecting technique
    (B) Paralleling technique
    (C) Occlusal technique
    (D) Buccal technique
    (E) Stillman technique

74. Each of the following is a measure included in the central tendency **EXCEPT** one. Which one is the **EXCEPTION**?
    (A) Average
    (B) Mean
    (C) Mode
    (D) Range
    (E) Median

75. Amides and esters are both types of local anesthetics used in dental offices. Why are amides used more often than esters in dental offices?
    (A) Amides are less expensive.
    (B) Amides are more readily available.
    (C) Amides cause fewer allergic reactions.
    (D) Amides are easier to administer.
    (E) Amides have fewer effects on the liver.

76. The body's immune system is responsible for causing inflammation after an injury or illness.

    Inflammation is a protective response meant to rid the body of whatever caused the injury or illness.
    (A) Both statements are true.
    (B) Both statements are false.
    (C) The first statement is true, the second is false.
    (D) The first statement is false, the second is true.

77. Which of these bony defects has the worst prognosis?
    (A) One-wall defect
    (B) Two-wall defect
    (C) Three-wall defect
    (D) Four-wall defect
    (E) Five-wall defect

78. Each of the following is a developmental tooth abnormality **EXCEPT** one. Which one is the **EXCEPTION**?
    (A) Hyperdontia
    (B) Concrescence
    (C) Erosion
    (D) Gemination
    (E) Anodontia

79. To anesthetize the mandibular anterior teeth and the first premolar on the side to be worked on, the anesthesia needle must be inserted
    (A) in the pterygomandibular triangle at the medial border of the coronoid notch.
    (B) near, or slightly anterior to, the depression of mental foramen between the mandibular first and second premolars.
    (C) in the mucobuccal fold distal to the last mandibular molar parallel to the retromolar pad of the anterior ramus.
    (D) near the depression of mental foramen between the mandibular first and second premolars.
    (E) slightly anterior to the mucobuccal fold distal to the first mandibular molar between the retromolar pad of the anterior ramus.

80. Each of the following is considered Gram-negative bacteria that inhabits the oral cavity **EXCEPT** one. Which one is the **EXCEPTION**?
    (A) Prevotella intermedia
    (B) Fusobacterium nucleatum
    (C) Capnocytophaga spirochetes
    (D) Actinomyces viscosus
    (E) Prevotella melaninogenica

81. Sucrose comes from maple syrup, cane sugar, and beet sugar. It is hydrolyzed into
    (A) lactose and fructose.
    (B) fructose and glucose.
    (C) glucose and galactose.
    (D) maltose and hexoses.
    (E) lactose and maltose.

82. Which two indices make up the simplified oral hygiene index (OHI-S)?
    (A) The plaque index (PI) and the calculus index (CI-S)
    (B) The calculus index (CI-S) and the debris index (DI-S)
    (C) The plaque index (PI) and the debris index (DI-S)
    (D) The pocket index and the plaque index (PI)
    (E) The calculus index (CI-S) and the pocket index

83. Epidemiology is the study of
    (A) behaviors.
    (B) oral hygiene practices.
    (C) disease prevalence.
    (D) population.
    (E) sterilization processes.

84. Which of these patients would most benefit from education about dental caries and preventing dental caries?
    (A) An overweight 6-year-old female
    (B) An 80-year-old male with no health problems
    (C) A 25-year-old male with HIV
    (D) An underweight 18-year-old female
    (E) A 55-year-old male with asthma

85. The scapula is considered a(an)
    (A) long bone.
    (B) short bone.
    (C) flat bone.
    (D) irregular bone.
    (E) sesamoid bone.

86. Each of the following is an advantage of digital radiography EXCEPT one. Which one is the EXCEPTION?
    (A) Digital radiography generates an image quickly for immediate evaluation.
    (B) Digital radiography uses less radiation than film-based imaging.
    (C) Digital radiography has advanced resolution, which allows for enhanced viewing.
    (D) Digital radiography initially costs less than film-based imaging systems.
    (E) Digital radiography reduces expenses associated with film and processing.

87. Nystatin, or Mycostatin, is considered to be which of the following types of medication?
    (A) Antibiotic
    (B) Antitubercular
    (C) Antiadrenergic
    (D) Antiviral
    (E) Antifungal

88. Each of the following is considered a semicritical or noncritical item to sterilize EXCEPT for one. Which one is the EXCEPTION?
    (A) Scalpels
    (B) Mirrors
    (C) Amalgam carriers
    (D) Counters
    (E) Blood pressure cuffs

89. Community water supplies are naturally fluoridated by water flowing over rock and soil containing fluoride BECAUSE optimum fluoride levels should be between 4–6 ppm.
    (A) Both the statement and reason are correct and related.
    (B) Both the statement and reason are correct but NOT related.
    (C) The statement is correct, but the reason is NOT.
    (D) The statement is NOT correct, but the reason is correct.
    (E) NEITHER the statement NOR the reason is correct.

90. Microleakage is the ability of materials to adequately seal margins by adhesion.

    Polyacrylic acid adheres sufficiently to avoid microleakage of saliva.
    (A) Both statements are true.
    (B) Both statements are false.
    (C) The first statement is true, the second is false.
    (D) The first statement is false, the second is true.

91. Each of the following is included under federally funded medical services EXCEPT one. Which one is the EXCEPTION?
    (A) Capitation plans
    (B) Maternal and Child Health Services
    (C) Medicaid
    (D) National Health Service Corps
    (E) Medicare

92. Each of the following is true of stannous fluoride EXCEPT one. Which one is the EXCEPTION?
    (A) It is an unstable fluoride.
    (B) It needs to be mixed before application.
    (C) It contains 5 percent sodium fluoride.
    (D) It has a harsh taste.
    (E) It can stain teeth.

93. One difference between the maximum permissible exposure (MPE) and the maximum permissible dose (MPD) in radiation levels is that the dose does not use an age-based formula.

    Another difference between the MPE and the MPD in radiation levels is that the MPD only applies to dental personnel, while the MPE is used in general settings.
    (A) Both statements are true.
    (B) Both statements are false.
    (C) The first statement is true, the second is false.
    (D) The first statement is false, the second is true.

94. You have planned and implemented a treatment plan for a middle-aged woman who suffers from severe dental caries. Which of these should you do after implementing the plan?
    (A) Identify any other major health issue the patient has.
    (B) Assess the value and success of the plan.
    (C) Consult with other dental professionals about the plan.
    (D) Research the patient's medical history.
    (E) Discuss the importance of managing the patient's dental health.

95. Each of the following is an example of connective tissue **EXCEPT** one. Which one is the **EXCEPTION**?
    (A) Sarcomeres
    (B) Blood
    (C) Adipose
    (D) Lymph
    (E) Collagen

96. On a prescription, what does the abbreviation tid mean?
    (A) Before meals
    (B) Three times a day
    (C) As needed
    (D) Twice a day
    (E) With food

Use the following scenario to answer questions 97–100.

Your patient is a 15-year-old who has been dropped off by his father, who says he will return shortly. He is running to the post office to mail a package. As you perform the examination, you notice that the patient needs to have bitewing radiographs taken. Your patient assures you that his father would give his permission to have the radiographs taken. Following the guidelines issued by your state regarding treatment of minors, you refuse to take the radiographs until the patient's father returns. The father returns expecting his son to be finished. When you inform the father that you had to wait to take the radiographs because his son is a minor, the father becomes irritated and starts yelling because he is now running late. After the patient leaves with his father, you call your friend to tell her what happened.

97. Taking radiographs of a minor without permission from his parents would be considered battery **BECAUSE** treatment was performed without parental consent.
    (A) Both the statement and reason are correct and related.
    (B) Both the statement and reason are correct but NOT related.
    (C) The statement is correct, but the reason is NOT.
    (D) The statement is NOT correct, but the reason is correct.
    (E) NEITHER the statement NOR the reason is correct.

98. By refusing to take the radiographs of the 15-year-old, you have
    (A) abandoned the patient.
    (B) committed malfeasance.
    (C) followed state regulations.
    (D) committed breach of duty.
    (E) violated HIPPA.

99. Which category would taking radiographs fall under?
    (A) Implied contract
    (B) Informed consent
    (C) Implied consent
    (D) Primary level of prevention
    (E) Tertiary level of prevention

100. By telling your friend about the incident, you have
    (A) committed negligence.
    (B) breached patient confidentiality.
    (C) breached an implied contract.
    (D) violated an unintentional tort.
    (E) committed fraud.

101. How long after collecting plaque accumulate does gingivitis occur?
    (A) 1 to 2 weeks
    (B) 2 to 3 weeks
    (C) 3 to 4 weeks
    (D) 1 to 2 months
    (E) 2 to 3 months

102. The third molars' roots are completed around age
    (A) 6–9.
    (B) 9–12.
    (C) 10–13.
    (D) 14–16.
    (E) 18–25.

Use the following scenario to answer questions 103–105.

A dental hygienist is working in a dental office and is scheduled to meet with a number of patients throughout the day. The first patient to arrive is a 30-year-old female who needs a root canal performed on one of her premolars. The woman is suffering from a bacterial respiratory infection. The second patient to arrive is a 75-year-old man who is undergoing a regularly scheduled cleaning and checkup.

103. The chain of infection has many links that must all be present for infection to pass from one person to another. Which of the following from the scenario is the susceptible host link in a possible chain of infection?
    (A) The female patient
    (B) The respiratory infection
    (C) The dental hygienist
    (D) The male patient
    (E) The bacteria causing the infection

104. While performing the root canal procedure on the patient, the provider notices that blood is oozing from the patient's mouth. What is most likely the cause of the bleeding?
    (A) An artery has been injured.
    (B) A capillary has been damaged.
    (C) A vein has been compromised.
    (D) A tooth's root has been broken.
    (E) A tendon has been nicked.

105. After noticing the bleeding during the procedure, the provider should
    (A) have the patient gently bite on a piece of folded gauze for about 10 minutes.
    (B) use suction to remove the excess blood from the patient's mouth.
    (C) have the patient rinse her mouth for about 10 minutes.
    (D) use a gentle stream of air to dry the tooth and the surrounding area.
    (E) have the patient rest and spit out excess blood for about 10 minutes.

106. Which one of the following topics should be discussed with the female patient who received the root canal?
    (A) Infection prevention through proper cleaning
    (B) Proper maintenance of implants
    (C) Removing tooth discoloration with bleach products
    (D) Living with and dealing with xerostomia
    (E) The ways proper diet can help avoid oral cancers

107. On a periodontal exam chart, tooth 32 on the mandibular right has an X on it. This indicates a
    (A) furcation.
    (B) healthy tooth.
    (C) clinically missing tooth.
    (D) through-and-through furcation.
    (E) clinically visible carious lesion.

108. What is the first step in community health planning?
    (A) Assessment of needs
    (B) Program formulation
    (C) Program financing
    (D) Implementation of program
    (E) Evaluation of success

109. Filtering blood and maintaining the body's pH balance are responsibilities of the
    (A) circulatory system.
    (B) digestive system.
    (C) respiratory system.
    (D) nervous system.
    (E) renal system.

110. Which of these bacteria exist on the tooth surface of a person with a high sugar diet?
    (A) *Streptococcus mutans*
    (B) *Prevotella histicola*
    (C) *Streptococcus sanguinis*
    (D) *Actinomyces viscosus*
    (E) *Streptococcus mitis*

111. Glucose is a monosaccharide that can be readily absorbed into the bloodstream for immediate use.

    Galactose is a monosaccharide that can be readily absorbed into the bloodstream for immediate use.
    (A) Both statements are true.
    (B) Both statements are false.
    (C) The first statement is true, the second is false.
    (D) The first statement is false, the second is true.

112. Which teeth are usually affected first by nursing-bottle decay?
    (A) Mandibular canines
    (B) Maxillary premolars
    (C) Mandibular molars
    (D) Maxillary incisors
    (E) Mandibular premolars

113. A hyoid bone is best described as a(an)
    (A) three-pronged bone.
    (B) Y-shaped bone.
    (C) U-shaped bone.
    (D) soft bone.
    (E) flat bone.

114. The application of statistics to a wide range of topics in biology is
    (A) statistical biology.
    (B) biostatistics.
    (C) pathology.
    (D) jurisprudence.
    (E) inferential statistics.

115. The metaphase stage of cell replication is best described as which of the following?
    (A) Chromatin compresses into chromosomes, and the centrioles assist in arranging the mitotic spindles as they move to opposite poles.
    (B) Chromosomes align centromeres at the center and mitotic spindles form.
    (C) Chromatids from each chromosome merge at the centromere and mitotic spindles move toward opposite poles.
    (D) Chromatids uncoil into two separate nuclei and are surrounded by nuclear membranes.
    (E) Chromatid pairs are surrounded by the nuclear envelope and the nucleoli reappear.

116. Each of the following should be inspected as part of an extraoral examination EXCEPT one. Which one is the EXCEPTION?
    (A) Labial and buccal mucosa
    (B) Head, face, and nose
    (C) Lips for cracks and dryness
    (D) Function of the temporomandibular
    (E) Lacrimation and dilation of pupils

117. Ramfjord's periodontal disease index (PDI) evaluates each of the following EXCEPT one. Which one is the EXCEPTION?
    (A) Gingival health
    (B) Probing depths
    (C) Dental biofilm
    (D) Calculus deposits
    (E) Dental caries

118. Each of the following is a part of the axial skeletal system EXCEPT one. Which one is the EXCEPTION?
    (A) Skull
    (B) Shoulders
    (C) Sternum
    (D) Ribs
    (E) Spinal cord

119. Which index is the one most widely used to measure fluorosis in a community?
    (A) Dean's fluorosis index
    (B) TSIF
    (C) CPITN
    (D) DMFT indices
    (E) PHP-M

120. Which piece of dental equipment is used for indirect vision, illumination, transillumination, and retraction?
    (A) Probe
    (B) Explorer
    (C) Tongue depressor
    (D) Mouth mirror
    (E) Periodontal scaler

121. Which of the following bodily function is aided by vitamin B2?
    (A) Heart function
    (B) Formation of red blood cells
    (C) Neural function
    (D) Digestion and absorption
    (E) Waste elimination

122. Each of the following is soluble in water **EXCEPT** one. Which one is the **EXCEPTION**?
    (A) Sugar alcohols
    (B) Lipoproteins
    (C) Fats
    (D) Carbohydrates
    (E) Ethanol

123. Sodium bicarbonate, which neutralizes pH, is an ingredient in
    (A) glucagon.
    (B) insulin.
    (C) hormones.
    (D) pancreatic fluid.
    (E) blood plasma.

124. Which of these gum disorders is characterized by white striae called Wickham's striae?
    (A) Lichen planus
    (B) Cicatricial pemphigoid
    (C) Pemphigus vulgaris
    (D) Desquamative gingivitis
    (E) Cheilitis granulomatosa

125. Which of the following is true of area-specific curettes?
    (A) They have two cutting edges per end.
    (B) Their edges are used for deposit removal.
    (C) The faces are set at a 70-degree angle to the terminal shank.
    (D) They adapt to any tooth surface in the oral cavity.
    (E) They are shaped like a knife.

126. Which phase of binary cell division takes place when the rate of cell growth is equal to the rate of cell death?
    (A) Lag phase
    (B) Log phase
    (C) Stationary phase
    (D) Decline phase
    (E) Replication phase

127. Antibiotics should be administered into pockets
    (A) 1.0–2.0 mm
    (B) 2.0–3.0 mm
    (C) 3.0–4.0 mm
    (D) 4.0–5.0 mm
    (E) 5.0–6.0 mm

128. How often should dental implants be checked for bone loss?
    (A) Every 3 months
    (B) Every 6 months
    (C) Annually
    (D) Every two years
    (E) As needed

129. Which of these cysts are benign, expansible lesions that are generally found over unerupted molars?
    (A) Ameloblastic fibroma
    (B) Cementoma
    (C) Lateral periodontal
    (D) Odontoma, comples
    (E) Ranula

130. According to the Controlled Substances Act, which of the following drugs may lead to moderate dependence or high psychological dependence?
    (A) Heroin
    (B) Oxycodone
    (C) Codeine
    (D) Valium
    (E) Bactrim

131. Ineffective endocarditis is an autogenious infection, which means it cannot pass from person to person.

    Ineffective endocarditis can spread to other parts of the body if vegetative growths of organisms destroy connective tissue and break free.
    (A) Both statements are true.
    (B) Both statements are false.
    (C) The first statement is true, the second is false.
    (D) The first statement is false, the second is true.

132. What is jurisprudence?
    (A) A judgment based on a moral evaluation
    (B) A disclosure of necessary information
    (C) An obligation to treat individuals fairly
    (D) A philosophy of law
    (E) An obligation to speak the truth

133. Each of the following is an ethical principle **EXCEPT** one. Which is the **EXCEPTION**?
    (A) Autonomy
    (B) Nonmaleficence
    (C) Justice
    (D) Informed refusal
    (E) Implied consent

134. A patient in a dental office suffers from sarcoidosis. About which of the following oral conditions should the patient most likely be educated?
(A) Xerostomia
(B) Dental caries
(C) TMJ
(D) Candidiasis
(E) Oral cancer

135. Erythrocytes do not circulate through the body after 120 days **BECAUSE** macrophages in the bone marrow, spleen, and liver remove them from the bloodstream.
(A) Both the statement and reason are correct and related.
(B) Both the statement and reason are correct but NOT related.
(C) The statement is correct, but the reason is NOT.
(D) The statement is NOT correct, but the reason is correct.
(E) NEITHER the statement NOR the reason is correct.

136. Dental practice acts are established by
(A) state dental boards.
(B) state legislatures.
(C) the federal government.
(D) individual practitioners.
(E) the American Dental Association.

137. People with low rates of caries are an example of a target group for a diet counseling community program **BECAUSE** they most likely do not eat sensibly or have good dietary habits.
(A) Both the statement and reason are correct and related.
(B) Both the statement and reason are correct but NOT related.
(C) The statement is correct, but the reason is NOT.
(D) The statement is NOT correct, but the reason is correct.
(E) NEITHER the statement NOR the reason is correct.

138. What is the name given to very thin shells of porcelain that are bonded to facial and incisal surfaces?
(A) Crowns
(B) Bridges
(C) Sealants
(D) Veneers
(E) Dentures

139. Which of the following are considered to be ideal for Class V restorations?
(A) Bonding agents
(B) Composites
(C) Glass ionomers
(D) Amalgams
(E) Porcelain

140. A patient who has slurred speech and no clear speech pattern as a result of damage to the CNS or peripheral nervous system might have
(A) aphasia.
(B) apraxia.
(C) dysarthria.
(D) dementia.
(E) autism.

Use the following scenario to answer questions 141–145.

A six-year veteran dental hygienist has volunteered to present an educational program to six classes of first graders at Cool Spring Elementary School. She has two children of her own, ages 8 and 10. One of the objectives of the program is, "After a demonstration of different tooth-brushing methods, students will be able to verbally describe one method of tooth brushing to a friend." During the presentation, the dental hygienist will relay experiences involving other young children about cavities and the results poor dental hygiene practices have had on their overall dental health.

141. The presenter is familiar with the subject matter, and the material is current and accurate.

    Information is appropriate to the level and needs of the audience.
    (A) Both statements are true.
    (B) Both statements are false.
    (C) The first statement is true, the second is false.
    (D) The first statement is false, the second is true.

142. The dental hygienist will evaluate the learning of the first-grade classes by
    (A) comparing the oral hygiene habits of the first graders to the habits of her children.
    (B) having the first-grade children demonstrate different methods of tooth brushing.
    (C) having the first-grade children verbally tell her how they brush their teeth.
    (D) having the first-grade children tell a friend one method of tooth brushing.
    (E) sharing experiences of other children she has worked with who have practiced poor oral hygiene.

143. Which part of a program presentation includes presenting major points and relating specific information to the audience's personal experiences?
    (A) The introduction
    (B) The body
    (C) The evaluation
    (D) The closure
    (E) The assessment

144. Each of the following areas of the presentation should be evaluated **EXCEPT** one. Which one is the **EXCEPTION**?
    (A) Audience's clarity of speech
    (B) Presenter's enthusiasm
    (C) Presenter's expressions
    (D) Audience behaviors
    (E) Eye contact

145. Which of the following might be an appropriate objective for this dental hygienist's particular program?
    (A) After the presentation, students will know how to screen themselves for signs of symptoms of oral cancer.
    (B) After the presentation, students will understand how to enroll in dental programs for people with financial difficulties.
    (C) After the presentation, students will understand how reducing the amount of sugary foods in their diet can help prevent tooth decay.
    (D) After the presentation, students will understand that the government has changed the suggested amount of fluoride in drinking water.
    (E) After the presentation, students will understand how particular drugs can affect saliva production in the oral cavity.

146. Which of the following radiographic techniques minimizes distortion by placing radiographic film at the same angulation as the long axis of the tooth?
    (A) Parallel technique
    (B) Bisecting technique
    (C) Horizontal angulation technique
    (D) Vertical angulation technique
    (E) The buccal object rule

147. What form of communication involves conveying a message within oneself?
    (A) Verbal
    (B) Nonverbal
    (C) Intrapersonal
    (D) Interpersonal
    (E) Paraphrasing

148. Each of the following should be described in the case presentation **EXCEPT** one. Which one is the **EXCEPTION**?
    (A) Treatment procedures
    (B) Time and money requirements for treatments
    (C) Risks and benefits of the possible treatments
    (D) Consequences of refusing the treatment
    (E) Evaluation of the plan's success

149. When should the oral hygiene index (OHI-S) be used?
    (A) To qualify dental biofilm
    (B) When a large population is being studied
    (C) To assist patients with improving their dental hygiene
    (D) To assess the thickness on dental biofilm
    (E) When the gingival index (GI) is also used

150. Which of the following would be a safely tolerated dose of fluoride for an 8-year-old child who weighs 45 pounds?
    (A) 164 mg
    (B) 193 mg
    (C) 233 mg
    (D) 301 mg
    (E) 334 mg

151. Debridement procedures are done on patients to
    (A) administer antibiotics into pockets that are 5.0–6.0 mm.
    (B) remove hard and soft deposits from coronal surfaces.
    (C) remove a thin layer of diseased cementum.
    (D) measure pocket depths and furcations.
    (E) determine whether a patient has periodontal disease.

152. Which of these is an example of a cholinergic drug?
    (A) Epinephrine
    (B) Clonidine
    (C) Pilocarpine
    (D) Atenolol
    (E) Malathion

153. Which of these best describes why a dental hygienist should plan to educate a patient with rheumatoid arthritis differently from a patient without this disease?
    (A) Patients with rheumatoid arthritis are prone to caries.
    (B) Patients with rheumatoid arthritis cannot be treated with antibiotics.
    (C) Patients with rheumatoid arthritis are prone to TMJ.
    (D) Patients with rheumatoid arthritis cannot be treated with nitrous oxide.
    (E) Patients with rheumatoid arthritis are prone to oral lesions.

154. You are examining a new patient and are looking for caries and evaluating a restoration. Which of these explorers is the best for this type of examination?
    (A) Shepherd's hook
    (B) #11/12
    (C) #17
    (D) Pigtail
    (E) #3A

155. Immunoglobulins can be divided into six work groups.

    Immunoglobulins can be found in tears and saliva.
    (A) Both statements are true.
    (B) Both statements are false.
    (C) The first statement is true, the second is false.
    (D) The first statement is false, the second is true.

156. All of the following fall under nonverbal behaviors **EXCEPT** one. Which one is the **EXCEPTION**?
    (A) Body orientation
    (B) Posture
    (C) Facial expressions
    (D) Reflective responding
    (E) Gestures

157. What is the maximum permissible dose of radiation a dental hygienist should be exposed to each year?
(A) 1 rem
(B) 2 rem
(C) 3 rem
(D) 4 rem
(E) 5 rem

158. Which of these is the main goal of patient education?
(A) Complying with regulation
(B) Preventing disease
(C) Meeting ethical standards
(D) Diagnosing disease
(E) Pleasing patients

159. Which of the following is considered an unintentional tort?
(A) Assault
(B) Battery
(C) Malpractice
(D) Defamation
(E) Slander

160. When preparing a tooth for restoration, what occurs after the tooth has been etched with 37 percent phosphoric acid?
(A) The tooth is etched with a less potent concentration of phosphoric acid a second time.
(B) A bonding material is applied to the tooth's surface and is cured with light.
(C) The surface of the tooth is primed with a hydrophilic resin that oozes into irregular surfaces.
(D) The restoration material is poured into the tooth and bonds to the dentin.
(E) Decay is removed from the surface of the tooth.

161. Which of the following is a hereditary bleeding disorder that can affect both men and women, but affects only about 1 percent of the population?
(A) Leukemia
(B) Hemophilia
(C) Prothrombin deficiency
(D) Christmas disease
(E) Von Willebrand disease

162. The nasal septum is a radiological landmark that can be identified by a
(A) radiolucent line between the maxillary incisors.
(B) radiopacity at the juncture of the anterior sinus with the floor of the nasal fossa.
(C) radiopaque area located between the central incisors that divides the nasal cavity into two parts.
(D) radiopaque area at the most posterior end of the maxilla.
(E) radiopaque area that is a thin, curved line of the medial pterygoid plate.

163. How often should radiographs of dental implants be taken?
(A) Every office visit
(B) Every two office visits
(C) Every two years
(D) Every year
(E) Every 6 months

164. Which one of the following phases of dental care planning focuses on controlling risk factors for disease?
(A) Preliminary phase
(B) Phase I therapy
(C) Phase II therapy
(D) Phase III therapy
(E) Phase IV therapy

165. The passageway for the spinal cord, accessory nerve, and vertebral arteries is the
(A) medulla oblongata.
(B) jugular foramen.
(C) paired parietal.
(D) sphenoid bones.
(E) foramen magnum.

166. According to G. V. Black, caries are organized using six classifications based on the location of caries on the tooth.

Root caries occur from xerostomia, radiation therapy, poor oral hygiene, recession, or a high-sugar diet.
(A) Both statements are true.
(B) Both statements are false.
(C) The first statement is true, the second is false.
(D) The first statement is false, the second is true.

167. Each of the following is true of compomers' **EXCEPT** one. Which one is the **EXCEPTION**?
    (A) They are able to bond to hard tooth structures easily.
    (B) They are a polyacid-modified composite resin.
    (C) They release fluoride into the surrounding teeth for about 300 days.
    (D) They have a low compressive and flexural strength.
    (E) They are available in various shades to match teeth.

168. How long should you dry the etched area before applying a pit-and-fissure sealant?
    (A) 5–10 seconds
    (B) 30–45 seconds
    (C) 1 minute
    (D) 3 minutes
    (E) 5 minutes

169. Infants suffering from Pierre Robin syndrome often face difficulties eating and breathing **BECAUSE** their tongues "ball up" in the back of their mouths and their jaws are small.
    (A) Both the statement and reason are correct and related.
    (B) Both the statement and reason are correct but NOT related.
    (C) The statement is correct, but the reason is NOT.
    (D) The statement is NOT correct, but the reason is correct.
    (E) NEITHER the statement NOR the reason is correct.

170. A patient's treatment plan should always include an education plan for the patient to follow **BECAUSE** the education plan explains the risk factors that accompany certain treatments.
    (A) Both the statement and reason are correct and related.
    (B) Both the statement and reason are correct but NOT related.
    (C) The statement is correct, but the reason is NOT.
    (D) The statement is NOT correct, but the reason is correct.
    (E) NEITHER the statement NOR the reason is correct.

171. Active listening requires eye contact.

    Active listening involves summarizing what the client has said.
    (A) Both statements are true.
    (B) Both statements are false.
    (C) The first statement is true, the second is false.
    (D) The first statement is false, the second is true.

172. About how many milligrams are in 1 grain?
    (A) 0.065
    (B) 1
    (C) 65
    (D) 100
    (E) 650

173. Mucogingival surgery is recommended for a patient with a diseased pocket that has moved beyond the mucogingival junction.

    Periodontal flap surgery is recommended for a patient who needs his or her gingival tissues reshaped.
    (A) Both statements are true.
    (B) Both statements are false.
    (C) The first statement is true, the second is false.
    (D) The first statement is false, the second is true.

174. Upon examination of a radiograph, you notice merged roots. This could be
    (A) dilaceration.
    (B) fusion.
    (C) gemination.
    (D) concrescence.
    (E) abscess.

175. How might pregnancy affect a woman's gingiva?
    (A) The gingiva takes longer to heal.
    (B) A dark-red hyperplasia may develop.
    (C) The gingiva become easily irritated.
    (D) Plaque retention is increased.
    (E) The gingiva recedes from the teeth.

176. Benzodiazepines are considered antineoplastic agents **BECAUSE** they reduce anxiety and bring about sleep.
    (A) Both the statement and reason are correct and related.
    (B) Both the statement and reason are correct but NOT related.
    (C) The statement is correct, but the reason is NOT.
    (D) The statement is NOT correct, but the reason is correct.
    (E) NEITHER the statement NOR the reason is correct.

177. Which type of microorganisms are normally contained in pit and fissure tooth surfaces?
    (A) *Actinomyces naeslundii*
    (B) *Streptococcus sanguinis*
    (C) *Actinomyces israelii*
    (D) *Lactobacillus acidophilus*
    (E) *Nocardia veterana*

178. A patient agreeing to a procedure after the health-care provider explains the risks involved in the procedure is an example of informed consent.

    A patient who attends an examination giving consent to have services performed based on the action of attending the examination is an example of a situation involving implied consent.
    (A) Both statements are true.
    (B) Both statements are false.
    (C) The first statement is true, the second is false.
    (D) The first statement is false, the second is true.

179. Enamel and dentin originate in the same area.

    Enamel and dentin proliferate in opposite directions.
    (A) Both statements are true.
    (B) Both statements are false.
    (C) The first statement is true, the second is false.
    (D) The first statement is false, the second is true.

180. Which of these is measured from the bottom of the sulcus to the mucogingival junction?
    (A) Periodontium
    (B) Attached gingiva
    (C) Clinical-attachment level (CAL)
    (D) Free gingival
    (E) Periodontal tissue

181. Each of the following statements about water is true **EXCEPT** one. Which one is the **EXCEPTION**?
    (A) Body temperature is regulated with water's assistance.
    (B) Water helps give the body energy.
    (C) Water aids in the transport of blood, nerve conduction, and nutrients.
    (D) Kidney function and blood pressure are affected by water intake.
    (E) Water assists in the processes of reparation and building of cells.

182. Each of the following statements about bacteria is true **EXCEPT** one. Which one is the **EXCEPTION**?
    (A) Bacteria are prokaryotes.
    (B) Some bacteria are classified as spirilli.
    (C) Bacteria divide by the process of mitosis.
    (D) Bacteria do not contain evidence of mitotic spindles.
    (E) All bacteria that form parasitic relationships are known as pathogens.

183. During a patient examination, it is possible to assume that your patient is suffering from bulimia nervosa **BECAUSE** you notice swelling of the parotid glands and erosion of the maxillary anterior teeth.
    (A) Both the statement and reason are correct and related.
    (B) Both the statement and reason are correct but NOT related.
    (C) The statement is correct, but the reason is NOT.
    (D) The statement is NOT correct, but the reason is correct.
    (E) NEITHER the statement NOR the reason is correct.

184. What do fremitus scores indicate?
(A) The amount of interradicular bone loss
(B) The amount of bone loss between roots
(C) The amount of lesions within the mouth
(D) The degree of bleeding during a periodontal screening
(E) The degree of vibration felt when teeth are tapped together

185. A patient suffering from diabetes mellitus should be monitored carefully for infected wounds **BECAUSE** the disease slows healing and increases chances of infection.
(A) Both the statement and reason are correct and related.
(B) Both the statement and reason are correct but NOT related.
(C) The statement is correct, but the reason is NOT.
(D) The statement is NOT correct, but the reason is correct.
(E) NEITHER the statement NOR the reason is correct.

186. When spraying air onto what appears to be abnormal epidermal tissue, you may create a blister **BECAUSE** the patient's outer layer of the epidermis separates from the basal layer.
(A) Both the statement and reason are correct and related.
(B) Both the statement and reason are correct but NOT related.
(C) The statement is correct, but the reason is NOT.
(D) The statement is NOT correct, but the reason is correct.
(E) NEITHER the statement NOR the reason is correct.

187. The correct angle for the oblique stroke used in calculus removal is a
(A) 25-degree angle.
(B) 45-degree angle.
(C) 50-degree angle.
(D) 75-degree angle.
(E) 90-degree angle.

188. Which of the following is true about the dentoperiosteal?
(A) It connects cementum to free gingiva and attached gingiva.
(B) It connects periosteum of bone to attached gingiva.
(C) It connects cementum at CEJ to alveolar crest.
(D) It connects interdental space to cementum.
(E) It connects alveolar mucosa to the free gingiva.

189. What must be avoided when caring for implants?
(A) Graphite dental tools
(B) Scratching the implant
(C) Strong mouthwashes
(D) Pocket probing
(E) Eating sticky foods

190. A double-blind study is a true reflection of an entire population.

Double-blind studies are performed over a long period of time.
(A) Both statements are true.
(B) Both statements are false.
(C) The first statement is true, the second is false.
(D) The first statement is false, the second is true.

191. What makes cleaning and polishing agents effective for removing stains, plaque, and debris on teeth?
(A) Foaming agent
(B) Abrasive agent
(C) Binding agent
(D) Moisture agent
(E) Thickening agent

192. What is significant to know about Down syndrome in relation to dentistry?
(A) Tooth eruption is often delayed and teeth are irregularly shaped.
(B) Patients usually have a large oral cavity and small, fissured tongue.
(C) Caries are uncommon, but gingivitis is common.
(D) Teeth often develop quickly, but are very prone to caries.
(E) Patients usually have a long, narrow palate.

193. An alloy composed of mercury mixed with a powder made mainly of silver and tin and other trace elements is called
    (A) amalgam.
    (B) creep.
    (C) cement.
    (D) varnish.
    (E) resin.

194. The frontal nerve, lacrimal nerve, and the nasocilary nerve are all afferent and part of the
    (A) trochlear.
    (B) mandibular nerve.
    (C) medial pterygoid.
    (D) tensor veli palatini.
    (E) trigeminal ophthalmic.

195. Which of these is true about B vitamins?
    (A) They support the body's metabolism.
    (B) They include beta-carotene and retinol.
    (C) They play a key role in scotopic and color vision.
    (D) They are water soluble and cannot be stored by the body.
    (E) They do not cause toxicity if consumed in excess.

196. Medical safety data sheets are a concern of
    (A) HIPAA.
    (B) OSHA.
    (C) PHI.
    (D) EPHI.
    (E) CDC.

Use the following scenario to answer questions 197–200.

Your new patient is a 23-year-old man. He says that he hasn't been to the dentist in several years. He is hoping to get a cleaning. You tell the patient that radiographs are taken for each new patient. He says that he worries about the effect radiation could have on his health. After much discussion, the patient agrees to have the radiographs taken.

197. Which of the following arguments most likely convinced the patient to have the radiographs taken?
    (A) Your cell phone admits more radiation than an X-ray machine.
    (B) People are constantly exposed to radiation from the sun.
    (C) The office uses digital radiography, which uses less radiation.
    (D) The lead apron worn during the exam protects from all radiation.
    (E) Today's faster film speeds require less radiation.

198. How often should you recommend that this patient have radiographs taken?
    (A) Every office visit
    (B) Every 6 months
    (C) Every year
    (D) Whenever the patient wants them
    (E) When the patient needs them

199. What is the minimum thickness required for a lead apron to protect the patient from radiation?
    (A) 0.25 mm
    (B) 0.50 mm
    (C) 0.75 mm
    (D) 1.00 mm
    (E) 1.25 mm

200. One of the radiographs that you've taken of a patient appears to have tree-like or root-like branches on it. What is the most likely cause?
    (A) The film was not placed at the proper angle.
    (B) Static electricity might have affected the film.
    (C) The film has been used in several locations.
    (D) Incorrect horizontal angulation was used.
    (E) The film may have been bent.

COMPONENT B

Directions: Study the case components and answer questions 1–10.

SYNOPSIS OF PATIENT HISTORY

CASE _DT-1_

Age ___20___

Sex ___Female___

Height _5'8"_

Weight _135_ lbs

_62.23_ kgs

Vital Signs

Blood pressure ___118/75___

Pulse rate ___75___

Respiration rate ___16___

---

1. Under Care of Physician
   Yes ☐ No ☑
   Condition: _____

2. Hospitalized within the last 5 years
   Yes ☐ No ☑
   Reason: _____
   _____

3. Has or had the following conditions:
   _Severe anxiety_____
   _____

4. Current medications:
   Discontinued anti-depression medication
   _____
   _____

5. Smokes or uses tobacco products
   Yes ☑ No ☐

6. Is pregnant
   Yes ☐ No ☑ N/A ☐

MEDICAL HISTORY:
The patient has acceptable health, but she is run down and not taking good care of herself. She does not eat right, does not exercise, and does not get enough sleep. She frequently goes out with friends and drinks too much alcohol.

DENTAL HISTORY:
Her last dental visit was 4 years ago for a cleaning and an exam. She has been advised to have partially impacted third molars removed.

SOCIAL HISTORY:
She is a second-year college student who is struggling to complete a difficult health technology program. She reports that at this time, she may have to drop out due to her poor financial situation, as well as her fear of not being able to keep up with the academics.

CHIEF COMPLAINT:
Generalized painful gums, metallic taste, and fetid odor from mouth. She is running a fever of 100°.

ADULT CLINICAL EXAMINATION

Case DT-1

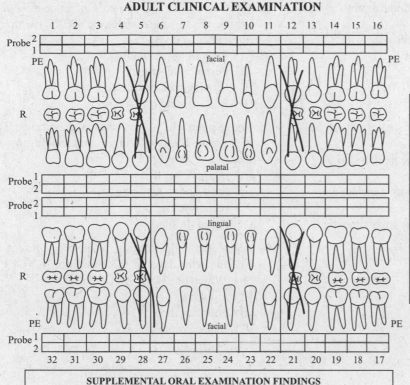

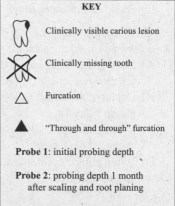

KEY

Clinically visible carious lesion

Clinically missing tooth

Furcation

"Through and through" furcation

Probe 1: initial probing depth

Probe 2: probing depth 1 month after scaling and root planing

SUPPLEMENTAL ORAL EXAMINATION FINDINGS

1. Grayish pseudomembrane generalized.
2. Severe halitosis.
3. Tissues generally inflamed.
4. Generalized moderate plaque and stain; poor oral hygiene.
5. Calculus deposits on lower anterior lingual and maxillary buccal.
6. Probing impossible due to patient's discomfort level.

---

1. Which of the following is **MOST LIKELY** the diagnosis for this patient's periodontal condition?
   (A) Chronic periodontitis
   (B) Necrotizing ulcerative periodontal disease
   (C) Primary herpetic gingivostomatitis
   (D) Necrotizing ulcerative gingivitis

2. Your patient has small grayish areas on her gums. These areas are
   (A) ulcers.
   (B) proteins.
   (C) bacteria.
   (D) plaque.

3. All of the following are clinical signs that distinguish this patient's condition from other conditions **EXCEPT** one. Which one is this **EXCEPTION**?
   (A) Punched-out papillae
   (B) Pseudomembrane
   (C) Involvement of deeper periodontium
   (D) Lymphadenopathy

4. The highest incidence of this patient's condition is seen in which of the following age ranges?
   (A) 20–30
   (B) 25–35
   (C) 30–40
   (D) 40–50

5. All of the following are part of the treatment of this patient's condition during the first appointment **EXCEPT** one. Which one is the **EXCEPTION**?
   (A) Remove pseudomembrane carefully with irrigation/moist cotton
   (B) Supragingival periodontal instrumentation
   (C) Gentle subgingival periodontal instrumentation
   (D) Patient self-care instruction

6. Which of the following is standard protocol in treating this patient's condition?
   (A) Three percent hydrogen peroxide with warm water every 3 hours
   (B) Antibiotic therapy
   (C) Gentle self-care regimen
   (D) Pseudomembrane removal

7. When should subgingival instrumentation be performed on your patient?
   (A) During the first visit, if the patient can tolerate it
   (B) During the second follow-up appointment, about 5 days later
   (C) During the third follow-up appointment, about 10 days later
   (D) When subgingival instrumentation is contraindicated

8. You can tell that your patient's infection is severe. Which of the following is the **BEST** treatment during her first visit?
   (A) Prescription of antibiotics
   (B) Periodontal surgery
   (C) Rinsing with warm salt water
   (D) Root planing and scaling

9. Your patient tells you that she realizes she needs to make some lifestyle changes. You should suggest that she
   (A) improve her diet.
   (B) limit or quit smoking.
   (C) reduce stress.
   (D) All of the above

10. All of the following are frequently present in patients who develop this condition **EXCEPT** one. Which one is the **EXCEPTION**?
    (A) Smoking
    (B) Poor nutrition
    (C) Impacted molars
    (D) Severe stress

Directions: Study the case components and answer questions 11–20.

SYNOPSIS OF PATIENT HISTORY

CASE _DT-2_

Age _6_

Sex _Male_

Height _3'5"_

Weight _60_ lbs

_27.22_ kgs

Vital Signs

Blood pressure _N/A_

Pulse rate _100_

Respiration rate _20_

1. Under Care of Physician
   Yes ☐ No ☑
   Condition: _____

2. Hospitalized within the last 5 years
   Yes ☐ No ☐
   Reason: _____ _N/A_ _____

3. Has or had the following conditions:
   Mild asthma _____
   _____

4. Current medications:
   _____
   _____
   _____

5. Smokes or uses tobacco products
   Yes ☐ No ☑

6. Is pregnant
   Yes ☐ No ☐ N/A ☑

MEDICAL HISTORY:
The patient is generally in good health. His mother reports that he has a fever during the last two days, a headache, and swollen lymph nodes. Overall, he does not feel well.

DENTAL HISTORY:
He has been coming to the dentist regularly since he was 3 years old. He has no decay and comes in twice a year for cleanings and exams.

SOCIAL HISTORY:
He is a well-adjusted first grader who does well in school, participates in sports, and has many friends.

CHIEF COMPLAINT:
He has severe oral pain, can't eat or drink easily, and his mouth has clusters of blisters on his gums.

CLINICAL EXAMINATION

Case DT-2

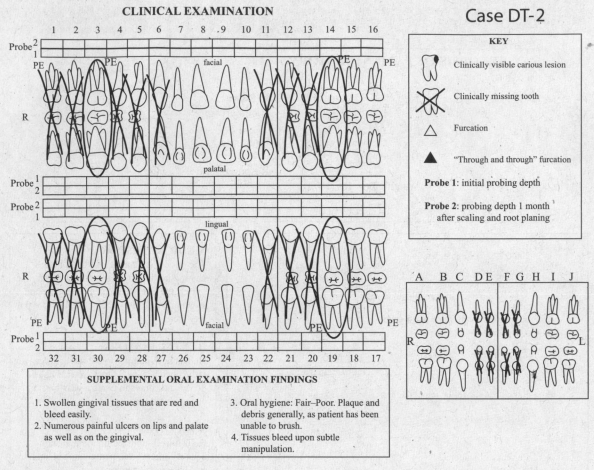

KEY

Clinically visible carious lesion

Clinically missing tooth

Furcation

"Through and through" furcation

Probe 1: initial probing depth

Probe 2: probing depth 1 month after scaling and root planing

SUPPLEMENTAL ORAL EXAMINATION FINDINGS

1. Swollen gingival tissues that are red and bleed easily.
2. Numerous painful ulcers on lips and palate as well as on the gingival.
3. Oral hygiene: Fair–Poor. Plaque and debris generally, as patient has been unable to brush.
4. Tissues bleed upon subtle manipulation.

11. This patient's condition is **MOST LIKELY** which of the following?
    - (A) Pre-pubertal gingivitis
    - (B) Acute gingivitis
    - (C) Primary herpetic gingivostomatitis
    - (D) Oral chicken pox

12. All of the following are characteristic of this patient's condition **EXCEPT** one. Which one is the **EXCEPTION**?
    - (A) Severe oral pain
    - (B) Difficulty in eating and drinking
    - (C) Skin rash on the arms and legs
    - (D) Painful oral ulcers

13. This patient may suffer ulcers in which of the following areas?
    - (A) Lips
    - (B) Palate
    - (C) Tongue
    - (D) All of the above

14. Which of the following is the etiology of this patient's condition?
    - (A) Bacterial
    - (B) Fungal
    - (C) Viral
    - (D) Autoimmune

15. To help this patient deal with the outbreak, you should recommend which of the following to his mother?
    - (A) Maintain proper hygiene.
    - (B) Increase fluid intake.
    - (C) Give analgesics to control pain.
    - (D) All of the above

16. This patient's condition is caused by which of the following?
    - (A) HSV-1
    - (B) HSV-2
    - (C) HSV-3
    - (D) HSV-4

17. All of the following are triggers that can cause this patient's condition to recur **EXCEPT** one. Which of the following is the **EXCEPTION**?
    (A) Sunlight
    (B) Malnutrition
    (C) Common cold
    (D) Dental caries

18. You should wear which of the following when treating this patient?
    (A) A mask
    (B) Gloves
    (C) Eye protection
    (D) All of the above

19. Which of the following is **NOT** commonly used to treat a patient with this condition?
    (A) Antiviral medications
    (B) Antipyretics
    (C) Localized gentle scaling
    (D) Topical oral anesthetics

20. This condition is most common among which of the following age groups?
    (A) Newborn to 1 year
    (B) 1 year to 6 years
    (C) 12 years to 18 years
    (D) Adults

Directions: Study the case components and answer questions 21–30.

SYNOPSIS OF PATIENT HISTORY

CASE _DT-3_

Age _24_

Sex _Male_

Height _5'11"_

Weight _175_ lbs

_79.38_ kgs

Vital Signs

Blood pressure _120/80_

Pulse rate _80_

Respiration rate _16_

1. Under Care of Physician
   Yes ☐ No ☑

   Condition: _____

2. Hospitalized within the last 5 years
   Yes ☑ No ☐

   Reason: _Emergency appendectomy 2 years prior_
   _____

3. Has or had the following conditions:

   Allergic to amoxicillin
   _____

4. Current medications:

   Has been on and off steroids for athletic gains;
   states he is not taking any now.

5. Smokes or uses tobacco products
   Yes ☑ No ☐   * _States he chews tobacco._

6. Is pregnant
   Yes ☐ No ☐ N/A ☑

MEDICAL HISTORY:
The patient is generally in good health and is an athlete, but has taken steroids to build body muscle for a weight-lifting competition.

DENTAL HISTORY:
His last dental visit was 18 months prior for a cleaning and an exam. The patient was told he should have his third molars removed.

SOCIAL HISTORY:
The patient is a part-time college student who also works as a delivery person. He is active in body-building and baseball. He said he would never smoke cigarettes but likes to chew tobacco.

CHIEF COMPLAINT:
"My gum is swollen on the lower left behind my last tooth, and it feels like it is on fire. My breath stinks."

ADULT CLINICAL EXAMINATION

Case DT-3

| | 1 | 2 | 3 | 4 | 5 | 6 | 7 | 8 | 9 | 10 | 11 | 12 | 13 | 14 | 15 | 16 |

Probe 2
1
| 323 | 323 | 323 | | 222 | 212 | 212 | 212 | 212 | 222 | | 222 | 323 | 323 |

facial

R

PE

palatal

Probe 1
2
| 323 | 323 | 323 | | 222 | 212 | 212 | 212 | 212 | 222 | | 222 | 323 | 323 |

Probe 2
1
| 323 | 323 | 323 | | 222 | 212 | 212 | 212 | 212 | 222 | | 222 | 323 | 323 |

lingual

R

PE

facial

Probe 1
2
| 323 | 323 | 323 | | 222 | 212 | 212 | 212 | 212 | 222 | | 222 | 323 | 323 |

| 32 | 31 | 30 | 29 | 28 | 27 | 26 | 25 | 24 | 23 | 22 | 21 | 20 | 19 | 18 | 17 |

KEY

Clinically visible carious lesion

Clinically missing tooth

Furcation

"Through and through" furcation

Probe 1: initial probing depth

Probe 2: probing depth 1 month after scaling and root planing

SUPPLEMENTAL ORAL EXAMINATION FINDINGS

1. Oral Hygiene: Fair, with moderate calculus deposits generally, and biofilm present on linguals of lower molars; no stain evident.
2. Localized area of swelling distal to #18 with exudates present
3. Patient is having difficulty opening mouth.
4. Patient has halitosis.
5. Bleeding in localized areas, especially lower left.
6. Deep pockct on #18 Dbu and DLi.
7. #16, #17, and #32 are partially erupted; probing at initial visit.

---

21. What type of anesthesia would you **MOST LIKELY** use to treat a patient with a pericoronal abscess?
(A) Topical local anesthesia
(B) Injected local anesthesia
(C) Analgesics
(D) General anesthesia

22. What is the most common site for a pericoronal abscess?
(A) Partially erupted maxillary third molar
(B) Partially erupted mandibular third molar
(C) Impacted mandibular third molar
(D) Impacted maxillary third molar

23. All of the following are signs of a pericoronal abscess **EXCEPT** one. Which one is the **EXCEPTION**?
(A) Pain at the site
(B) Lymphadenopathy

(C) Blanching of the flap of soft tissue covering the tooth
(D) Limited mouth opening

24. The flap of soft tissue covering a portion of a partially erupted tooth is known as which of the following?
(A) Opercula vitale
(B) Pericoronal flap
(C) Operculum
(D) Retromolar extension

25. Your patient is having difficulty opening his mouth. This is known as
(A) lymphadenopathy.
(B) lockjaw.
(C) trismus.
(D) TMJ crepitation.

26. Treating a periocoronal abscess differs from treating other types of abscesses because periocoronal abscesses
    (A) are difficult to diagnose.
    (B) typically heal on their own.
    (C) are difficult to access.
    (D) require a specific antibiotic.

27. All of the following are part of the treatment of a periocoronal abscess **EXCEPT** one. Which one is the **EXCEPTION**?
    (A) Place a local antibiotic inside the infected area.
    (B) Establish a path of drainage for the pus.
    (C) Irrigate the undersurface of the operculum.
    (D) Thorough periodontal debridement of the tooth surfaces in the area.

28. When treating this patient, you should use which of the following to irrigate the area under the operculum?
    (A) Chlorhexadine
    (B) Sterile saline
    (C) Hydrogen peroxide
    (D) Listerine®

29. Which of the following should you use to puncture the soft-tissue wall of the pocket to allow drainage?
    (A) Sterile cotton pliers
    (B) A shepherd's hook explorer
    (C) Sterile curet
    (D) Never puncture the soft tissue wall

30. X-rays of a pericoronal abscess usually indicate which of the following?
    (A) A light area around the pulp
    (B) A dark area around the root
    (C) An absence of a root canal
    (D) A blurry area around the abscess

Directions: Study the case components and answer questions 31–40.

SYNOPSIS OF PATIENT HISTORY

CASE _DT-4_

Age _50_

Sex _Female_

Height _5'3"_

Weight _165_ lbs

_74.84_ kgs

Vital Signs

Blood pressure _140/85_

Pulse rate _78_

Respiration rate _14_

---

1. Under Care of Physician
   Yes ☑ No ☐

   Condition: _Cholesterol, fatigue, arthritis_

2. Hospitalized within the last 5 years
   Yes ☑ No ☐

   Reason: _Hysterectomy_

3. Has or had the following conditions:

   Latex allergy, depression, arthritis, high cholesterol

4. Current medications:

   Aleve p.r.n. (1–2 tablets) most days for arthritis

5. Smokes or uses tobacco products
   Yes ☑ No ☐

6. Is pregnant
   Yes ☐ No ☐ N/A ☑

MEDICAL HISTORY:
The patient is attempting to control her cholesterol with weight loss. She is depressed but trying to exercise more and feels that this helps her mood. She has cut back her smoking to six cigarettes a day. She is trying to use her anti-inflammatory arthritis meds minimally.

DENTAL HISTORY:
The patient had not had a cleaning in 5 years and recently went to a different dental office, where the doctor began a "gross scaling." She was scheduled for another visit but did not return as she did not like the dentist.

SOCIAL HISTORY:
The patient works part-time as a secretary at her local church office. She is divorced with one child in high school. She has recently lost weight and is feeling better about herself.

CHIEF COMPLAINT:
"I know my cleaning did not get finished, but I now have swelling on my lower right gums in the middle area with a bad taste in my mouth. I don't want to go back to that dentist."

ADULT CLINICAL EXAMINATION

Case DT-4

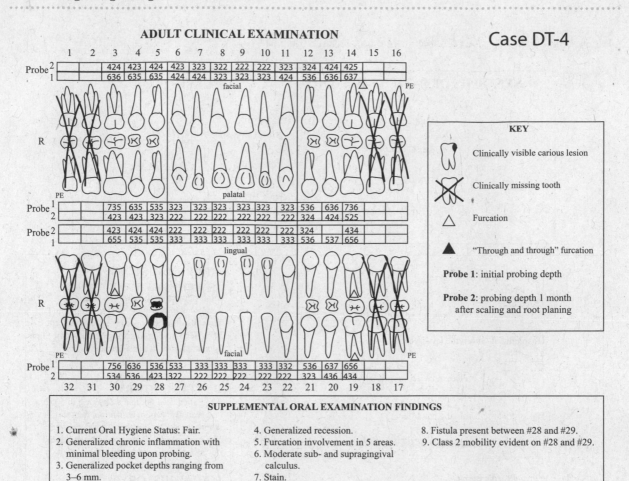

SUPPLEMENTAL ORAL EXAMINATION FINDINGS

1. Current Oral Hygiene Status: Fair.
2. Generalized chronic inflammation with minimal bleeding upon probing.
3. Generalized pocket depths ranging from 3–6 mm.
4. Generalized recession.
5. Furcation involvement in 5 areas.
6. Moderate sub- and supragingival calculus.
7. Stain.
8. Fistula present between #28 and #29.
9. Class 2 mobility evident on #28 and #29.

31. Based on the patient's clinical presentation without X-rays, what is the **MOST LIKELY** diagnosis?
(A) Advanced periodontitis
(B) Moderate chronic generalized periodontitis
(C) Necrotizing ulcerative periodontitis
(D) Aggressive adult periodontitis

32. What is the American Dental Association (ADA) classification of this patient's periodontitis?
(A) Type 1
(B) Type 2
(C) Type 3
(D) Type 4

33. What is the probable diagnosis for the fistula/swelling between #28 and #29?
(A) Periapical abscess
(B) Periodontal abscess
(C) Pericoronitis
(D) RAU

34. All of the following may have contributed to the patient's fistula/swelling between #28 and #29 **EXCEPT** one. Which one is the **EXCEPTION**?
(A) History of smoking
(B) Gross scaling treatment one week prior
(C) Periodontal pocketing #28 and #29 buccal aspects
(D) An old amalgam on #28 that is breaking down at margins

35. Which of the following is **NOT** a treatment for the swelling between #28 and #29?
(A) Establishment of a path of drainage for the pus
(B) Thorough periodontal debridement of the tooth surface in area
(C) Relief of pain
(D) Extraction of the tooth that is infected

36. Which of the following **BEST** describes the pain that is felt with this patient's condition?
    (A) Constant, and easy to localize
    (B) Intermittent, brought on by heat
    (C) Intermittent, brought on by pressure
    (D) Instigated by pressure from mastication

37. All of the following may occur during a follow-up for your patient once her condition has been resolved **EXCEPT** one. Which one is the **EXCEPTION**?
    (A) Complete periodontal exam and assessment
    (B) Completion of the gross scaling
    (C) Quadrant or half-mouth debridement with pain control
    (D) Self-care instruction

38. After reevaluation, which of the following will be most effective for your patient to use to maintain her interproximal areas?
    (A) Toothpicks
    (B) Rubber tip
    (C) Proxy brush and floss
    (D) End tuft brush and water pik

39. Which of the following is the appropriate recare frequency for this patient after reevaluation?
    (A) 6 months
    (B) 4 months
    (C) 3 months
    (D) 2months

40. Which of the following is the **BEST** mouth rinse for the patient to use on a regular basis?
    (A) Chlorhexidine
    (B) Any OTC fluoride rinse
    (C) Hydrogen peroxide diluted to 2 percent
    (D) An antimicrobial rinse that does not contain alcohol

Directions: Study the case components and answer questions 41–50.

SYNOPSIS OF PATIENT HISTORY

CASE _DT-5_

Age _10_

Sex _Male_

Height _4'6"_

Weight _70_ lbs

_37.5_ kgs

Vital Signs

Blood pressure _100/60_

Pulse rate _100_

Respiration rate _20_

1. Under Care of Physician
   Yes ☑ No ☐

   Condition: _For seizure disorder_

2. Hospitalized within the last 5 years
   Yes ☑ No ☐

   Reason: _For grand mal seizure 2 years prior_

3. Has or had the following conditions:

   Seizure disorder, and mold, dust, and pollen allergies

4. Current medications:

   Phenytoin

5. Smokes or uses tobacco products
   Yes ☐ No ☑

6. Is pregnant
   Yes ☐ No ☐ N/A ☑

MEDICAL HISTORY:
The patient was diagnosed 2 years ago with a seizure disorder. The seizures are under control with phenytoin.

DENTAL HISTORY:
The patient's last cleaning was 1½ years prior. The family is low income.

SOCIAL HISTORY:
The patient is a friendly child, but he is shy and apprehensive about professional care.

CHIEF COMPLAINT:
The patient's mother states, "My son's gums have become so swollen they are 2/3 of the way up the teeth."

CLINICAL EXAMINATION

Case DT-5

KEY

Clinically visible carious lesion

Clinically missing tooth

Furcation

"Through and through" furcation

Probe 1: initial probing depth

Probe 2: probing depth 1 month after scaling and root planing

All pseudopocketing

SUPPLEMENTAL ORAL EXAMINATION FINDINGS

1. No periodontal charting.
2. Oral hygiene: Fair.
3. Tissue overgrowth generalized through mouth.
4. Moderate plaque, no calculus.
5. Bleeding easily upon gentle manipulation of gums.

41. Your patient's gingival enlargement is **MOST LIKELY** caused by which of the following?
    (A) Poor dental care
    (B) Nutritional deficiencies
    (C) Seizures
    (D) Phenytoin

42. The American Dental Association (ADA) classification for this disease is
    (A) Type 1.
    (B) Type 2.
    (C) Type 3.
    (D) Type 4.

43. All of the following drugs **EXCEPT** one may cause gingival enlargement. Which one is the **EXCEPTION**?
    (A) Cyclosporine A
    (B) Certain calcium channel blockers
    (C) Azathioprine erplasia
    (D) Procardia

44. Gingival enlargement occurs **MOST** often in which of the following age groups?
    (A) Children and infants
    (B) Children and young adults
    (C) Equally among all age groups
    (D) Middle-aged persons

45. If your patient's gingival enlargement is drug influenced, which of the following is the **BEST** action to take regarding his medication?
    (A) Alternate weeks of taking the drug.
    (B) Prescribe an adjunct drug to counteract effects.
    (C) Continue the drug but rinse with antimicrobials.
    (D) Discontinue the drug, if possible.

46. Which of the following is true if your patient undergoes surgery to eliminate drug-influenced gingival enlargement?
    (A) The patient may suffer rapid weight loss.
    (B) The overgrowth will likely reoccur.
    (C) The drug will no longer be needed.
    (D) The condition will be permanently eliminated.

47. All of the following should be included in your patient's meticulous plaque control **EXCEPT** one. Which one is the **EXCEPTION**?
    (A) Education on self-care
    (B) Frequent professional care
    (C) Periodontal debridement of tooth surfaces
    (D) Increased fluid intake to prevent dehydration

48. Which of the following may be a valuable adjunct to mechanical plaque control for this patient?
    (A) Fluoride mouth rinses
    (B) Antimicrobial mouth rinses
    (C) Saltwater rinses
    (D) Hydrogen peroxide rinse

49. In addition to medication, which of the following increases a patient's risk of an outbreak of gingival enlargement?
    (A) Family history
    (B) Poor oral hygiene
    (C) Braces
    (D) All of the above

50. Which of the following is the **BEST** recall frequency for this patient?
    (A) 2 months
    (B) 4 months
    (C) 6 months
    (D) 1 year

Directions: Study the case components and answer questions 51–60.

SYNOPSIS OF PATIENT HISTORY

CASE   _DT-6_

Age   _27_

Sex   _Female_

Height _5'8"_

Weight _145_ lbs

_65.77_kgs

Vital Signs

Blood pressure   _130/82_

Pulse rate   _90_

Respiration rate   _19_

1. Under Care of Physician
   Yes ☑ No ☐

   Condition: _Routine physicals_

2. Hospitalized within the last 5 years
   Yes ☐ No ☑

   Reason: _____

3. Has or had the following conditions:

   _____
   _____

4. Current medications:

   _____
   _____

5. Smokes or uses tobacco products
   Yes ☐ No ☑

6. Is pregnant
   Yes ☐ No ☑ N/A ☐

MEDICAL HISTORY:
The patient states that she is in excellent health.

DENTAL HISTORY:
The patient has regular cleanings, but her periodontal health has deteriorated rapidly over the past year. Her mother lost all her teeth when she was the patient's age.

SOCIAL HISTORY:
She is a stay-at-home mother who helps her husband with their pest-control business. She has two children.

CHIEF COMPLAINT:
"I am so afraid I am going to lose my teeth just like my mother did."

ADULT CLINICAL EXAMINATION

Case DT-6

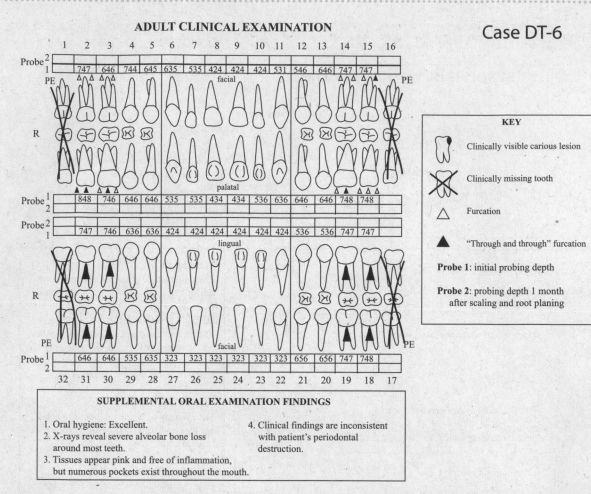

KEY

tooth	Clinically visible carious lesion
X	Clinically missing tooth
△	Furcation
▲	"Through and through" furcation

Probe 1: initial probing depth

Probe 2: probing depth 1 month after scaling and root planing

---

SUPPLEMENTAL ORAL EXAMINATION FINDINGS

1. Oral hygiene: Excellent.
2. X-rays reveal severe alveolar bone loss around most teeth.
3. Tissues appear pink and free of inflammation, but numerous pockets exist throughout the mouth.
4. Clinical findings are inconsistent with patient's periodontal destruction.

---

51. Your patient's diagnosis is **MOST LIKELY** which of the following?
(A) Generalized aggressive periodontitis
(B) Chronic generalized periodontitis
(C) Localized aggressive periodontitis
(D) Localized chronic periodontitis

52. This condition occurs **MOST** often in patients who are
(A) under 20 years old.
(B) under 30 years old.
(C) over 35 years old.
(D) over 55 years old.

53. All of the following are primary features of your patient's condition **EXCEPT** one. Which one is the **EXCEPTION**?
(A) Heavy generalized calculus deposits.
(B) Rapid destruction of the attachment.
(C) No obvious signs or symptoms of systemic disease.
(D) A family history of aggressive periodontitis.

54. Your patient's condition is characterized by a generalized interproximal attachment loss affecting how many permanent teeth other than the first molars and incisors?
(A) 0
(B) 1
(C) 2
(D) 3

55. Treatment of your patient's condition may involve which of the following?
    - (A) Oral hygiene instruction
    - (B) Frequent evaluation of the patient's plaque control
    - (C) Supra- and subgingival scaling
    - (D) All of the above

56. Which of the following is true of your patient's condition?
    - (A) It is more common than chronic perodontitis.
    - (B) It is less common than chronic periodontitis.
    - (C) It is equally as common as chronic periodontitis.
    - (D) It is extremely rare.

57. Which of the following are desired outcomes for periodontal therapy in this patient?
    - (A) Reduction of probing depths
    - (B) Progression toward occlusal stability
    - (C) Reduction of gingival inflammation
    - (D) All of the above.

58. The treatment of your patient's condition is **MOST** similar to the treatment of which of the following?
    - (A) Gingivitis
    - (B) Acute periodontal abscesses
    - (C) Chronic periodontitis
    - (D) Diabetic periodontitis

59. Which is **NOT** part of a care plan for your patient's condition?
    - (A) Evaluation of her biofilm control skills
    - (B) Periodontal instrumentation of tooth surfaces along with antimicrobial therapy
    - (C) Gingivectomy
    - (D) Surgical debridement of the soft tissue

60. Your patient's condition is usually associated with which of the following pathogens?
    - (A) *Actinobacillus actinomycetemcomitans*
    - (B) *Tannerella forsythensis*
    - (C) *Lactococcus lactis*
    - (D) *Streptococcus mutans*

Directions: Study the case components and answer questions 61–70.

SYNOPSIS OF PATIENT HISTORY

CASE _DT-7_

Age _12_

Sex _Male_

Height _5'5"_

Weight _110_ lbs

_49.9_ kgs

Vital Signs

Blood pressure _100/65_

Pulse rate _90_

Respiration rate _20_

---

1. Under Care of Physician
   Yes ☐ No ☑

   Condition: _____

2. Hospitalized within the last 5 years
   Yes ☐ No ☑

   Reason: _____
   _____

3. Has or had the following conditions:

   acne _____
   _____

4. Current medications:

   low-dose antibiotics for the acne — does not know name

5. Smokes or uses tobacco products
   Yes ☐ No ☑

6. Is pregnant
   Yes ☐ No ☐ N/A ☑

MEDICAL HISTORY:
The patient's mother says that he is in good health and only is taking a low-dose antibiotic for his acne.

DENTAL HISTORY:
The patient has regular dental checkups and cleanings. He has had orthodontic braces for the past year. He is fully banded. He sees the orthodontist every 6 weeks.

SOCIAL HISTORY:
The patient enjoys school and plays sports. He says he enjoys spending time with his friends and family — all normal.

CHIEF COMPLAINT:
Both he and his mother state that his gums are up close to the ortho wires and bleeding. He is showing signs of demineralization around his maxillary anterior brackets.

CLINICAL EXAMINATION

Case DT-7

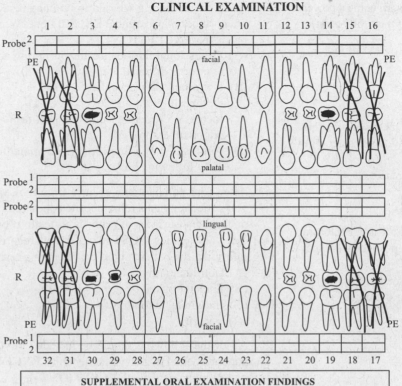

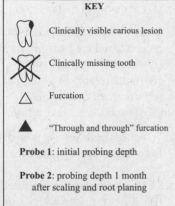

KEY

	Clinically visible carious lesion
	Clinically missing tooth
△	Furcation
▲	"Through and through" furcation

Probe 1: initial probing depth

Probe 2: probing depth 1 month after scaling and root planing

SUPPLEMENTAL ORAL EXAMINATION FINDINGS

1. Generalized gingival edema and inflammation.
2. Tissues swollen up close to ortho wire on both arches.
3. Tissues bleed easily.
4. Oral hygiene: Poor with debris, plaque biofilm, and food visibly present.
5. Demineralization present around some anterior brackets.
6. Patient has 4 to 5 areas of active decay diagnosed.

61. All of the following are risk factors for decay in this patient **EXCEPT** one. Which one is the **EXCEPTION**?
(A) Age group
(B) Position of teeth
(C) Problems with appliances
(D) Medication

62. Which part of the gingiva is **MOST** susceptible to gingival enlargement during orthodontic treatment?
(A) Facial and lingual aspects
(B) Marginal tissue
(C) Subgingival tissues
(D) Interdental

63. All of the following are significant factors in determining the selection of biofilm-control procedures for a patient undergoing orthodontic treatment **EXCEPT** one. Which one is the **EXCEPTION**?
(A) Anatomic feature of the gingival
(B) Orthodontist's philosophy regarding hygiene
(C) Position of the teeth
(D) Type of orthodontic appliance

64. Which type of toothbrush is **NOT** effective for self-care of orthodontic patients?
(A) Power brush
(B) Soft brush with end-rounded filaments
(C) Bilevel orthodontic brush
(D) Hard brush

65. Your patient says he plans to begin using a power brush. Which speed is safest for an orthodontic patient?
(A) Low
(B) Medium
(C) High
(D) It does not matter.

66. Which of the following is the best way for this patient to reduce gum inflammation and bleeding?
(A) Increase dental visits.
(B) Seek treatment for dental caries.
(C) Improve oral hygiene.
(D) Discontinue medication.

67. Which of the following is the **BEST** interdental aid for your patient to clean between adjacent contact areas?
(A) Floss threader with tufted dental floss
(B) Floss threader with regular dental floss
(C) Interdental brush
(D) Single tuft brush

68. All of the following will aid in remineralization after orthodontic treatment **EXCEPT** one. Which one is the **EXCEPTION**?
(A) Professional fluoride treatments during and after orthodontic therapy
(B) Use of an ADA-accepted fluoride toothpaste
(C) Increasing water consumption post-orthodontic therapy
(D) Application of a fluoride varnish immediately following bonding

69. After your patient's braces have been removed, you notice remnants of composite adhesive resin on the facial surfaces of many of his teeth. Which core value comes **MOST** into play with regard to informing the patient about the remaining resin?
(A) Confidentiality
(B) Societal trust
(C) Individual autonomy
(D) Veracity

70. All of the following should be included in your patient's dental hygiene treatment plan **EXCEPT** one. Which one is the **EXCEPTION**?
(A) Tongue deplaquing
(B) Partial mouth debridement
(C) Application of 5 percent NaF fluoride varnish
(D) Use of calcium phosphate systems

Directions: Study the case components and answer questions 71–80.

SYNOPSIS OF PATIENT HISTORY

CASE _DT-8_

Age ___72___

Sex ___Female___

Height _5'3"_

Weight _170_ lbs

_77.11_ kgs

Vital Signs

Blood pressure ___135/88___

Pulse rate ___78___

Respiration rate ___15___

---

1. Under Care of Physician
   Yes ☐   No ☑
   Condition: _____

2. Hospitalized within the last 5 years
   Yes ☐   No ☑
   Reason: _____

3. Has or had the following conditions:
   Allergic to sulfa drugs
   _____

4. Current medications:
   Diltiazem 120 mg
   _____

5. Smokes or uses tobacco products
   Yes ☑   No ☐

6. Is pregnant
   Yes ☐   No ☑   N/A ☐

MEDICAL HISTORY:
The patient reports no known medical problems, but says she enjoys desserts and eats more sugar than she should.

DENTAL HISTORY:
The patient comes in regularly for dental checkups and cleanings. She has been wearing a maxillary denture for 8 years.

SOCIAL HISTORY:
She is widowed and retired but leads a happy and fulfilling life. She smokes a pack of cigarettes a day. She is low income.

CHIEF COMPLAINT:
"I want to make sure I do not lose my lower teeth."

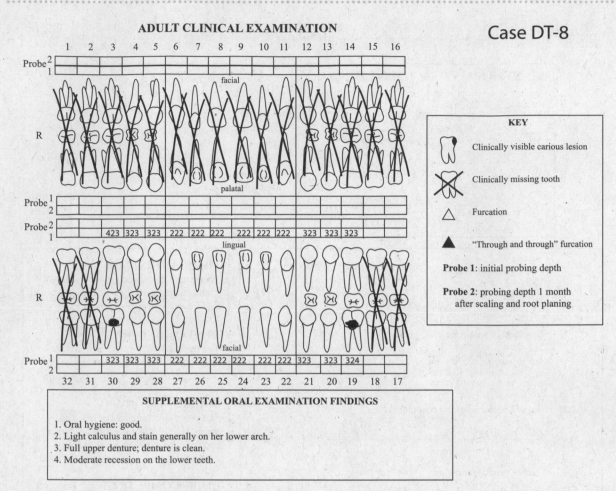

ADULT CLINICAL EXAMINATION

Case DT-8

KEY

⬜ Clinically visible carious lesion

❌ Clinically missing tooth

△ Furcation

▲ "Through and through" furcation

Probe 1: initial probing depth

Probe 2: probing depth 1 month after scaling and root planing

SUPPLEMENTAL ORAL EXAMINATION FINDINGS

1. Oral hygiene: good.
2. Light calculus and stain generally on her lower arch.
3. Full upper denture; denture is clean.
4. Moderate recession on the lower teeth.

71. Your patient has not had X-rays in 7 years. What films should be taken?
    (A) Bitewings and three periapicals on the maxillary arch
    (B) A panograph
    (C) FMX with the maxillary arch films modified in number
    (D) Periapicals on the mandibular arch only

72. Who should ideally remove the patient's denture at the hygiene visit?
    (A) The patient
    (B) The hygienist
    (C) The doctor
    (D) The dental assistant

73. All of the following may include denture deposits **EXCEPT** one. Which one is the **EXCEPTION**?
    (A) Mucin and food debris on the surface
    (B) Residue from daily denture cleaner

(C) Denture pellicle and denture biofilm
(D) Denture calculus

74. Which of the following is the **BEST** way to professionally clean the denture?
    (A) Brush the denture with a toothbrush and toothpaste.
    (B) Hand-scale the denture with a sharp, modified sickle scaler.
    (C) Polish the denture with prophy paste and immerse in an ultrasonic cleaning device.
    (D) Place the denture in a sealed bag filled with denture cleaner and immerse in an ultrasonic cleansing device.

75. Which of the following guidelines should you give the patient for self-cleaning her denture?
    (A) Brush the denture each day.
    (B) Immerse the denture each night.
    (C) Rinse the denture, immerse it, and brush it daily.
    (D) Rinse each day, and brush at least twice a week.

76. Which of the following are soft-tissue changes associated with wearing a removable prostheses?
    (A) Traumatic ulcerations
    (B) Denture stomatitis
    (C) Angular cheilitis
    (D) All of the above

77. Suppose your patient does not want to remove her denture during the hygiene visit. Which of the following is the **BEST** response?
    (A) "No problem. We will check it at your next visit."
    (B) "We need to check your soft tissue to make sure it is healthy, and I would also like to clean it for you."
    (C) "If you do not want to remove it, the dentist will do it for you."
    (D) "I understand, but this is not in the best interest of your health."

78. Which of the following is the appropriate recall frequency for this patient?
    (A) Once a year
    (B) Every 6 months
    (C) Every 4 months
    (D) Every 3 months

79. All of the following risk factors for periodontal disease appear in this patient **EXCEPT** one. Which one is the **EXCEPTION**?
    (A) Gender
    (B) Cigarette smoking
    (C) Socioeconomic status
    (D) Diet

80. Which of the following is your patient's blood-pressure category?
    (A) Hypertension
    (B) Normal
    (C) Prehypertension
    (D) Hypotension

Directions: Study the case components and answer questions 81–90.

SYNOPSIS OF PATIENT HISTORY

CASE _DT-9_

Age _52_

Sex _Male_

Height _5'9"_

Weight _170_ lbs

_77.1_ kgs

Vital Signs

Blood pressure _130/79_

Pulse rate _90_

Respiration rate _16_

1. Under Care of Physician
   Yes ☑ No ☐

   Condition: _Sjogren's Syndrome_

2. Hospitalized within the last 5 years
   Yes ☑ No ☐

   Reason: _Acute depression_

3. Has or had the following conditions:

   Allergies to cats, pollen; previously suffered
   from depression; Sjogren's syndrome

4. Current medications:

   N/A; Prescribed pilocarpine therapy
   but discontinued it

5. Smokes or uses tobacco products
   Yes ☐ No ☑

6. Is pregnant
   Yes ☐ No ☐ N/A ☑

MEDICAL HISTORY:
The patient was diagnosed with Sjogren's syndrome three years ago. Six months later, he was admitted to acute care for depression after suffering a nervous breakdown. He has rebounded well, sees a psychologist, and is doing well.

DENTAL HISTORY:
He has not had routine cleanings but is in the dental office today for a checkup and maintenance visit. He has all his teeth.

SOCIAL HISTORY:
He is married, with four children, and self-employed as a landscaper. During the winter, he does snow removal.

CHIEF COMPLAINT:
"I see holes in many of my teeth, and my mouth is dry."

ADULT CLINICAL EXAMINATION

Case DT-9

	1	2	3	4	5	6	7	8	9	10	11	12	13	14	15	16
Probe 2/1		323	323	323	322	212	212	212	212	212	212	222	222	323	323	

facial

PE · R · PE

palatal

Probe 1/2		323	323	212	212	212	212	212	212	212	212	222	223	323	323
Probe 2/1		323	323	222	222	212	212	212	212	322	322	223	323	323	323

lingual

R

facial

PE · PE

Probe 1/2		323	323	323	322	212	212	212	212	212	212	222	223	323	323

| | 32 | 31 | 30 | 29 | 28 | 27 | 26 | 25 | 24 | 23 | 22 | 21 | 20 | 19 | 18 | 17 |

KEY

Clinically visible carious lesion

Clinically missing tooth

Furcation

"Through and through" furcation

Probe 1: initial probing depth

Probe 2: probing depth 1 month after scaling and root planing

SUPPLEMENTAL ORAL EXAMINATION FINDINGS

1. Generalized slight recession 1–2 mm.
2. Moderate calculus generally.
3. Light to moderate plaque and stain.
4. Tissues inflamed interproximally.

81. Your patient is suffering from which of the following conditions?
(A) Xerostomia
(B) Xerostitis
(C) Xerostenatia
(D) Xerostatin

82. If the patient's dry mouth is not addressed, he will **MOST LIKELY** develop
(A) gingivitis.
(B) periodontitis.
(C) gastric enteritis.
(D) increased caries.

83. Which of the following has predisposed this patient for having dry mouth?
(A) His age and gender
(B) His having Sjogren's syndrome
(C) His infrequent dental cleanings
(D) His occupation keeping him out in the elements

84. All of the following should be included in your patient's personal care program **EXCEPT** one. Which one is the **EXCEPTION?**
(A) A return to his pilocarpine therapy
(B) A rigorous biofilm control effort
(C) Multiple fluorides (dentifrice, rinse, brush-on gel, or trays)
(D) Avoidance of tobacco and alcohol

85. Which of the following is true of a saliva substitute?
(A) It has chemical and physical properties similar to saliva.
(B) It coats the mouth and teeth and helps to remineralize and prevent biofilm.
(C) It contains carboxymethylcellulose.
(D) It is free of calcium, phosphorous, and fluoride.

86. All of the following drugs decrease salivary function **EXCEPT** one. Which one is the **EXCEPTION**?
    (A) Antihistamines
    (B) Antihypertensives
    (C) Aspirin
    (D) Diuretics

87. All of the following may be clinical symptoms of dry mouth **EXCEPT** one. Which one is the **EXCEPTION**?
    (A) Lower G.I. tract burning
    (B) Oral dryness
    (C) Impaired taste
    (D) Difficulty with mastication, swallowing, or speech

88. Which of the following adjuncts should you recommend to this patient to clean his interproximal surfaces?
    (A) Toothpick
    (B) Dental floss
    (C) Rubber tip
    (D) Proxy brush

89. What type of toothbrush should you recommend for this patient?
    (A) Power brush
    (B) Hard manual toothbrush
    (C) Medium toothbrush
    (D) Soft toothbrush

90. What is the appropriate recall frequency for this patient?
    (A) 2 months
    (B) 3 months
    (C) 4 months
    (D) 6 months

Directions: Study the case components and answer questions 91–100.

SYNOPSIS OF PATIENT HISTORY

CASE _DT-10_

Age _49_

Sex _Male_

Height _6'0"_

Weight _220_ lbs

_99.8_ kgs

Vital Signs

Blood pressure _132/90_

Pulse rate _80_

Respiration rate _18_

1. Under Care of Physician
   Yes ☑ No ☐
   Condition: _____

2. Hospitalized within the last 5 years
   Yes ☐ No ☑
   Reason: _____
   _____

3. Has or had the following conditions:
   Hypertension, rheumatoid arthritis
   _____

4. Current medications:
   Vasotec for HBP
   _____
   _____

5. Smokes or uses tobacco products
   Yes ☐ No ☑

6. Is pregnant
   Yes ☐ No ☐ N/A ☑

MEDICAL HISTORY:
The patient was diagnosed with high blood pressure five years ago and takes Vasotec daily. He has rheumatoid arthritis and takes 600 mg of ibuprofen daily.

DENTAL HISTORY:
The patient is of record but has not been in the office in five years. He brushes once a day and does not floss. He is very fearful of any discomfort whatsoever during dental visits. He has had discomfort when the dentist administered anesthesia.

SOCIAL HISTORY:
The patient is a police officer in the local township. He is divorced and does not have custody of his two children.

CHIEF COMPLAINT:
He notices that his gums have been bleeding whenever he brushes his teeth.

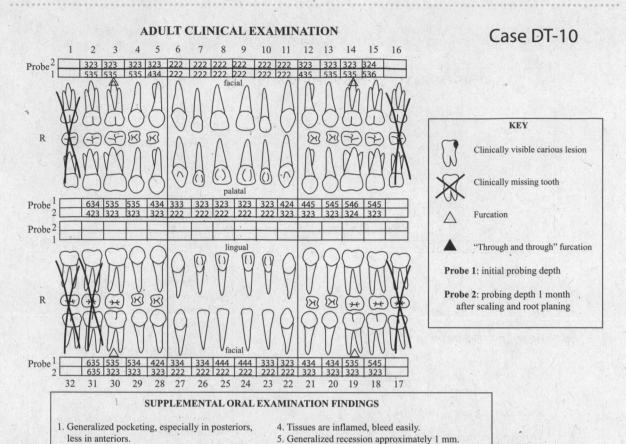

ADULT CLINICAL EXAMINATION

Case DT-10

	1	2	3	4	5	6	7	8	9	10	11	12	13	14	15	16
Probe 2		323	323	323	323	222	222	222	222	222	222	323	323	323	324	
Probe 1		535	535	535	434	222	222	222	222	222	222	435	535	535	536	

facial

R

palatal

Probe 1		634	535	535	434	333	323	323	323	323	424	445	545	546	545	
Probe 2		423	323	323	323	222	222	222	222	222	323	323	323	324	323	
Probe 2																
Probe 1																

lingual

R

facial

Probe 1		635	535	534	424	334	334	444	444	333	323	434	434	535	545	
Probe 2		635	323	323	323	222	222	222	222	222	222	323	323	323	323	
	32	31	30	29	28	27	26	25	24	23	22	21	20	19	18	17

KEY

Clinically visible carious lesion

Clinically missing tooth

Furcation

"Through and through" furcation

Probe 1: initial probing depth

Probe 2: probing depth 1 month after scaling and root planing

SUPPLEMENTAL ORAL EXAMINATION FINDINGS

1. Generalized pocketing, especially in posteriors, less in anteriors.
2. Heavy calcium deposits.
3. Minimal biofilm present today.
4. Tissues are inflamed, bleed easily.
5. Generalized recession approximately 1 mm.
6. Radiographs reveal horizontal bone loss generally.
7. #3 and #14 have type 1 mobility.

91. Which of the following is **MOST LIKELY** the diagnosis for this patient's periodontal condition?
    (A) Moderate, chronic localized periodontitis
    (B) Moderate chronic generalized periodontitis
    (C) Severe, acute localized periodontitis
    (D) Generalized aggressive periodontitis

92. The patient's clinical presentation, symptoms, and time last seen at the dental office support the need for which of the following films?
    (A) Vertical bitewings only
    (B) A panograph
    (C) A full-mouth series
    (D) Horizontal bitewings and anterior periapicals

93. Phase 1 nonsurgical periodontal therapy for this patient should consist of which of the following?
    (A) Gross scaling with a follow-up cleaning appointment
    (B) Quadrant debridement with a follow-up cleaning appointment
    (C) Quadrant debridement with placement of arestin in #14 Mesial and #3 Mesial
    (D) Prophylaxis and topical fluoride treatment

94. What is the American Dental Association (ADA) periodontal classification of this patient's periodontitis?
    (A) Type 1
    (B) Type 2
    (C) Type 3
    (D) Type 4

95. Pain management for this patient is **BEST** achieved with
    (A) an attempt to tolerate.
    (B) topical anesthetic.
    (C) oraqix.
    (D) a local anesthesia by quadrant.

96. According to the clinical exam, this patient has furcation on which of the following teeth?
    (A) 21
    (B) 28
    (C) 29
    (D) 30

97. Which of the following is **BEST** for this patient to clean his posterior interproximal contact areas after tissue resolution if he has Type 2 embrasures?
    (A) Dental floss
    (B) A proxi brush
    (C) A water pik
    (D) Toothpicks

98. Your patient has halitosis. What should you recommend that he do in addition to his normal brushing routine?
    (A) Brush his tongue and use a chlorine dioxide rinse.
    (B) Use dental floss and a fluoride rinse.
    (C) Use a cosmetic breath rinse, such as Scope.
    (D) Use a water pik and then a fluoride rinse.

99. Upon completion of nonsurgical therapy, the patient asks you to go out with him. Which of the following is the **BEST** response?
    (A) "Call me at home, and we will discuss it."
    (B) "I'm sorry, but I am already seeing someone."
    (C) "Thank you, but I try to keep my social life separate from my work."
    (D) "No thank you! Asking me out is inappropriate."

100. At the 6-week reevaluation, your patient has demonstrated good tissue resolution. Which of the following is the appropriate recall frequency?
    (A) 3 months
    (B) 4 months
    (C) 6 months
    (D) Annually

Directions: Study the case components and answer questions 101–110.

SYNOPSIS OF PATIENT HISTORY   CASE *DT-11*

Age _____ *53* _____

Sex _____ *Female* _____

Height *5'5"*

Weight *175* lbs

79.38 kgs

Vital Signs

Blood pressure _____ *130/87* _____

Pulse rate _____ *20* _____

Respiration rate _____ *18* _____

---

1. Under Care of Physician
   Yes ☑ No ☐

   Condition: *Diabetes, depression, arthritis*

2. Hospitalized within the last 5 years
   Yes ☑ No ☐

   Reason: *Gall bladder removed 2 years prior;*
   hysterectomy 6 months ago

3. Has or had the following conditions:

   Diabetes, depression, arthritis

   _____

4. Current medications:

   Insulin, Elavil, Naproxen

   _____

   _____

5. Smokes or uses tobacco products
   Yes ☐ No ☑

6. Is pregnant
   Yes ☐ No ☑ N/A ☐

MEDICAL HISTORY:
The patient has had a history of medical issues. She is an insulin-dependent diabetic who controlled her diabetes with oral medication up to 6 months ago. She suffers from depression, and takes Elavil. She takes Naproxen regularly for arthritic joint pain in her legs. She has had two surgical procedures in the past 2 years. She is overweight and has not had success in losing weight.

DENTAL HISTORY:
She came in regularly for checkups and cleanings up to 2 years ago but has not been in since then. She has many fillings and crowns on her teeth, and has had four root canals.

SOCIAL HISTORY:
The patient is divorced and has been unemployed for 10 months and is unable to find work.

CHIEF COMPLAINT:
"I know I need my teeth cleaned, and my teeth are sensitive to cold much of the time."

ADULT CLINICAL EXAMINATION

Case DT-11

KEY

- Clinically visible carious lesion
- Clinically missing tooth
- Furcation
- "Through and through" furcation

Probe 1: initial probing depth

Probe 2: probing depth 1 month after scaling and root planing

	SUPPLEMENTAL ORAL EXAMINATION FINDINGS
1. Generalized recession, 1 mm.	4. Bite-wing X-rays show no significant attachment loss.
2. Tissues marginally inflamed, pocket depths 2–3 mm on average.	5. Teeth show evidence of bruxism.
3. Moderate calculus interproximally and lower anterior linguals.	

101. Which of the following is **MOST LIKELY** the diagnosis for this patient's periodontal condition?
(A) Generalized acute gingivitis
(B) Generalized mild periodontitis
(C) Acute necrotizing ulcerative gingivitis (ANUG)
(D) Localized chronic periodontitis

102. Which of the following is the **BEST** treatment protocol to return this patient's tissues to optimum periodontal health?
(A) Half-mouth debridement with local anesthesia, two appointments to complete
(B) Prophylaxis and professional fluoride treatments, three appointments to complete
(C) Generalized debridement to remove all deposits, followed by a fine scale and polish at a second appointment
(D) Referral to periodontist for a treatment protocol because of patient's diabetes

103. What is the **BEST** time of day to schedule this patient's appointments?
(A) Late afternoon, about two hours before dinner
(B) First appointment, before breakfast
(C) It does not matter.
(D) Morning appointments, about an hour after breakfast

104. Which of the following is a reaction in which a diabetic patient has too much insulin and abnormally low blood glucose?
(A) Hyperglycemia
(B) Ketoacidosis
(C) Hypoglycemia
(D) Diabetic coma

105. Based on the American Diabetes Association classification system, this patient has which of the following types of diabetes?
    (A) Chemically induced
    (B) Type 1
    (C) Gestational
    (D) Type 2

106. All of the following are signs of hyperinsulinism **EXCEPT** one. Which one is the **EXCEPTION**?
    (A) Confusion
    (B) Incoherence
    (C) Hunger, weakness
    (D) "Fruity" breath odor

107. If your patient has an insulin reaction, what should you do?
    (A) Discontinue dental care and take her to a hospital.
    (B) Give her a sugary drink or sugar and then send her home.
    (C) Give a sugar drink or sugar and encourage the patient to eat a complex carbohydrate with protein.
    (D) Stop the treatment and let the patient take a break.

108. Which of the following is true of the results of a fasting-plasma glucose test (FPG)?
    (A) < 126mg/dL is considered well controlled; >160mg/dL is considered uncontrolled.
    (B) >160mg/dL is considered well controlled; <126mg/dL is considered uncontrolled.
    (C) >160mg/dL is considered moderately controlled.
    (D) <126mg/dL is considered moderately controlled.

109. All of the following are true of diabetes **EXCEPT** one. Which one is the **EXCEPTION**?
    (A) Diabetes is a significant risk factor for periodontal infections.
    (B) Periodontal infections also affect control of blood glucose levels in diabetic patients.
    (C) Inadequate dental biofilm control contributes to more severe tissue response because of decreased resistance.
    (D) Patients with well-controlled diabetes are treated the same as patients with uncontrolled diabetes.

110. Which of the following is an important question to ask a diabetic patient prior to treatment?
    (A) "When have you last eaten?"
    (B) "Did you get a good night's sleep?"
    (C) "How many times did you exercise this week?"
    (D) "Are you nervous about this appointment?"

Directions: Study the case components and answer questions 111–120.

SYNOPSIS OF PATIENT HISTORY

CASE *DT-12*

Age   *25*

Sex   *Female*

Height *5'7"*

Weight *135* lbs

61.23 kgs

Vital Signs

Blood pressure   *120/79*

Pulse rate   *80*

Respiration rate   *15*

1. Under Care of Physician
   Yes ☑ No ☐
   Condition: *Routine checkups*

2. Hospitalized within the last 5 years
   Yes ☐ No ☑
   Reason: _____
   _____

3. Has or had the following conditions:
   _____
   _____

4. Current medications:
   _____
   _____
   _____

5. Smokes or uses tobacco products
   Yes ☑ No ☐

6. Is pregnant
   Yes ☐ No ☑ N/A ☐

MEDICAL HISTORY:
The patient has a history of excellent health with one exception. She has smoked a pack of cigarettes a day since she was a teenager.

DENTAL HISTORY:
The patient comes in regularly for dental cleanings and checkups. She has never had a restoration or decay of any type. She uses a power brush and flosses a few times a week.

SOCIAL HISTORY:
She is attractive and well-educated. She works as a human resources manager for a large company.

CHIEF COMPLAINT:
No complaints. "I'm due for my cleaning!"

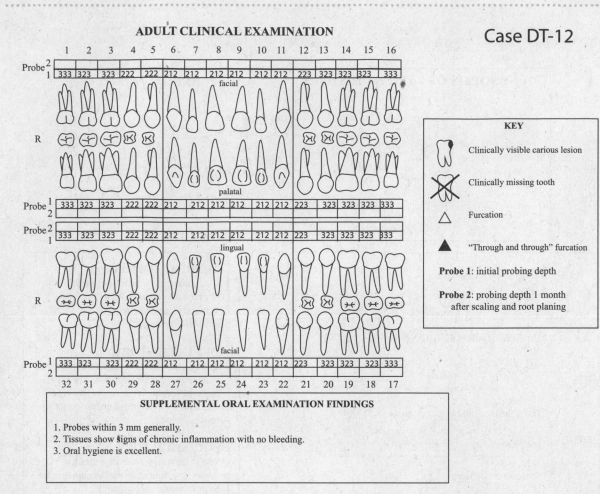

ADULT CLINICAL EXAMINATION

Case DT-12

KEY

Clinically visible carious lesion

Clinically missing tooth

Furcation

"Through and through" furcation

Probe 1: initial probing depth

Probe 2: probing depth 1 month
after scaling and root planing

SUPPLEMENTAL ORAL EXAMINATION FINDINGS

1. Probes within 3 mm generally.
2. Tissues show signs of chronic inflammation with no bleeding.
3. Oral hygiene is excellent.

---

111. What should be your main priority during this patient's recare visit?
(A) Getting her to floss every day, instead of every other
(B) Getting her to stop eating chocolate periodically
(C) Encouraging her to stop smoking
(D) Encouraging her to brush more frequently

112. Which of the following explains why this patient does not show more signs of bleeding if she flosses only a few days per week?
(A) Even though she only flosses a few days per week, her flossing and brushing are very effective.
(B) She uses a power brush, which compensates for her lack of flossing.
(C) She has remarkably good tissue resistance.
(D) Her smoking constricts her blood vessels and masks the impact of pathogens on the tissues.

113. All of the following evidence of smoking will be noted in an extraoral examination of a smoker **EXCEPT** one. Which one is the **EXCEPTION**?
(A) Breath and body odor
(B) Eyes
(C) Fingers
(D) Skin

114. Which of the following is **NOT** an oral consequence of tobacco use?
(A) Localized recession and clinical attachment loss
(B) Nicotine stomatitis
(C) Delayed wound healing
(D) Increased cervical caries

115. Your patient is **MOST** at risk for developing which of the following conditions?
    (A) Heart disease
    (B) Dementia
    (C) Cancer
    (D) Diabetes

116. Which of the following is a form of nicotine replacement therapy?
    (A) Nicotine gum
    (B) Nicotine patch
    (C) Nicotine inhaler
    (D) All of the above

117. Which of the following is **NOT** an option for nicotine-free therapy?
    (A) Bupropion SR
    (B) Varenicline tartrate
    (C) Clonidine
    (D) Serum IgG

118. All of the following are components of the 5 As in tobacco cessation programs **EXCEPT** one. Which one is the **EXCEPTION**?
    (A) Ask
    (B) Advise
    (C) Analyze
    (D) Assist

119. According to the dental chart, this patient has decay on which of the following teeth?
    (A) Second mandibular right molar
    (B) First maxillary left molar
    (C) Left maxillary lateral incisor
    (D) This patient does not have any decay.

120. If your patient has a relapse in trying to quit smoking, what should you do?
    (A) Ask her to recall and record the circumstances that led to reuse, and then set another quit date.
    (B) Clean the patient's teeth again immediately to give her a fresh start.
    (C) Ask her to consider smokeless tobacco as an alternative.
    (D) Give her another lecture on the pitfalls of smoking.

Directions: Study the case components and answer questions 121–130.

SYNOPSIS OF PATIENT HISTORY

CASE *DT-13*

Age ___*80*___

Sex *Female*

Height *5'1"*

Weight *160* lbs

72.6 kgs

Vital Signs

Blood pressure *130/86*

Pulse rate *100*

Respiration rate *17*

---

1. Under Care of Physician
   Yes ☑ No ☐
   Condition: *Hypothyroidism*

2. Hospitalized within the last 5 years
   Yes ☑ No ☐
   Reason: *Kidney stones*

3. Has or had the following conditions:
   Hypothyroidism

4. Current medications:
   Levothyroxine (Synthroid)

5. Smokes or uses tobacco products
   Yes ☐ No ☑

6. Is pregnant
   Yes ☐ No ☑ N/A ☐

MEDICAL HISTORY:
This elderly patient has a history of kidney stones and hypothyroidism, which she takes Synthroid for. Beyond that, she enjoys good health.

DENTAL HISTORY:
The patient comes in regularly for check-ups. She has all her teeth, some posterior restorations, and is in good periodontal health. She uses a medium toothbrush twice daily.

SOCIAL HISTORY:
She is a cheerful widow who lives with her daughter and family.

CHIEF COMPLAINT:
"My teeth are very sensitive to cold and I am dreading this cleaning."

ADULT CLINICAL EXAMINATION

Case DT-13

KEY

	Clinically visible carious lesion
	Clinically missing tooth
	Furcation
	"Through and through" furcation

Probe 1: initial probing depth

Probe 2: probing depth 1 month after scaling and root planing

SUPPLEMENTAL ORAL EXAMINATION FINDINGS

1. Generalized recession, 2 mm around all teeth.
2. Moderate plaque and calculus.
3. Pocket depths 1–3 mm.
4. Oral hygiene is fair.

---

121. All of the following are recommended during this patient's cleaning appointment **EXCEPT** one. Which one is the **EXCEPTION**?
(A) Use oraqix.
(B) Polish with a desensitizing agent prior to cleaning.
(C) Use an ultrasonic scaler.
(D) Apply fluoride varnish at the end of the visit.

122. All of the following should be recommended to help this patient with her sensitivity to cold outside the dental office **EXCEPT** one. Which one is the **EXCEPTION**?
(A) Brush with a desensitizing toothpaste.
(B) Use a fluoride rinse before bed at night.
(C) Keep contact with extreme cold liquids and foods to a minimum.
(D) Regularly chew a gum containing xylitol.

123. This patient has which of the following conditions?
(A) Hypotension
(B) Hypertension
(C) Chronic periodontitis
(D) Advanced periodontitis

124. Your patient has hypothyroidism, which
(A) is also known as Grave's disease.
(B) may lead to a partial thyroidectomy.
(C) is more common in women than in men.
(D) results in excessive production of thyroid hormones.

125. Patients with hypothyroidism often have which of the following?
(A) Low metabolism
(B) Artrial fibrillation
(C) Low tolerance for heat
(D) Ocular symptoms

126. The sensitivity your patient is experiencing is **MOST LIKELY** caused by her
     (A) imagination.
     (B) age.
     (C) recession.
     (D) thyroid disease.

127. You should recommend that this patient clean her teeth with a
     (A) soft toothbrush.
     (B) hard toothbrush.
     (C) child-size toothbrush.
     (D) tooth wipe.

128. All of the following ingredients in dentifrices are helpful in reducing sensitivity **EXCEPT** one. Which one is the **EXCEPTION**?
     (A) Potassium nitrate
     (B) Potassium chloride
     (C) Potassium citrate
     (D) Sodium monofluorophosphate

129. In terms of radiographs, the patient's hypothyroidism necessitates
     (A) the need to take less-routine X-rays.
     (B) no special consideration with regard to taking films.
     (C) the importance of using a double thyroid collar.
     (D) no need to reduce exposure time.

130. The patient's sensitivity to cold necessitates which of the following?
     (A) More frequent hygiene visits
     (B) Less frequent hygiene visits
     (C) Shorter hygiene visits
     (D) Normal scheduling

Directions: Study the case components and answer questions 131–140.

SYNOPSIS OF PATIENT HISTORY

CASE *DT-14*

Age ___5___

Sex ___Male___

Height _4'4"_

Weight _46_ lbs

_20.89_kgs

Vital Signs

Blood pressure _N/A_

Pulse rate _119_

Respiration rate _20_

---

1. Under Care of Physician

   Yes ☑ No ☐

   Condition: _Asthma, allergies to be determined_

2. Hospitalized within the last 5 years

   Yes ☐ No ☑

   Reason: _____

3. Has or had the following conditions:

   Asthma, excema

4. Current medications:

   Albuterol (Inhaler form)

5. Smokes or uses tobacco products

   Yes ☐ No ☑

6. Is pregnant

   Yes ☐ No ☐ N/A ☑

MEDICAL HISTORY:

The patient is a 5-year-old boy with a history of asthma that is controlled with an albuterol inhaler as needed. He is currently undergoing testing to determine what he is allergic to. He recently had to be on two rounds of antibiotics for an ear infection.

DENTAL HISTORY:

He went to a dentist once at the age of 3, but has not been back since. This is his second visit and the first at this office. His mother brushes his teeth once daily, after breakfast.

SOCIAL HISTORY:

The patient is well behaved and shy. He has friends and is active in school. He lives with his two parents and an older sister.

CHIEF COMPLAINT:

His mother wants his teeth cleaned and checked.

CLINICAL EXAMINATION

Case DT-14

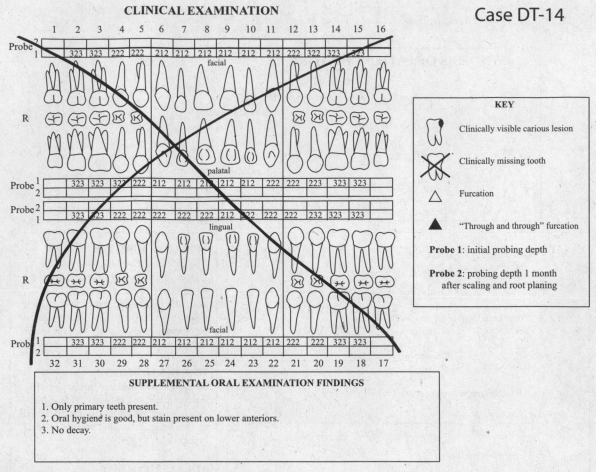

KEY

Clinically visible carious lesion

Clinically missing tooth

△ Furcation

▲ "Through and through" furcation

Probe 1: initial probing depth

Probe 2: probing depth 1 month after scaling and root planing

SUPPLEMENTAL ORAL EXAMINATION FINDINGS

1. Only primary teeth present.
2. Oral hygiene is good, but stain present on lower anteriors.
3. No decay.

131. Which of the following is **MOST LIKELY** the cause of the stain on the patient's lower anteriors?
(A) Chocolate
(B) Second-hand smoke
(C) Antibiotic therapy
(D) Lack of flossing

132. Your patient's mother asks how often her son should brush his teeth. What should you recommend?
(A) Once a day
(B) 2–3 times a day
(C) 4–5 times a day
(D) 6–7 times a day

133. Your patient is 5 years old. In regards to self-care, all of the following are true **EXCEPT** one. Which one is the **EXCEPTION**?
(A) His parents should help with brushing.
(B) His parents should floss for him.
(C) He should do most of the brushing himself.
(D) He should be instructed not to swallow the toothpaste.

134. What is the minimum amount of time that this child should spend having his teeth brushed?
(A) 1 minute
(B) 2 minutes
(C) 3 minutes
(D) As long as it takes to sing "Happy birthday"

135. Which of the following is the **BEST** recommendation regarding your patient's self-care with the use of his inhaler?
(A) He should brush the inhaler after each use.
(B) He should rinse, swish, and expectorate after each use.
(C) He should keep the inhaler in a cup filled with water.
(D) All of the above

136. If the child's asthma continues into adulthood, it is important to take his blood pressure and pulse before dental treatment to prevent
(A) xerostomia.
(B) dieresis.
(C) tachycardia.
(D) bronchodilation.

137. What is the recommended fluoride application for this child at the end of the visit?
(A) 1.23 percent acidulated phosphate fluoride gel in a tray
(B) 1.23 percent APF foam in a tray
(C) 2.0 percent sodium fluoride gel in a tray
(D) 5 percent neutral sodium varnish

138. All of the following are delivery systems for disclosants **EXCEPT** one. Which one is the **EXCEPTION**?
(A) Direct application
(B) Rinsing
(C) Tablets or wafers
(D) Trays

139. How often should the patient's mother replace his toothbrush?
(A) Every 3 months
(B) Every 4 months
(C) Every 6 months at the dental visit
(D) When the bristles get splayed

140. Your patient's mother asks if her son should have sealants. He should have sealants on the
(A) first and second primary molars.
(B) second primary molar.
(C) first and second permanent molars, when they erupt.
(D) second permanent molars, when they erupt.

Directions: Study the case components and answer questions 141–150.

SYNOPSIS OF PATIENT HISTORY

CASE _DT-15_

Age _____16_____

Sex _____Female_____

Height _5'6"_

Weight _125_ lbs

_56.70_kgs

Vital Signs

Blood pressure _____110/72_____

Pulse rate _____70_____

Respiration rate _____15_____

1. Under Care of Physician
   Yes ☑ No ☐

   Condition: _Psychiatrist, for bulimia nervosa_

2. Hospitalized within the last 5 years
   Yes ☐ No ☑

   Reason: _____

3. Has or had the following conditions:

   Bulimia nervosa _____

   _____

4. Current medications:

   _____

   _____

   _____

5. Smokes or uses tobacco products
   Yes ☐ No ☑

6. Is pregnant
   Yes ☐ No ☑ N/A ☐

MEDICAL HISTORY:
This teenage female patient has been bulimic for 2 years. She is seeing a psychiatrist for cognitive behavioral therapy to control the disorder. She was previously on an antidepressant but no longer is.

DENTAL HISTORY:
Her parents have always brought her in regularly for dental visits. Her caries rate has increased significantly over the past year.

SOCIAL HISTORY:
She is popular at school and does very well academically. She lives with her two parents and a younger sister.

CHIEF COMPLAINT:
Cleaning and checkup

CLINICAL EXAMINATION

Case DT-15

SUPPLEMENTAL ORAL EXAMINATION FINDINGS

1. Oral hygiene: good.
2. Light calculus present.
3. Tissues are relatively healthy.
4. Note incidence of caries on charting.
5. Maxillary anterior lingual are translucent and glass-like.
6. Teeth show evidence of erosion on cervical areas.
7. Probes within 3 mm.

141. All of the following methods are used by patients with purging-type bulimia to control weight gain **EXCEPT** one. Which one is the **EXCEPTION**?
(A) Self-induced vomiting
(B) Laxatives or diuretics
(C) Diuretics
(D) Fasting

142. In which teeth is perimylolysis first seen?
(A) Maxillary anterior linguals
(B) Maxillary posterior buccals
(C) Mandibular anterior linguals
(D) Mandibular posterior occlusals

143. What part of the mouth is **MOST LIKELY** to be traumatized by the item used to initiate the vomiting?
(A) Throat
(B) Hard palate
(C) Soft palate
(D) Gingival

144. An increase in caries incidence is sometimes found in bulimics on what areas of the teeth?
(A) Occlusal
(B) Cervical
(C) Facial
(D) Lingual

145. Which of the following are common oral findings in bulimic patients?
(A) Eroded tooth enamel
(B) Xerostomia
(C) Hypersensitive teeth
(D) All of the above

146. Expensive dental care, such as using caps or crowns to repair damaged teeth, should be performed
(A) on a first visit.
(B) on a second or third visit.
(C) when the bulimia is cured.
(D) at any time.

147. Your patient should be instructed not to brush after vomiting because brushing may
    (A) cause enamel erosion.
    (B) loosen fillings and crowns.
    (C) decrease the amount of saliva.
    (D) increase tooth sensitivity.

148. All of the following should be recommended to this patient to reduce hypersensitivity and build resistance to acid demineralization **EXCEPT** one. Which one is the **EXCEPTION**?
    (A) Fluoride dentifrice
    (B) Neutral pH sodium fluoride mouth rise
    (C) Higher protein diet
    (D) Custom-fitted tray for daily home fluoride application

149. Which of the following would **NOT** be useful in treating your patient's xerostomia?
    (A) Chewing gum containing sugar
    (B) Chewing gum containing xylitol as its sweetener
    (C) Using saliva substitutes containing fluoride
    (D) Eating sugar-free mints

150. Which of the following is **MOST LIKELY** seen in a bulimic patient?
    (A) Over-exercising
    (B) Tooth discoloration
    (C) Repeated tooth brushing
    (D) All of the above

ANSWER KEY AND EXPLANATIONS
Component A

1. A	41. C	81. B	121. B	161. E
2. A	42. C	82. B	122. C	162. B
3. B	43. C	83. C	123. D	163. D
4. D	44. A	84. A	124. A	164. B
5. B	45. A	85. C	125. C	165. E
6. C	46. C	86. D	126. C	166. A
7. C	47. E	87. E	127. E	167. A
8. B	48. B	88. A	128. C	168. A
9. C	49. B	89. C	129. A	169. A
10. C	50. B	90. A	130. C	170. E
11. D	51. B	91. A	131. A	171. C
12. D	52. A	92. C	132. D	172. C
13. D	53. A	93. C	133. D	173. C
14. D	54. B	94. B	134. A	174. D
15. C	55. B	95. A	135. A	175. B
16. E	56. C	96. B	136. B	176. D
17. C	57. A	97. A	137. E	177. A
18. B	58. C	98. C	138. D	178. A
19. B	59. D	99. D	139. C	179. A
20. B	60. C	100. B	140. C	180. B
21. A	61. D	101. B	141. A	181. B
22. A	62. C	102. E	142. D	182. C
23. D	63. E	103. D	143. B	183. A
24. E	64. D	104. C	144. D	184. E
25. B	65. C	105. A	145. C	185. A
26. D	66. A	106. A	146. A	186. A
27. B	67. C	107. C	147. C	187. B
28. B	68. B	108. A	148. E	188. C
29. D	69. D	109. E	149. B	189. B
30. D	70. A	110. A	150. A	190. B
31. C	71. A	111. A	151. B	191. B
32. E	72. A	112. D	152. C	192. A
33. B	73. B	113. C	153. C	193. A
34. B	74. D	114. B	154. A	194. E
35. D	75. C	115. B	155. D	195. D
36. B	76. A	116. A	156. D	196. B
37. B	77. A	117. E	157. E	197. C
38. A	78. C	118. B	158. B	198. E
39. D	79. B	119. A	159. C	199. A
40. B	80. D	120. D	160. C	200. B

1. **The correct answer is (A).** Asthma is an inflammatory disorder that occurs when the bronchi constrict and mucous plugs block the alveoli. Symptoms include wheezing, coughing, chest tightness, shortness of breath, and anxiety.

2. **The correct answer is (A).** Periodontal disease is unrelated to consuming a high-fat diet, and eating fattening foods can keep food particles from sticking to teeth. Diets high in carbohydrates can sometimes cause dental problems because the sugars can promote bacteria growth on tooth surfaces.

3. **The correct answer is (B).** The white areas on a radiograph are radiopaque. These are areas where less radiation has reached the radiographic film due to a harder substance preventing possible radiation penetration.

4. **The correct answer is (D).** The two-provider wheelchair transfer is used for both heavier and fragile wheelchair-bound patients. In order to perform this transfer, one clinician stands behind the patient while the patient crosses his or her arms across his or her chest. Next, the clinician places his or her arms under the patient's upper arms and grasps the patient's wrists. The second clinician then places both hands under the patient's thighs and counts to coordinate the lift between the two clinicians.

5. **The correct answer is (B).** The mean is the average number. Occasionally, the mean and the median will be the same number.

6. **The correct answer is (C).** Ceramic and Arkansas sharpening stones are used for routine instrument sharpening. India stones are used to sharpen very dull edges, and Composition stones are used to reshape improperly sharpened instruments and damaged cutting edges.

7. **The correct answer is (C).** While candidiasis does present itself with lesions, this condition causes white, rather than red, lesions. Candidiasis is an infectious condition caused by the Candida fungus.

8. **The correct answer is (B).** OSHA requires that dental personnel be offered a hepatitis B immunization within 10 days of employment. If an employee refuses the immunization, it must be documented and the documentation should be kept in the employee's confidential medical file.

9. **The correct answer is (C).** After performing a Gram stain procedure, bacteria may change to a violet color, but only they have tested as Gram-positive, rather than Gram-negative. Bacteria that tests as Gram-negative will appear as a red or pink color after the Gram stain procedure. This procedure also helps determine the thickness of cell walls, the chemical composition of the bacteria, and the sensitivity of the bacteria to penicillin.

10. **The correct answer is (C).** The dentoperiosteal fiber anchors teeth. This connective tissue connects cementum at the cementoenamel junction (CEJ) to the alveolar crest.

11. **The correct answer is (D).** The primary difference between hyperglycemia and hypoglycemia is the amount of sugar in a patient's blood. Patients with hyperglycemia have too much glucose in their blood. Patients with hypoglycemia, however, have low blood sugar.

12. **The correct answer is (D).** The masseter muscle is the largest and strongest of the muscles of mastication. It originates in several places from the zygomatic arch. The masseter muscle's main function is to close or elevate the mandible to centric occlusion.

13. **The correct answer is (D).** Several events occur during the cap stage. Initially, however, tissues start to morphodifferentiate into ectoderm and mesenchyme. After that, the ectoderm becomes the enamel organ and the mesoderm develops into the dental papilla and dental sac.

14. **The correct answer is (D).** Written and verbal consent do not need to be attained during an emergency situation. Dental personnel must do all they can to save the patient's life in the case of a medical emergency.

15. **The correct answer is (C).** General tonic-clonic seizures, also known as grand mal seizures, cause a loss of consciousness; muscle stiffening; convulsions; and periods of temporary confusion, headache, and extreme fatigue. However, these seizures are not generally accompanied by a prolonged coma.

16. **The correct answer is (E).** Periodontal diseases result in bone loss. The bones lost due to periodontal disease will not grow back; therefore, periodontal diseases are irreversible. Also, the gingival tissues are not easy to repair and are unrelated to periodontal diseases.

17. **The correct answer is (C).** It is recommended that 2.0 grams of amoxicillin be administered orally to adults 1 hour before any oral procedure. Although this is the standard regimen, the dosage and type of medication given to a patient always depends on a patient's medical history, allergies, and ability to take medications.

18. **The correct answer is (B).** Enamel pearls occur due to too much enamel formed by ameloblasts. Excess enamel can be seen on root surfaces near CEJ, or the cementoenamel junction, and near maxillary molars.

19. **The correct answer is (B).** Although debridement is necessary to treat periodontal diseases, chemotherapeutic agents help to eliminate potentially pathogenic organisms that could be causing or irritating periodontal diseases.

20. **The correct answer is (B).** Intradermal is a parenteral route of administering medication, meaning it is not injected into the digestive tract. Instead, it is slowly injected into the dermal layer. Introdermal injections are used in allergy testing and in skin testing. Enteral routes are those that lead directly to the intestine.

21. **The correct answer is (A).** Instruments must be exposed to all three parameters of sterilization including time, temperature, and steam pressure. In addition, instruments should be tested weekly for spores to ensure the sterilization methods are effective.

22. **The correct answer is (A).** You are showing the client empathy by listening to her concerns and understanding the emotions she's feeling related to the procedure. Empathy helps build trust between the client and the dental hygienist.

23. **The correct answer is (D).** Preservatives prolong dentifrice shelf-life and deter the growth of bacteria. Dentifrices may include toothpaste and mouthwash.

24. **The correct answer is (E).** Over-the-counter bleaching strips typically contain 6.5–14 percent hydrogen peroxide. Home bleaching kits typically contain 10, 15, or 22 percent hydrogen peroxide. Kits used in dental offices include 30–35 percent hydrogen peroxide and are often activated using heat or light.

25. **The correct answer is (B).** The mesiobuccal surface and distolingual surface converge at a line angle. A point angle is a point where three surfaces converge.

26. **The correct answer is (D).** The Occupational Safety and Health Administration (OSHA) requires employers to supply dental professionals with eyewear, face masks, outerwear or protective clothing, and gloves. Employers do not need to supply hygienists with antibacterial soap.

27. **The correct answer is (B).** When assessing the attached gingiva (AG), the second measurement, the measurement of the CEJ to the base of the pocket, is subtracted from the first measurement, the measurement of the CEJ to the mucogingival junction. In this example, $5 - 2 = 3$.

28. **The correct answer is (B).** Plastic curettes will not scratch the titanium surface of dental implants. Air abrasive powders, ultrasonic tips, metal instruments, and coarse prophylaxis pastes will scratch the surface, which could lead to the accumulation of bacteria.

29. **The correct answer is (D).** The mandibular tori is identified by a radiopaque area on the lingual surfaces of the mandible where additional bone growth happened. Other mandibular radiopaque landmarks include genial tubercles, interior oblique ridge, exterior oblique ridge, inferior border, and mandibular tori.

30. **The correct answer is (D).** Although cements are used for a variety of dental purposes, liners are used for pulp capping. They are applied in a thin layer to seal dentin. Cements are also poor thermal conductors.

31. **The correct answer is (C).** AVPU is an acronym that stands for "alert, verbal, pain, and unresponsive." This acronym helps people remember they can recognize an emergency by noticing if the patient is alert, assessing the patient's level of

consciousness through verbal responses, assessing whether the patient responds to painful stimuli, and determining if the patient is unresponsive.

32. **The correct answer is (E).** The patient has taken the action of informed refusal. The patient has been informed of all the risks of refusing treatment and made the informed decision to refuse treatment based on all the information available.

33. **The correct answer is (B).** Self-disclosure promotes trust between the dental hygienist and client because the dental hygienist reveals personal experiences to the client. This shows the client that the dental hygienist can relate to the client.

34. **The correct answer is (B).** Aspirin is not an essential component of a Basic Life Support (BLS) kit. Oxygen, epinephrine, diphenhydramine, albuterol, glucose, and nitroglycerine should all be included in a BLS kit.

35. **The correct answer is (D).** Herpes simplex virus type 1 appears as a clear fluid-like blister or cold sore on the lips or face. Herpes simplex virus type 2 appears as sores only in the genital area. They are both transmitted through physical contact. Someone suffering from herpes simplex virus type 1 may show symptoms similar to the flu.

36. **The correct answer is (B).** Analgesic drugs, both non-opioids and opioids, treat pain. Examples of analgesic drugs include nonsteroidal anti-inflammatory drugs, COX-2 inhibitors, and opiates.

37. **The correct answer is (B).** The acronym CAB stands for circulation, airway, breathing. When performing CPR, it is important to check for circulation. If the patient's heart is not beating, an individual should perform chest compressions. He or she should also check the person's airway and breathing. Although the CPR guidelines previously suggested that people blow two breaths into individuals who were not breathing, the guidelines now indicate that giving chest compressions should be the first area of focus.

38. **The correct answer is (A).** Both of these statements are true. Saliva acts as a buffer and slows the formation of caries; therefore, as the flow of saliva increases, the oral cavity becomes less acidic.

39. **The correct answer is (D).** Sodium fluoride, stannous fluoride, and acidulated phosphate fluoride are most often administered topically in the dentist's office. Fluoride can also be found in toothpastes and mouthwashes over the counter.

40. **The correct answer is (B).** Many active desensitizing agents and brands of toothpaste exist. Potassium nitrate, calcium hydroxide, strontium chloride, sodium citrate, potassium oxalate, and ferric oxalate are active ingredients used in desensitizing toothpastes. Desensitizing agents are not a one-size-fits-all solution, so suggesting another brand of toothpaste might work for the patient.

41. **The correct answer is (C).** A carious lesion begins as a demineralized area that enters the tooth structure and later gives way to a white spot on the tooth's enamel. As time passes, the area might become stained, remineralize, or be arrested before cavitation can take place. If remineralization occurs, the tooth is saved, and cavitation does not occur.

42. **The correct answer is (C).** The chi-square test compares the observed measurement of a given characteristic with the expected measurement for a sample. It is usually used to study categorical information. The standard deviation is the positive square root of variance. It is a measure of variability. Standard deviation is the most useful when measuring variability in descriptive statistics. It also considers all the scores in a distribution.

43. **The correct answer is (C).** Many vitamins have chemical names as well as common names. The chemical name for vitamin D is calciferol.

44. **The correct answer is (A).** Custom mouth guards are molded to the athlete's mouth, and therefore, ensure the best fit. This custom fit allows athletes to talk and breathe comfortably, and it reduces athlete's tendency to gag from the guard.

45. **The correct answer is (A).** Acidulated fluorides are not recommended for patients who have dental implants because the acid will etch the implants' surface and the scratches will attract bacteria. Ultrasonic cleaning is also not recommended for patients with implants because it will cause severe scratching.

46. **The correct answer is (C).** Beta-adrenergic blocking agents block catecholamine stimulation

of the beta-receptors of the heart. Some of these drugs can cause gingival hyperplasia.

47. **The correct answer is (E).** Meckel's cartilage first develops in the mandible before intramembranous ossification occurs and forms the bone of the mandible.

48. **The correct answer is (B).** Assessing the functional level of those with disabilities includes evaluating one's ability to perform activities of daily living (ADL). Categories include high functioning, moderate functioning, and low functioning. High functioning individuals are able to attend to most activities of daily living with some supervision. Moderate functioning individuals need assistance and supervision with some activities of daily living. They are not able to give informed consent. Low functioning individuals have little or no ability to perform activities of daily living independently.

49. **The correct answer is (B).** Normally, sealants are put on children's teeth when their 6-year and 12-year molars erupt. Therefore, you should check to see if the child has her 6-year molars before you make a decision about giving the child the treatment.

50. **The correct answer is (B).** Panoramic radiographs do not have good definition and detail and should be used with periapicals X-rays. Panoramic radiographs are quite useful for an edentulous patient, when checking for pathology, for a patient with a strong gag reflex, and when orthodontics are to be performed. Panoramic radiographs do not require more radiation than normal radiographs do.

51. **The correct answer is (B).** Self-curing sealants require a minimum of 1–3 minutes to set and cure and should remain on teeth undisturbed during this time.

52. **The correct answer is (A).** The tongue begins to develop in the fourth week. It forms from the first through fourth branchial arches. The first branchial arch forms the body of the tongue, while the second and third arches form the base of the tongue.

53. **The correct answer is (A).** Over-the-counter teeth whitening products do not have the ability to reduce deep stains and only have slight whitening results. Results of extrinsic stains are better than those for intrinsic stains, and yellow teeth have better results than brownish or gray teeth.

54. **The correct answer is (B).** The normal heart rate for an average adult is 60–100. Infants have a heart rate of 120–160, toddlers have a heart rate of 80–130, and school-age children have a heart rate of 70–110.

55. **The correct answer is (B).** Research shows that allergies to foods such as shellfish, bananas, and pineapples could trigger latex allergies. Based on this information, the dental hygienist may wish to use another type of glove when examining the patient.

56. **The correct answer is (C).** It is important for the dental hygienist to know if a patient is on birth-control pills because certain medications, such as antibiotics, can make birth-control pills less effective. Patients who use birth-control pills and require antibiotics should use another form of birth control while taking the antibiotics.

57. **The correct answer is (A).** A PRS score of 0 indicates that the patient has no deposits. The PRS scale is used to determine if periodontal disease is present. The scale ranges from 0 to 4.

58. **The correct answer is (C).** Chronic periodontitis is an inflammation of the periodontium that involves alveolar bone loss. Root planing, gingival curettage, bone grafting, and implants are all appropriate treatments for patients suffering from periodontal disease. Fissure sealants are not appropriate treatments for periodontal disease because dental professionals generally want to remove infected gum and bone in patients with periodontal disease, rather than cover and seal the areas.

59. **The correct answer is (D).** Adrenergic drugs stimulate adrenergic receptors to produce effects similar to those of the sympathetic nervous system. The sympathetic nervous system is the system responsible for the fight-or-flight response, which dilates the bronchi and the pupils, accelerates heart rate and respiration, and increases perspiration and blood pressure. Antiadrenergic drugs, not adrenergic drugs, block adrenergic receptors.

60. **The correct answer is (C).** Excessive salivation, abdominal pain, and vomiting are signs of acute fluoride toxicity. In severe cases, cardiac arrest

may occur. Bleeding is not usually a sign of acute fluoride toxicity.

61. **The correct answer is (D).** The state board of dental examiners does not usually inspect dental practices. They do, however, regulate, grant, and revoke dental licenses and institute continuing education standards.

62. **The correct answer is (C).** Many advantages for using a power-driven ultrasonic scaler exist. The disadvantages are that they need constant water management to control heat and clear areas of debris, they often produce aerosols, and access is sometimes unachievable such as in the contact areas of mandibular anteriors.

63. **The correct answer is (E).** Implementing the plan with the patient is not a part of the planning process for educating patients. The implementation phase of educating patients occurs after the planning phase.

64. **The correct answer is (D).** A patient's medical history should be updated every office visit, without fail. This should be done at every visit because patients do not often remember to inform dental hygienists or dentists about changes in their medical status.

65. **The correct answer is (C).** Most of the tissue tooth structure is composed of dentin. It is 70 percent inorganic, 18 percent organic, and 12 percent water. Enamel has the highest composition of inorganic material, being 95 percent inorganic, 1 percent organic, and 4 percent water.

66. **The correct answer is (A).** Nitrous oxide allows a patient to be consciously sedated, which means they are awake, but cannot feel pain.

67. **The correct answer is (C).** It takes about 2–5 minutes for an alginate hydrocolloid impression to set, depending on water temperature. The impression must then be removed quickly to prevent distortion.

68. **The correct answer is (B).** Oral ectoderm gives rise to enamel. Bone is a connective tissue that arises from cartilage.

69. **The correct answer is (D).** To receive the maximum benefits from optimally fluoridated water, children should begin ingesting the water at the onset of tooth development. Children should continue drinking optimally fluoridated water until tooth eruption is complete.

70. **The correct answer is (A).** The vagus, cranial nerve X, is an afferent nerve. Its function is to control sensation in the ear and epiglottis. This nerve helps humans develop their sense of taste. It is also responsible for controlling the muscles needed to produce voice. If this nerve is damaged, it may inhibit the ability to swallow.

71. **The correct answer is (A).** Nitrous oxide is stored in a blue tank, and oxygen is stored in a green tank. Because these gases are used for different purposes, it is important to know the difference between the tanks.

72. **The correct answer is (A).** A good community dental plan includes a lesson plan with defined goals and objectives. A good lesson plan includes an instructional set, which introduces content and states objectives. A good lesson plan also includes a body and a closure segment. The body of the plan includes the bulk of the information. The closure segment sums up the major points of the presentation.

73. **The correct answer is (B).** The paralleling technique requires that the film be placed parallel to the long axis of the tooth in a film holder to ensure proper film placement, and that the X-ray beam be placed perpendicular to the film and the long axis of the tooth.

74. **The correct answer is (D).** Central tendency measures the average score. It is also a summary or typical distribution of scores. The mean and average are the same values. They are both found by adding a certain number of values, then dividing by the number of values added together. The median is the center score in a distribution of scores arranged from least to greatest. The mode is the value that occurs most often in a set of scores. The mean, median, and mode are all segments that fall within the central tendency.

75. **The correct answer is (C).** Amides are used in dental offices more often than esters because amides cause fewer allergic reactions than esters. Although amides are frequently used, they can be dangerous for people with liver complications as

individuals with such conditions cannot properly metabolize these compounds.

76. **The correct answer is (A).** Inflammation is the body's way of healing after injury and protecting itself from further injury. When inflammation occurs, fluid, blood, and chemicals flow to the affected area to help rid the area of the harmful object or illness and heal the area.

77. **The correct answer is (A).** Bone defects are named based on the number of walls remaining due to the defect. One-wall defect has the worst prognosis because there is only one wall remaining.

78. **The correct answer is (C).** Erosion is considered an environmental tooth abnormality since the tooth is lost due to chemical forces. Hyperdontia, concrescence, gemination, and anodontia are naturally occurring abnormalities.

79. **The correct answer is (B).** To anesthetize the mandibular anterior teeth and the first premolar on the side to be worked on, the anesthesia needle must be inserted near, or slightly anterior to, the depression of mental foramen between the mandibular first and second premolars. By penetrating this area, the incisive nerve will be affected. The incisive nerve connects with the mental nerve at the mental foramen near the roots of the mandibular premolars to become the IA nerve.

80. **The correct answer is (D).** Actinomyces viscosus is a type of Gram-positive bacteria that attaches to tooth surfaces and eventually attracts Gram-negative bacteria.

81. **The correct answer is (B).** Fructose is the sweetest sugar derived from fruits and honey. Glucose is absorbed in the small intestine by the hepatic portal system and then moves to the liver where it is stored as glycogen. Sucrose hydrolyzes into both of these.

82. **The correct answer is (B).** The calculus index and the debris index combined yield the simplified oral hygiene index (OHI-S). The calculus index measures calculus on teeth surfaces.

83. **The correct answer is (C).** Epidemiology is the study of disease prevalence using systematic observation in medicine, science, and statistics. In dentistry, it is used to evaluate the specific disease patterns and needs of a community.

84. **The correct answer is (A).** Although all patients will benefit from education about dental caries, an overweight 6-year-old female would most benefit. Dental caries are one of the biggest oral health issues faced by children. Because dental caries can be caused by sugary foods, overweight children are more at risk for dental caries than other children.

85. **The correct answer is (C).** There are four types of bones in the human body: (1) long bones, (2) short bones, (3) irregular bones, and (4) cranial bones. The femur and humerus are examples of long bones. The carpals and tarsals are examples of short bones. Short bones may also be called sesamoid bones. Vertebrae are examples of irregular bones, and cranial bones and the scapula are examples of flat bones.

86. **The correct answer is (D).** Digital radiography initially costs more than film-based imaging systems. However, digital radiography does allow for immediate evaluation of images, uses less radiation than film-based radiography, and has advanced resolution. It also reduces costs associated with film and development over time.

87. **The correct answer is (E).** Nystatin is the generic name for Mycostatin, which is an antifungal medication. Doctors typically prescribe antifungal medications to those patients with fungal infections of the skin, intestinal tract, vagina, or mouth.

88. **The correct answer is (A).** Dental items that must be sterilized or disinfected are broken down into three categories: (1) critical, (2) semicritical, and (3) noncritical. Scalpels are considered to be critical and must be heat-sterilized or placed in a high-level disinfectant.

89. **The correct answer is (C).** Community water supplies are naturally fluoridated by water flowing over rock and soil containing fluoride, but optimum fluoride levels should be between 0.7–1.2 parts per million (ppm) and not 4–6 ppm.

90. **The correct answer is (A).** Microleakage is the ability of materials to adequately seal margins by adhesion. Polyacrylic acid is used to avoid microleakage of saliva, dental biofilm, and by-products into the area.

91. **The correct answer is (A).** Capitation plans are plans created between a dentist and an insurance provider, and are not federally funded medical

services. Capitation plans include fixed, monthly payments made to the dentist regardless of whether a patient is seen during a particular month. The amount the dentist is paid is based on the number of patients assigned to the dentist by the program. Capitation plans include co-payments and yearly maximums.

92. **The correct answer is (C).** Varnish contains 5 percent fluoride, not stannous fluoride. Stannous fluoride comes in either a 0.4 percent gel or a 0.63 percent solution. Its purpose is to reduce gingival inflammation and can also be used as an antimicrobial agent.

93. **The correct answer is (C).** The maximum permissible dose (MPD) uses the whole anatomy to prevent genetic alterations, while the maximum permissible exposure (MPE) uses the formula $5(N-18)R$, where N = the patient's age. The second statement is false because MPD does not only apply to dental personnel, as radiation does not affect only those in the dental field.

94. **The correct answer is (B).** After implementing any dental treatment plan, a provider should always assess the plan's success. In the case of this patient, the treatment plan should attempt to manage and treat the patient's dental caries. It should also aim to prevent the patient from developing more dental caries.

95. **The correct answer is (A).** Connective tissues include blood, bone, cartilage, lymph, adipose, elastic, fibrous (or collagen), and reticular connective tissue. Sarcomeres are found in skeletal and cardiac muscle tissue and are also known as the contractile units of muscle or myofibrils.

96. **The correct answer is (B).** Pharmacology abbreviations used on prescription medications appear as abbreviations for Latin words. In Latin, the phrase "three times per day" is translated to "ter in die." This phrase is abbreviated as tid, TID, or t.i.d on prescription labels.

97. **The correct answer is (A).** Taking radiographs on a minor without parental permission would be considered battery. Although the minor said that his father wouldn't mind, the minor cannot provide consent for the procedure in this case.

98. **The correct answer is (C).** Your refusal to take the radiographs follows state regulations. This action does not equal abandonment, malfeasance, or breach of duty. It also does not violate any part of HIPPA.

99. **The correct answer is (D).** The primary level of prevention is to hinder the beginning of disease. Radiographs are taken to detect issues before they develop into major problems.

100. **The correct answer is (B).** Revealing information about a patient to your friend is a breach of patient confidentiality. State and federal laws prevent medical providers from revealing information about patients to people unconnected with the patient's care. It is never appropriate for a medical professional to discuss a patient with a friend.

101. **The correct answer is (B).** Different forms of bacteria accumulate on tooth surfaces. A matrix protects the microcolonies of bacteria and eventually they merge. Gingivitis occurs about two to three weeks (10 to 20 days) after collecting plaque accumulate on tooth surfaces.

102. **The correct answer is (E).** The third molars are part of the permanent dentition. Both the maxillary and manibular third molars erupt around age 17–21. The roots of these molars are completed around age 18–25, depending on when the molars erupted.

103. **The correct answer is (D).** In chains of infection that spread disease from human to human, susceptible hosts include people with weak immune systems including children, elderly people, and immunosuppressed people. In the scenario, the elderly man is the susceptible host.

104. **The correct answer is (C).** When blood begins to ooze, most likely a vein has been compromised. If blood begins to spurt, most likely an artery has been injured.

105. **The correct answer is (A).** The intraoral injury should be treated as an extraoral injury by applying pressure to the bleeding area. The best way to accomplish this is to have the patient bite on a folded piece of gauze gently for approximately 10 minutes. Do not have the patient rinse or forcefully spit as this may aggravate the injured area.

106. **The correct answer is (A).** The female patient from the scenario was treated with a root canal. Since root canals occur because of infections inside teeth, the patient should be educated about infection prevention through proper cleaning.

107. **The correct answer is (C).** An X over a tooth on a periodontal exam chart indicates a clinically missing tooth. A clinically visible carious lesion is shown as a portion of the tooth shaded in on the periodontal exam chart. White triangles represent furcations and black triangles represent through-and-through furcations. Healthy teeth are left unmarked on the chart.

108. **The correct answer is (A).** The first step in community health planning is the assessment of needs. This is followed by program formulation, program financing, and implementation of the program. After this is complete, the success of the program can be evaluated.

109. **The correct answer is (E).** The renal system involves the kidney, which helps filter blood and maintain the body's pH balance. The circulatory system maintains homeostasis by supplying nutrients to cells and transporting away waste materials. The respiratory system involves breathing and the lungs. The nervous system controls and coordinates functions by maintaining homeostasis. The digestive system breaks down food and provides the body with nutrients.

110. **The correct answer is (A).** *Streptococcus mutans* bacteria is more prevalent in the mouths of people who eat high-sugar diets, and *Streptococcus sanguinis* bacteria is more prevalent in the mouths of people who eat low-sugar diets.

111. **The correct answer is (A).** Glucose is also known as dextrose and is absorbed in the small intestine. Galactose is the by-product of the breakdown of lactose and can also be readily absorbed into the bloodstream.

112. **The correct answer is (D).** Milk tends to pool in the maxillary anterior teeth when the child falls asleep drinking a bottle or breast-feeding and, therefore, these teeth are affected first by nursing-bottle decay. This decay is typically seen in 15 percent of children.

113. **The correct answer is (C).** The hyoid bone moves upward when food is swallowed. It is a U-shaped bone that is responsible for supporting the tongue.

114. **The correct answer is (B).** Biostatistics is the use of statistics procedures and analysis in the study and practice of biology. It is used to analyze and define research data. Normally, a sample of the population is taken, statistics are gathered, and generalizations and conclusions are drawn based on the data.

115. **The correct answer is (B).** Metaphase is the second stage of mitosis, or cell division. During metaphase, the chromosomes align centromeres and mitotic spindles begin to form.

116. **The correct answer is (A).** During an extraoral examination, functions and parts outside the mouth are inspected. The extraoral examination starts as soon as the patient arrives; the patient's attentiveness, handshake, appearance, and emotional state are important aspects to observe during the extraoral examination. When performing an intraoral examination, labial and buccal mucosa should be inspected.

117. **The correct answer is (E).** Ramfjord's periodontal disease index (PDI) evaluates gingival health, probing depths, dental biofilm, and calculus deposits—not dental caries. It is used for teeth #3, #9, #12, #19, #25, and #28, usually in clinical studies to represent a sample of the entire dentition.

118. **The correct answer is (B).** The shoulders are part of the appendicular skeletal system. Parts of the axial skeletal system include the skull, spinal column, sternum, and ribs.

119. **The correct answer is (A).** Both Dean's index and tooth surface index of fluorosis (TSIF) are indices that measure fluorosis. Dean's fluorosis index is most widely used in community studies, even though TSIF is more sensitive. In Dean's fluorosis index, the fluorosis score is based on the most severe form of fluorosis found on at least two teeth.

120. **The correct answer is (D).** The mouth mirror can have flat, concave, or frontal surfaces. Since the mouth is a very small and tight space, the use of a mouth mirror is essential.

121. **The correct answer is (B).** Vitamin B2, or riboflavin, is essential for metabolism of carbohydrates, fats and protein, and red blood cell formation. Humans receive riboflavin and other vitamins through proper nutrition, as humans do not produce their own vitamins.

122. **The correct answer is (C).** Fats, or lipids, are materials that are insoluble in water. Because they are not water soluble, they congeal into masses and must be broken down by bile.

123. **The correct answer is (D).** The pancreas is responsible for both endocrine and exocrine functions. The exocrine produces a pancreatic fluid consisting of sodium bicarbonate, pancreatic lipase, pancreatic amylase, and proteases.

124. **The correct answer is (A).** Lichen planus is a chronic disease. Lichen planus erodes the gingival mucosa. Wickham's striae, or white keratotic lines, may be present.

125. **The correct answer is (C).** The faces of area-specific curettes are set at a 70-degree angle to the terminal shank. On the other hand, universal curettes are set at a 90-degree angle from the terminal shank.

126. **The correct answer is (C).** The stationary phase is the phase in which cell growth equals cell death. The lag phase is the first phase, and it occurs when the cells begin to grow in size. The log phase is the phase during which binary fission occurs. During the final, or decline, phase the cells die off because all of the nutrients have been depleted. Binary fission does not include a replication phase.

127. **The correct answer is (E).** Antibiotics should be administered into pockets 5.0–6.0 mm. A periodontal probe should be used to measure and determine pocket depth.

128. **The correct answer is (C).** It is best to use annual radiographs to assess any bone loss of dental implants. An implant may be loose because the prosthesis is loose, not the implant itself.

129. **The correct answer is (A).** Ameloblastic fibroma are benign and expansible lesions found mainly over unerupted molars. They originate on the odontogenic epithelium and connective tissue.

130. **The correct answer is (C).** Codeine, which is also called methylmorphine, has a medium potential for abuse according to the Controlled Substances Act. Codeine can be refilled only for medical use.

131. **The correct answer is (A).** Autogenious infections are those that cannot spread from person to person. They may spread throughout the body, but they cannot spread from physical contact with another person. Ineffective endocarditis is spread throughout the body when vegetative growths or clumps of organisms break through connective tissue and move throughout the rest of the body.

132. **The correct answer is (D).** Jurisprudence is the philosophy of law, which includes civil law and tort law. Civil law involves crimes against a person, while tort law involves a civil wrong or injury to another person.

133. **The correct answer is (D).** Informed refusal against dental advice occurs when a dentist informs a patient of his or her treatment plan and the patient refuses treatment. It is not an ethical principle.

134. **The correct answer is (A).** Sarcoidosis is an inflammatory disease that can cause patients to suffer from xerostomia. If a patient has this condition, he should be instructed about xerostomia, its effects, and possible treatments.

135. **The correct answer is (A).** Both the statement and reason are correct and related because erythrocytes, or red blood cells, do not flow through the bloodstream after 120 days. At this point, the bone marrow, spleen, or the liver may remove the red blood cells from the bloodstream.

136. **The correct answer is (B).** Dental practice acts are established by state legislatures. These rules and regulations are then adopted by the state board of dental examiners.

137. **The correct answer is (E).** People with low rates of caries usually eat sensibly and have good dietary habits, which leads to good overall dental health. People with high rates of caries, however, are a good target group for a diet counseling community program because improved dietary habits can also improve their overall dental health.

138. **The correct answer is (D).** Veneers are used to hide stains, fractures, and other tooth defects. They are normally very thin shells of porcelain laminate that are bonded to the appropriate teeth.

139. **The correct answer is (C).** Glass ionomers contain ground fluoride. The fluoride is absorbed into neighboring teeth for about two years. In addition, research has shown that fewer *Streptococcus mutans* live on tooth surfaces treated with glass ionomers.

140. **The correct answer is (C).** Dysarthria is a communication disorder in which the patient has no clear speech pattern and slurs his words because of damage to the CNS, or peripheral nervous system.

141. **The correct answer is (A).** When evaluating a plan, two of the areas take the presenter's familiarity with the subject matter into account and whether the information being presented is appropriate to the level and the needs of the audience. The presenter is a six-year veteran, and she has two children of her own who are older than the audience. She, therefore, has experience both professionally and personally on the topic of oral hygiene for children. The information being presented is on the level of first graders and is applicable to their current needs. Many first graders have lost at least one tooth and are growing new adult teeth. They are old enough, and mature enough, to receive information about the best and correct ways to brush their teeth in order to achieve the best oral hygiene possible.

142. **The correct answer is (D).** Successful dental programs should evaluate the audience's understanding of the information. Because the hygienist in the scenario is having the audience members explain what they've learned to each other, she can be sure the students comprehended the information she told them.

143. **The correct answer is (B).** The body of a presentation includes the bulk of the information being presented. Major points and related experiences are generally part of the body of a quality presentation. Other parts of a presentation include the introduction in which the topic and objectives are introduced, and the closure, in which the entire presentation is summed up.

144. **The correct answer is (D).** Presenters should be evaluated based on their speech clarity, enthusiasm, body and facial expressions, responses to questions, and eye contact. In addition, presenters can be evaluated of their success using audiovisual equipment and their ability to manage time. Presenters can often evaluate the success of their presentation by administering tests, quizzes, and exams.

145. **The correct answer is (C).** Children are the age group that is most likely to contract dental caries from sugary foods. By teaching children about how reducing sugary foods may reduce their likelihood of cavities, the dental hygienist is teaching the audience something that is important to them. The other objectives are geared toward older audiences, not young students.

146. **The correct answer is (A).** The parallel technique has the tooth and the radiograph at the same angle. The central ray of the tube head is then directed perpendicular to both. This technique minimizes distortion.

147. **The correct answer is (C).** Intrapersonal communication involves conveying a message within oneself. Interpersonal communication is communication between two or more people.

148. **The correct answer is (E).** Since the case presentation occurs before the plan is implemented, it cannot contain an evaluation of the plan's success. Nevertheless, all treatment plans should be evaluated after they have been implemented.

149. **The correct answer is (B).** Dental indices are used to study caries and periodontal disease. The oral hygiene index (OHI-S) was developed by Greene and Vermillion and is mainly used for large populations. This index adds the debris index and calculus index together to arrive at a final score. Other indices include the O'Leary plaque index, personal hygiene performance index-modified (PHP-M), plaque index (PI), gingival index (GI), gingival bleeding index, Russell's periodontal index (PI), Ramfjord's periodontal disease index (PDI), Plaque Assessment Scoring System (PASS), and community periodontal index of treatment needs (CPITN).

150. The correct answer is (A). The maximum safely tolerated dose for an 8-year-old child who weighs 45 pounds would be 164 mg. Anything above this number is not recommended for a child of this age and weight.

151. The correct answer is (B). For patients with moderate or advanced periodontal disease, debridement may be the initial therapy prescribed. The patient should then be evaluated again in six weeks. The procedure should begin with a full mouth debridement. Then, two weeks after the first appointment, debridement and scaling should be done on the worst areas. Two weeks later, antibiotics should be administered.

152. The correct answer is (C). Pilocarpine is a cholinergic drug. Cholinergic drugs stimulate cholinergic receptors. These drugs mimic the effects of acetylcholine, a neurohormone of the parasympathetic nervous system. The parasympathetic nervous system is responsible for everyday bodily activities such as salivation, muscle relaxation, and digestion.

153. The correct answer is (C). Patients with rheumatoid arthritis (RA), which is an autoimmune disease that causes inflammation, are prone to temporomandibular joint disorder (TMJ). Patients with RA should be educated about the possible occurrence of TMJ and possible treatments for the condition.

154. The correct answer is (A). Five basic types of explorers exist: Shepherd's hook, pigtail, which is also known as the cowhorn, the #17, the #3A, and the #11/12. The Shepherd's hook should be used to detecting caries and evaluate restorations.

155. The correct answer is (D). Immunoglobulins are found in tears, saliva, and other parts of the human body, but they are typically divided into five, not six, work groups. These work groups include A or (lgA), D or (lgD), E or (lgE), G or (lgG), and M (or lgM).

156. The correct answer is (D). Reflective responding is a verbal behavior. Reflective responding addresses the actual feelings of the client.

157. The correct answer is (E). The maximum permissible dose of radiation a dental hygienist should be exposed to each year is 5 rem. This number has nothing to do with the age of the dental hygienist.

158. The correct answer is (B). The main goal of patient education is preventing disease. By educating patients about oral hygiene and specific methods of oral care, providers can help prevent disease in patients.

159. The correct answer is (C). Malpractice is considered an unintentional tort. Assault, battery, and defamation are intentional torts. Slander is verbal defamation, so it is considered an intentional tort.

160. The correct answer is (C). Bonding materials and techniques have greatly improved over the past few years, and newer bonding materials have primers and adhesives that do not require the etching step. After the tooth has been etched, the tooth surface must be primed with hydrophilic resin.

161. The correct answer is (E). Von Willebrand disease is a hereditary bleeding disorder that affects roughly 1 percent of the population. The Von Willebrand factor is a protein found in the blood that allows platelets to adhere together and assists in clotting. The Von Willebrand factor is defective in people who have this condition.

162. The correct answer is (B). The nasal septum is above the incisive foramen, another radiological landmark located between the maxillary incisors. The nasal septum divides the nasal cavity into two parts.

163. The correct answer is (D). Radiographs of the dental implants should be taken every year. This will help the dentist identify any problems with the dental implants.

164. The correct answer is (B). Phase I therapy focuses on controlling risk factors for disease. This phase could include educating patients about diet and self-care. It can also include cleaning and antimicrobial treatments.

165. The correct answer is (E). The foramen magnum is located in the occipital bone that forms the base or back of the cranium and houses the cerebellum and the occipital lobes of the brain. The medulla oblongata also enters and exits the skull via this opening.

166. The correct answer is (A). G. V. Black listed six classifications of caries based on the location of caries on the tooth. These classifications are simply named Class I through VI. This classification system is used during a dentition assessment to assess caries. Root caries are sometimes called cemental or cervical caries and occur from xerostomia, radiation therapy, poor oral hygiene, recession, or a high-sugar diet.

167. **The correct answer is (A).** Compomers do not bond to hard tooth structures; therefore, they are best used in areas that bear little to no stress. Compomers are relatively new materials that have the advantages of composites and glass ionomers.

168. **The correct answer is (A).** You should dry the etched area with clean air spray for 5–10 seconds before applying the sealant. This occurs after the occlusal surfaces have been thoroughly washed.

169. **The correct answer is (A).** Pierre Robin syndrome is a birth defect that results in the lower jaw appearing smaller than normal. It also causes the tongue to "ball up" in the back of the mouth. Infants may have difficulties eating and breathing due to this condition.

170. **The correct answer is (E).** The information gathered about the patient to form a treatment plan can also be used to compile an educational oral hygiene plan for the patient to follow; however, an educational plan is not a necessary part of a treatment plan, so the statement is incorrect. The reason is also incorrect because the education plan does not explain the risk factors that accompany certain treatments.

171. **The correct answer is (C).** Active listening requires eye contact and focusing on what the client is communicating. Paraphrasing involves summarizing what the client has said.

172. **The correct answer is (C).** In pharmacology, 1 grain ≈ 0.065g (and 0.065g = 65mg). In 1958, The International System of Units defined the measurement of a grain to be 64.79891 milligrams.

173. **The correct answer is (C).** Mucogingival surgery corrects mucogingival defects, but excisional surgery, which is known as gingivectomy, is used when the gingival tissues need to be reshaped. Periodontal flap surgery allows underlying bone to be exposed so that it can be corrected or modified.

174. **The correct answer is (D).** Concrescence is a condition that occurs after root formation is complete and two roots have joined together. This condition normally occurs after a traumatic incident.

175. **The correct answer is (B).** Hormonal fluctuations, such as those caused by pregnancy, can cause patients' gums to become inflamed. Especially when a woman is pregnant, gums will initially bleed a little and might advance to produce a dark-red pregnancy tumor.

176. **The correct answer is (D).** The statement is incorrect because benzodiazepines are considered anxiety agents, not antineoplastic agents. Benzodiazepines do, however, help to reduce anxiety and bring about sleep. Antineoplastic agents are cancer drugs.

177. **The correct answer is (A).** Microorganisms accumulate on different tooth surfaces. Pit and fissures mostly contain *Actinomyces naeslundii* and *Streptococcus mutans*. *Streptococcus sanguinis*, *Actinomyces israelii*, and *Lactobacillus acidophilus* are usually found on interproximal surfaces of the teeth. *Nocardia veterana* is a type of bacteria that is often found on healthy gingiva.

178. **The correct answer is (A).** When a patient gives a health-care provider permission to perform a procedure and he or she understands the risks involved, this is an example of informed consent. When patients come in for examinations and consultations, they are giving their consent to have services performed based on their actions. This is an example of implied consent.

179. **The correct answer is (A).** Enamel, dentin, and cementum are all part of tooth composition, but the layers are not necessarily equal on each tooth. The enamel organ determines the shape of the crown, and enamel rods have a prism-like appearance when viewed under a microscope. It takes four ameloblasts to form one enamel rod.

180. **The correct answer is (B).** The attached gingiva measures the bottom of the sulcus to the mucogingival junction. To measure the attached gingiva, two measurements are required. The first measurement should be taken from the CEJ to the mucogingival line. The second is the measurement from the CEJ

to the base of the pocket. Once these measurements are determined, the second measurement is subtracted from the first to yield the amount of attached gingiva.

181. **The correct answer is (B).** Water is an essential nutrient for the human body, and the body cannot survive without water for more than 3 days. A healthy intake of water keeps blood pressure and body temperature regulated, blood clots from forming, and kidneys functioning. It is also responsible for the healthy appearance of skin and hair.

182. **The correct answer is (C).** Bacteria are prokaryotes that divide by binary fission, not by mitosis. Eukaryotes divide by mitosis, where mitotic spindles appear just before cell division occurs.

183. **The correct answer is (A).** Patients who suffer from bulimia nervosa generally binge and purge. The purging can cause sufferers' knuckles to be calloused and their maxillary anterior teeth to be eroded. Furthermore, the parotid glands and the esophagus of people with bulimia nervosa may become swollen or inflamed.

184. **The correct answer is (E).** Fremitus is a vibration-like sensation that occurs when teeth close together. Fremitus can be measured by having the patient tap his or her teeth together while resting a finger on each maxillary tooth. A fremitus score measures whether the vibration was seen, felt, or both.

185. **The correct answer is (A).** Patients who have diabetes mellitus should be monitored carefully because their condition makes them more prone to infections and wounds that heal slowly.

186. **The correct answer is (A).** You may create a blister when spraying air onto abnormal epidermal tissue if you have witnessed Nikolsky's sign, which is the separation of the outer layer of the epidermis from the basal layer. The air pressure from the air-water syringe can create blisters.

187. **The correct answer is (B).** The oblique stroke, which is used to scale the majority of a tooth's surface, is used at a 45-degree angle to the long axis of the tooth.

188. **The correct answer is (C).** The dentoperiosteal is a primary gingival fiber group that attaches cementum at CEJ to the alveolar crest in order to anchor teeth.

189. **The correct answer is (B).** When caring for implants, dental personnel and patients must take care not to scratch the implant. Scratches harbor bacteria.

190. **The correct answer is (B).** A double-blind study is a study in which neither the examiner nor the participant knows which is the control or experimental group. Cross-sectional studies are considered true reflections of an entire population, and longitudinal studies are performed over a long period of time.

191. **The correct answer is (B).** Cleaning and polishing agents contain an abrasive agent that removes stains, plaque, and debris from teeth. They are very effective when combined with the appropriate brushing technique.

192. **The correct answer is (A).** Those with Down syndrome often have delayed tooth eruption, and when the teeth do come in, they are small and irregularly shaped. Other dental issues common to those with Down syndrome is that they tend to breathe through their mouths, have cracked lips, are at an increased risk for gingivitis and periodontal disease, and have short, arrow palates.

193. **The correct answer is (A).** An amalgam is an alloy composed of mercury mixed with a powder made mainly of silver and tin. It is a common filling used for dental restorations.

194. **The correct answer is (E).** The trigeminal ophthalmic includes the frontal nerve, which controls sensation in the scalp and forehead, the lacrimal nerve, which controls sensation in the lacrimal glands and eyelids, and the nasocillary nerves, which control sensation in the nose and nasal mucosa.

195. **The correct answer is (D).** B vitamins are water soluble so they are flushed out of the body and cannot be stored there. Other vitamins, such as vitamins E and K, are fat soluble. Fat-soluble vitamins are stored in fat deposits in the body.

196. **The correct answer is (B).** Some may think that medical safety data sheets are a concern of HIPAA. However, Title II of HIPAA Administrative Simplification provision states that the use of

medical safety data sheets is a concern of the Occupational Safety and Health Administration (OSHA).

197. The correct answer is (C). Digital radiography requires less radiation than film-based systems. This argument would most likely convince the patient to have the radiographs taken. Although some of the other arguments are valid, they would most likely do little to convince the patient to have the radiographs taken.

198. The correct answer is (E). The American Dental Association recommends taking radiographs based on the patient's individual health needs. The dental hygienist and dentist will be able to determine when they are necessary.

199. The correct answer is (A). The lead in the apron should be at least 0.25 mm thick in order to protect the patient from radiation. This protects organs and tissues that are sensitive to free radicals.

200. The correct answer is (B). Sometimes when the film is removed too quickly from the packaging, dry, static electric air compromises the integrity of the film and branch or root-like images appear on the developed film. To correct this problem, remove film slowly from the packaging in a controlled environment.

Component B

1. D	31. B	61. D	91. B	121. C
2. A	32. C	62. D	92. C	122. D
3. C	33. B	63. B	93. C	123. A
4. A	34. D	64. D	94. B	124. C
5. C	35. D	65. A	95. D	125. A
6. C	36. A	66. C	96. D	126. C
7. B	37. B	67. A	97. B	127. A
8. A	38. C	68. C	98. A	128. D
9. D	39. C	69. D	99. C	129. B
10. C	40. D	70. B	100. A	130. D
11. C	41. D	71. C	101. A	131. C
12. C	42. A	72. A	102. C	132. B
13. D	43. C	73. B	103. D	133. C
14. C	44. B	74. D	104. C	134. B
15. D	45. D	75. C	105. B	135. B
16. A	46. B	76. D	106. D	136. C
17. D	47. D	77. B	107. C	137. D
18. D	48. B	78. B	108. A	138. D
19. C	49. D	79. A	109. D	139. A
20. B	50. B	80. D	110. A	140. D
21. B	51. A	81. A	111. C	141. D
22. B	52. B	82. D	112. D	142. A
23. C	53. A	83. B	113. B	143. A
24. D	54. D	84. A	114. D	144. B
25. C	55. D	85. C	115. A	145. D
26. C	56. B	86. C	116. D	146. C
27. A	57. D	87. A	117. D	147. A
28. B	58. C	88. B	118. C	148. C
29. C	59. C	89. A	119. D	149. A
30. B	60. A	90. B	120. A	150. D

1. **The correct answer is (D).** The patient's symptoms, which include painful gums, a metallic taste, and severe halitosis, are characteristic of necrotizing ulcerative gingivitis (NUG).

2. **The correct answer is (A).** The small grayish areas on the patient's gums are ulcers. The gum tissue in these areas has become so inflamed that it has died.

3. **The correct answer is (C).** Involvement of the deeper periodontium is a clinical sign of NUP, or necrotizing ulcerative periodontal disease.

4. **The correct answer is (A).** The age group most associated with necrotizing ulcerative gingivitis (NUG) is ages 20 to 30.

5. **The correct answer is (C).** A gentle subgingival periodontal instrumentation might be performed on this patient, but not during the first visit. Careful

removal of the pseudomembrane with irrigation, supragingival periodontal instrumentation, and patient self-care are more likely to take place during a first appointment.

6. **The correct answer is (C).** Gentle self-care regimen is standard protocol in any case of NUG.

7. **The correct answer is (B).** Subgingival instrumentation should be performed during the follow-up appointment.

8. **The correct answer is (A).** If the NUG is severe, the patient should be prescribed antibiotics.

9. **The correct answer is (D).** NUG is caused by stress, poor dental habits, and an imbalanced diet. The patient should also refrain from drinking alcohol.

10. **The correct answer is (C).** Impacted molars are not a factor in this patient's condition.

11. **The correct answer is (C).** The patient's clinical signs and symptoms indicate that he has primary herpetic gingivostomatitis. The patient has numerous painful ulcers on the lips and palate. These ulcers are called vesicles and are characteristic of this condition.

12. **The correct answer is (C).** A skin rash on the arms and legs is not characteristic of primary herpetic gingivitis (PHG). Other symptoms of PHG include the presence of vesicles, malaise, fever, and swollen lymph nodes.

13. **The correct answer is (D).** Ulcers associated with primary herpetic gingivostomatitis (PHG), which are commonly called cold sores or fever blisters, often occur on the lips and in the oral cavity.

14. **The correct answer is (C).** Primary herpetic gingivostomatitis (PHG) is of viral origin. It is caused by the type 1 herpes simplex virus and is highly contagious. It is often contracted by coming into contact with an infected person's saliva.

15. **The correct answer is (D).** While it is difficult to maintain proper oral hygiene during an outbreak, the mother should attempt to do this. Increasing the boy's fluids will prevent dehydration and giving him an analgesic such as ibuprofen or Tylenol will control pain.

16. **The correct answer is (A).** Type 1 herpes simplex virus, or HSV-1, is the virus that causes cold sores, as this patient has.

17. **The correct answer is (D).** Common triggers that can cause a recurrence of primary herpetic gingivostomatitis (PHG) include sunlight, malnutrition, the common cold or flu, and stress. Dental caries are not associated with this condition.

18. **The correct answer is (D).** This patient's condition is highly contagious; some dentists will not treat a child with an active infection. If you do treat a patient with primary herpetic gingivostomatitis (PHG), you should wear a mask, gloves, and eye protection.

19. **The correct answer is (C).** Localized gentle scaling is not indicated for primary herpetic gingivostomatitis (PHG). While there is no cure for this condition, its symptoms are treated with antibiotics.

20. **The correct answer is (B).** This condition is most common among children, ages 1 to 6 years old. It can also occur in older children.

21. **The correct answer is (B).** While topical local anesthesia may be used to numb the site of an injection, injected local anesthesia is most often used to limit patient discomfort during the treatment of a periocoronal abscess.

22. **The correct answer is (B).** The most common site for a pericoronal abscess, also known as pericoronitis, is a partially erupted mandibular third molar. As the dental chart indicates, this is the case with this patient.

23. **The correct answer is (C).** Blanched tissue is not a sign of pericoronal abscess. Other symptoms include swollen lymph glands, a fever, and swelling around the affected tooth.

24. **The correct answer is (D).** The anatomical definition for a flap that covers a partially erupted tooth is the operculum.

25. **The correct answer is (C).** A difficulty in opening the mouth is called trismus, which may be a symptom of an abscess. Trismus might also be a symptom of lockjaw (tetanus) or may be caused by a muscle spasm.

26. **The correct answer is (C).** Periocoronal abscesses typically occur in the mandibular third molar area, making them difficult to access.

27. **The correct answer is (A).** Placing a local antibiotic inside the infected area is not part of the standard treatment protocol for a periocoronal abscess. Prescribing medication to relieve pain is also part of the treatment of a periocoronal abscess.

28. **The correct answer is (B).** Sterile saline is the safest liquid to use to irrigate the area under the operculum. Saline also does not irritate infected tissue.

29. **The correct answer is (C).** A sterile curet is the instrument of choice to allow drainage of the abscess.

30. **The correct answer is (B).** X-rays of a pericoronal abscess show a dark area around the apex, or tip, of the root.

31. **The correct answer is (B).** Based on the patient's history and clinical examination, the patient most likely has moderate chronic generalized periodontitis. X-rays showing bone loss will confirm this diagnosis.

32. **The correct answer is (C).** Based on the patient's generalized pocketing and bone loss, the classification of her condition is Type 3, early periodontitis. The ADA classifies patients as Type 3 if they have attachment loss of 4 to 6 mm.

33. **The correct answer is (B).** The signs and symptoms of this patient indicate that she has a periodontal abscess. The signs include tooth mobility, moderate gingival calculus, and pocket depths. The symptoms include swollen and bleeding gums and a bad taste in the mouth.

34. **The correct answer is (D).** While the restoration (old amalgam on #28) may require updating, it has nothing to do with the swelling.

35. **The correct answer is (D).** Extraction of the infected tooth should not be necessary.

36. **The correct answer is (A).** The patient has a periodontal abscess. The pain characterized by this condition is constant, intense, and easy to localize.

37. **The correct answer is (B).** In the Dental History, the patient indicated that she went to a different dentist who began a gross scaling. Gross scaling is never appropriate for periodontal patients. Always scale to completion.

38. **The correct answer is (C).** Your patient should use a proxy brush and floss, since these items will effectively clean areas with more and less space.

39. **The correct answer is (C).** The appropriate recare frequency for this patient after reevalution is 3 months, since periodontal pathogens recolonize after 9 to 12 weeks.

40. **The correct answer is (D).** An antimicrobial rinse that does not contain alcohol is most appropriate for long-term maintenance for periodontal patients.

41. **The correct answer is (D).** Phenytoin (Dilantin™) is responsible for about half the cases of gingival enlargement. This is most likely the cause of your patient's gingival enlargement, which is called drug-influenced gingival enlargement or Dilantin™ hyperplasia. Other causes of gingival enlargement include braces, plaque, and other drugs.

42. **The correct answer is (A).** Gingival enlargement is considered a gingival disease, so the classification is Type 1. With this classification, there is no attachment loss, and bleeding may or may not be present. Only the gingival tissues are inflamed.

43. **The correct answer is (C).** Azathioprine is a drug that suppresses the immune system. It does not cause gingival enlargement.

44. **The correct answer is (B).** Gingival enlargement occurs most often in children and young adults, mainly because it can be caused by hormonal changes experienced during puberty.

45. **The correct answer is (D).** Ideally, the drug should be discontinued. This is the best course of treatment. If this is not possible, an alternate drug may be prescribed.

46. **The correct answer is (B).** In the majority of cases, overgrowth of the gums will likely recur in patients who undergo surgery to treat gingival enlargement.

47. **The correct answer is (D).** Increasing the amount of fluids the patient drinks is irrelevant to the regimen of controlling plaque.

48. **The correct answer is (B).** Antimicrobial mouth rinses may be beneficial to this patient's mechanical plaque control because it may reduce enlargement. A mouth rinse containing .12 percent chlorhexidine is usually recommended.

49. **The correct answer is (D).** Heredity, poor oral hygiene, and braces all increase a patient's risk of developing gingival enlargement.

50. **The correct answer is (B).** A more frequent debridement than average is recommended for this patient.

51. **The correct answer is (A).** Clinical and radiographic findings, which include bone loss and pockets, are consistent with generalized aggressive periodontitis (GAP), which affects individuals who are otherwise healthy.

52. **The correct answer is (B).** Generalized aggressive periodontitis (GAP) most often occurs in patients who are under 30 years old.

53. **The correct answer is (A).** Heavy generalized calculus deposits are not consistent with GAP. In addition to the other answer options, rabid bone loss is also a primary feature of this condition.

54. **The correct answer is (D).** Generalized aggressive periodontitis (GAP) is characterized by a generalized interproximal attachment loss affecting at least three permanent teeth other than the first molars and incisors.

55. **The correct answer is (D).** Your patient's GAP should be treated with oral hygiene instruction, frequent evaluation of plaque, and supra- and subgingival scaling. Other treatments include root scaling to remove microbial plaque and occlusal therapy. The patient may also need periodontal surgery.

56. **The correct answer is (B).** Your patient's condition is generalized aggressive periodontitis (GAP), which is less common than chronic periodontitis.

57. **The correct answer is (D).** Reduction of probing depths, progression toward occlusal stability, and reduction of gingival inflammation are all desired outcomes for periodontal therapy. Other desired outcomes include gain of clinical attachment, resolution of osseous lesions, and reduction of plaque.

58. **The correct answer is (C).** The treatment of generalized aggressive periodontitis (GAP) and chronic periodontitis are very similar. Treatment includes oral hygiene instruction, plaque control, supra- and subgingival scaling, and root planing.

59. **The correct answer is (C).** Gingivectomy, which is the removal of gingival tissue, is not a recognized treatment protocol for generalized aggressive periodontitis (GAP).

60. **The correct answer is (A).** Generalized aggressive periodontitis is usually associated with the pathogens *Actinobacillus actinomycetemcomitans* and *Porphyromonas gingivalis* and neutrophil-function abnormalities.

61. **The correct answer is (D).** The patient is taking a low-dose antibiotic. Antibiotics are used to treat bacterial infections. They do not cause tooth decay.

62. **The correct answer is (D).** Interdental tissue is the gum tissue between the teeth. It is the most susceptible to gingival enlargement during orthodontic treatment. If the tissue enlarges, it may cover the appliance and create pockets that retain biofilm.

63. **The correct answer is (B).** The orthodontist's philosophy regarding hygiene is the least significant factor in determining the selection of biofilm-control procedures. The position of the orthodontic appliance is also an important factor.

64. **The correct answer is (D).** A hard toothbrush may damage appliances, tissues, and teeth and is the least effective for cleaning.

65. **The correct answer is (A).** A low speed is safest for an orthodontic patient. This speed and a light stroke are effective for maintenance.

66. **The correct answer is (C).** This patient's gums are most likely inflamed and bleeding because of his poor oral hygiene. Supplemental oral findings include food that is visibly present.

67. **The correct answer is (A).** The best interdental aid for an orthodontic patient is a floss threader with tufted dental floss. Tufted dental floss can remove biofilm more efficiently than regular dental floss.

68. **The correct answer is (C).** Increasing water consumption post-orthodontic therapy is not likely to

aid in remineralization after orthodontic treatment. While water containing fluoride may have a slight topical benefit, the other answer choices are much more likely to aid in remineralization.

69. **The correct answer is (D).** The core value of veracity involves an obligation to tell the truth and maintain honesty in relationships. As a professional dental hygienist, you must inform your patient of the problem.

70. **The correct answer is (B).** Your dental hygiene treatment plan for this patient should include full mouth debridement/instrumentation with hand instruments. Your plan should also include recare visits at least every 6 months and oral hygiene instruction.

71. **The correct answer is (C).** An FMX, full-mouth radiographic survey, should be taken of this patient. This radiograph allows for a new baseline with a view of the maxilla while conserving the number of films due to fewer teeth being present.

72. **The correct answer is (A).** It is usually the most comfortable for the patient to remove his or her own dentures.

73. **The correct answer is (B).** Residue from daily denture cleaner is not a typical denture deposit. Denture deposits might also include stains.

74. **The correct answer is (D).** Placing the denture in a sealed bag filled with denture cleaner and then immersing the bag in an ultrasonic cleaning device is a highly effective technique to clean the denture.

75. **The correct answer is (C).** The optimum regimen for cleaning the denture is to rinse, immerse, and brush the denture daily.

76. **The correct answer is (D).** All of the following are soft-tissue changes associated with wearing a denture. Epulis formation is another soft-tissue change.

77. **The correct answer is (B).** The best response is to explain to the patient why you would like her to remove her denture. An ideal response is given in choice (B).

78. **The correct answer is (B).** Because her lower dentition is healthy, a 6-month recall is adequate.

79. **The correct answer is (A).** The patient's gender is not a risk factor in her development of periodontal disease. Men are more likely to develop periodontal disease than women.

80. **The correct answer is (D).** This patient's blood pressure is below normal, so it is categorized as hypotension.

81. **The correct answer is (A).** The correct terminology for dry mouth is xerostomia.

82. **The correct answer is (D).** Patients with dry mouth, or xerostomia, are at a high risk of developing dental caries.

83. **The correct answer is (B).** This patient has Sjorgren's syndrome, a chronic autoimmune disorder that causes dry mouth.

84. **The correct answer is (A).** While it may be a good idea for your patient to return to his pilocarpine therapy, this is not a dental hygienist's decision.

85. **The correct answer is (C).** A saliva substitute contains carboxymethylcellulose, as well as other minerals typical of normal saliva.

86. **The correct answer is (C).** Aspirin is not known to decrease salivary function. Antihistamines, antihypertensives, and diuretics as well as anticonvulsants decrease salivary function.

87. **The correct answer is (A).** A patient with dry mouth is more likely to experience a burning sensation on the tongue or in the mouth than in the lower G.I. tract. The patient would also be very thirsty.

88. **The correct answer is (B).** This patient has sulcus depths within 3mm with normal embrasure spaces, so you should recommend dental floss.

89. **The correct answer is (A).** You should recommend a power brush for this patient, as this type of toothbrush aids in stimulating saliva.

90. **The correct answer is (B).** This patient should be seen more frequently than most other patients due to his history of decay and ongoing xerostomia.

91. **The correct answer is (B).** The most likely diagnosis for this patient is moderate chronic generalized periodontitis based on pocket depths, furcation, and bone loss.

92. **The correct answer is (C).** A full-mouth series, or FMX, is necessary to appropriately diagnose the patient's periodontal condition.

93. **The correct answer is (C).** Heavy calculus deposits and deep pockets require quadrant scaling. Isolated sites will benefit from local antibiotic delivery.

94. **The correct answer is (B).** The Type 2 periodontal classification includes chronic periodontitis. This patient has some bone loss and moderate pocketing, which are characteristic of Type 2 periodontitis.

95. **The correct answer is (D).** This patient's dental history indicates that he is fearful of discomfort. He should therefore have a local anesthesia by quadrant to keep him relaxed and comfortable.

96. **The correct answer is (D).** According to the dental chart, the patient has furcation on tooth 30.

97. **The correct answer is (B).** A proxy brush cleans effectively when there is more spacing, as is the case with this patient.

98. **The correct answer is (A).** In addition to his normal brushing routine, this patient should take part in extra mouth debridement and use an agent, such as a chlorine dioxide rinse, that works directly on sulfa compounds.

99. **The correct answer is (C).** It is best to handle the situation graciously and professionally. Answer choice (C) is the best response.

100. **The correct answer is (A).** Periodontal pathogens recolonize every 9 to 11 weeks; therefore, the patient should be seen more often than usual because maintaining debridement is especially important.

101. **The correct answer is (A).** This patient has no bone or attachment loss; therefore, she most likely has generalized acute gingivitis.

102. **The correct answer is (C).** Because the patient has no significant pocketing or bone or attachment loss, generalized debridement to remove all deposits followed by a fine scale and polish at a second appointment is recommended.

103. **The correct answer is (D).** Because she is a diabetic, it is best to schedule this patient's appointments in the morning after breakfast. She will be rested at this time, and her meal and medication schedules will not be interrupted.

104. **The correct answer is (C).** If a diabetic patient has too much insulin and abnormally low blood glucose, it is referred to as hypoglycemia. This can happen to a diabetic patient if he or she skips a meal, exercises excessively, or vomits.

105. **The correct answer is (B).** Since this patient takes insulin, she has Type 1 diabetes.

106. **The correct answer is (D).** A "fruity" breath odor is not a symptom of hyperinsulinism, a condition in which a person has too much insulin. In addition to confusion, incoherence, and hunger/weakness, moist skin is also a symptom of this condition.

107. **The correct answer is (C).** Giving a patient a sugary drink or sugar and encouraging her to eat a complex carbohydrate with protein usually elicits a rapid recovery and prevents a recurrence.

108. **The correct answer is (A).** Note that the values <126 mg/dL (well controlled) and >160 mg/dL (uncontrolled) are considered the end points of each range.

109. **The correct answer is (D).** Answer choice (D) is not true. If a patient's diabetes is well controlled, he or she can be treated the same as a patient without diabetes.

110. **The correct answer is (A).** Knowing when a diabetic patient has last eaten decreases the risk of a hypoglycemic incident.

111. **The correct answer is (C).** Since smoking puts this patient's general and oral health at risk, you should encourage her to stop smoking.

112. **The correct answer is (D).** Even though the woman flosses only a few days per week, her gums do not bleed. This is most likely because smoking constricts her blood vessels and masks the impact of pathogens on the tissues.

113. **The correct answer is (B).** No evidence of smoking is discerned in the eyes. In addition to the breath, fingers, and skin, evidence of smoking can be found in the mouth.

114. **The correct answer is (D).** An Increase in cervical caries is not an oral consequence of tobacco use.

115. **The correct answer is (A).** Because your patient smokes, she has a higher-than-average chance of developing heart disease. Surprisingly, heart disease is more common in smokers than cancer.

116. **The correct answer is (D).** Nicotine gum, a nicotine patch, and a nicotine inhaler are all options for nicotine replacement therapy. Nicotine nasal spray is also available.

117. **The correct answer is (D).** Serum IgG is not a pharmacotherapy.

118. **The correct answer is (C).** The other components are assess and arrange. Analyze is not a component.

119. **The correct answer is (D).** No dental caries are indicated on this patient's dental chart. It is also indicated in her dental history that she has never had any type of decay.

120. **The correct answer is (A).** You should approach the relapse as a learning experience. Help her understand the reasons for the relapse so it does not happen again in the future.

121. **The correct answer is (C).** An ultrasonic scaler is not necessary and will make this patient uncomfortable.

122. **The correct answer is (D).** Chewing a gum containing xylitol would have no impact on this patient's sensitivity to cold.

123. **The correct answer is (A).** The patient's blood pressure is lower than normal. This means that she has hypotension.

124. **The correct answer is (C).** Hyothyroidism is more common in women than in men.

125. **The correct answer is (A).** Patients with hypothyroidism often have a low metabolism and tend to be tired due to deficient thyroid activity.

126. **The correct answer is (C).** The patient's sensitivity is most likely caused by her recession. She has generalized root surface exposure 1–2 mm.

127. **The correct answer is (A).** You should recommend that this patient clean her teeth with a soft toothbrush because it is the least abrasive to the teeth and tissues.

128. **The correct answer is (D).** Sodium monofluorophosphate reduces incidence of dental caries. It does not reduce sensitivity.

129. **The correct answer is (B).** No special consideration is needed in taking films of patients with hypothyroidism. Simply follow the standard of care.

130. **The correct answer is (D).** There is no correlation to duration or frequency regarding this patient's sensitivity to cold.

131. **The correct answer is (C).** The patient recently had antibiotic therapy, which is most likely the cause of the stain on his teeth.

132. **The correct answer is (B).** You should recommend that he brush his teeth 2 to 3 times a day, especially after meals.

133. **The correct answer is (C).** Your patient does not yet have adequate motor skills to do most of the brushing himself. Therefore, answer choice (C) is correct.

134. **The correct answer is (B).** The minimal recommended duration for tooth brushing is 2 minutes.

135. **The correct answer is (B).** Your patient should rinse, swish, and expectorate each time he uses his inhaler. This is recommended to avoid xerostomia.

136. **The correct answer is (C).** It is important to take his blood pressure and pulse before treatment to prevent tachycardia, which can be caused by adrenergic agonists.

137. **The correct answer is (D).** The ADA recommends varnish for children at risk for caries under age 6 because of the risk of over ingestion.

138. **The correct answer is (D).** Trays are not a delivery system for disclosants.

139. **The correct answer is (A).** Bacteria will build up on the child's toothbrush after about 3 months, so his mother should replace his toothbrush around this time.

140. **The correct answer is (D).** The patient should have sealants on the first and second permanent molars. However, he has only primary teeth present.

141. **The correct answer is (D).** Patients with the purging-type bulimia usually do not fast. They typically binge eat, and then purge.

142. **The correct answer is (A).** Perimylolysis is the first incidence of the chemical erosion caused by vomiting. It is usually first seen in the maxillary anterior linguals.

143. **The correct answer is (D).** The soft palate is the part of the mouth most likely to be injured by the item used to initiate vomiting. It is the most likely site to initiate the gag reflex.

144. **The correct answer is (B).** Caries are usually seen on the cervical area of the teeth. However, tooth erosion is a better indicator that a patient may be bulimic.

145. **The correct answer is (D).** Eroded tooth enamel, xerostomia, and hypersensitive teeth are all common findings in bulimic patients. Other oral findings include cavities, tooth discoloration, and bleeding gums.

146. **The correct answer is (C).** Most dentists recommend waiting until the bulimia has been cured and the vomiting has stopped to perform expensive dental care to repair extremely damaged teeth.

147. **The correct answer is (A).** Demineralization starts immediately upon contact, and brushing may cause demineralization to occur in unaffected areas.

148. **The correct answer is (C).** There is no direct correction between a high-protein diet and reduced tooth sensitivity.

149. **The correct answer is (A).** Gum with sugar can worsen her teeth and her xerostomia.

150. **The correct answer is (D).** Over-exercising, tooth discoloration, and repeated tooth brushing are commonly seen in bulimic patients. Other characteristics include excessive vomiting, tooth decay, hiding or stealing food, and excessive use of laxatives.

PART III

NBDHE COMPONENT A QUESTIONS

CHAPTER 5

Scientific Basis Questions

OVERVIEW

- **Histology and embryology**
- **Atomic sciences**
- **Biochemistry and nutrition**
- **Microbiology and immunology**
- **General and oral pathology**
- **Pharmacology**
- **Four tips for answering scientific basis questions**
- **Practice questions**
- **Answer key and explanations**
- **Summing it up**

You learned earlier that the National Board Dental Hygiene Examination (NBDHE) is a computer-based test containing 350 multiple-choice questions. The first part of the examination, Component A, includes 200 multiple-choice questions covering three areas: (1) Scientific Basis for Dental Hygiene Practice, (2) Provision of Clinical Dental Hygiene Services, and (3) Community Health and Research Principles. The second part of the examination, Component B, contains questions about patient cases. In this chapter, you'll learn about questions assessing your knowledge of the basic sciences. About 30 percent of the questions (or 60 test questions) on the NBDHE deal with Scientific Basis questions, which include the following topics.

- Histology and embryology

- Anatomic sciences, including general anatomy and physiology, anatomy of the head and neck, dental anatomy, and root anatomy

- Biochemistry and nutrition

- Microbiology and immunology

- General and oral pathology

- Pharmacology

Although this chapter does not review every detail of the subjects that you learned in school, it highlights some very important information and provides you with practice questions to test your knowledge in these areas. If you are having trouble remembering the information in this chapter or answering the practice questions, review your textbooks and notes from school.

HISTOLOGY AND EMBRYOLOGY

Histology is the study of tissues and cells that can be seen under a microscope. Embryology is the study of human development beginning with egg fertilization until birth. To pass the NBDHE, you need to have a solid grasp of both histology and embryology.

Histology

Cells are the smallest units in the body and the building blocks of tissues. Healthy cells recognize each other and group together to form tissues. Unhealthy cells, such as cancer cells, do not recognize other cells in this manner. Understanding cells and their functions helps dental hygienists detect diseases and disorders in the tissues and gums.

Embryology

> **NOTE**
>
> At five weeks of gestational development, a cleft lip may result if the maxillary and medial nasal processes do not fuse.

Human development begins with fertilization, which is the union of a female egg, called an ovum, and a male sperm. Both the egg and the sperm are referred to as germ cells. Each germ cell contains 23 chromosomes. After fertilization, a zygote develops containing 46 chromosomes. The zygote develops an outer shell called the morula and an inner shell called the blastocyst. The embryonic period begins when the blastocyst implants in the uterine wall. The blastocyst becomes an embryo that starts to develop different body parts. This is the period when most congenital malformations will occur. The structures of the mouth begin to develop in the fourth week of embryonic development as the face and neck start to take shape. Facial and neck structures develop from five branchial arches. During the ninth week of development, the embryo becomes a fetus that continues to develop until birth.

Review these topics related to histology and embryology before taking the NBDHE:

- Definition of a cell
- Functions of cells
- Common properties of cells
- Cell replication
- Types of cell junctions, including the following:
  - Desmosomes
  - Tight junctions
  - Gap functions
- Types of cells in the body

- Characteristics of the following tissues in the oral cavity:
  - Epithelial tissue
  - Connective tissue
  - Muscle tissue
  - Nerve tissue
- Facial development
- Palatal development
- Tongue development
- Tooth development
  - Morphodifferentiation and cytodifferentiation
  - Development of the dentin and enamel
- Development of the soft tissue of the oral cavity
- Development of tissues of the tooth
  - Dentin
  - Pulp
  - Enamel
  - Cementum
  - Root Formation
- Development of supporting tissues

EXERCISES: HISTOLOGY AND EMBRYOLOGY

Directions: Choose the option that best answers the question.

1. During which stage of cell division do chromosomes align their centromeres?
   (A) Prophase
   (B) Metaphase
   (C) Anaphase
   (D) Telophase
   (E) Interphase

   Mitosis is the process of cell division. There are several stages of mitosis. Metaphase is the second stage of mitosis. During this stage, chromosomes align their centromeres at the midpoint. **The correct answer is (B).**

2. Which one of the following is the structure that is formed from the first branchial arch?
   (A) Hyoid bone
   (B) Thymus hypopharynx
   (C) Frontonasal process
   (D) Pharyngeal muscles
   (E) Styloid process

   The first branchial arch forms the frontonasal process. This arch is also responsible for the formation of two mandibular processes and two maxillary processes. **The correct answer is (C).**

ATOMIC SCIENCES

As a dental hygienist, it's important for you to understand various anatomical structures. The structures of the mouth are connected to other organ systems, such as the digestive system, so you must learn how all the body systems are related to one another. In this section, you'll review general anatomy and physiology, anatomy of the head and neck, dental anatomy, and root anatomy.

General Anatomy and Physiology

Many body systems work together to keep the human body functioning. These include the digestive system, skeletal system, muscular system, endocrine system, renal system, cardiovascular system, respiratory system, integumentary system, immune system, reproductive system, and nervous system.

The *digestive system* is responsible for breaking down food into nutrients, water, and electrolytes that provide the body with energy. Digestion begins in the mouth. Other structures and organs of the digestive tract include the esophagus, the stomach, the small intestine, the large intestine, the rectum, and the anus. The liver, pancreas, and gallbladder are also involved in digestion.

The *skeletal system* supports and protects the body. The skeletal system includes a variety of bones, including long bones, short bones, flat bones, and irregular bones. Cartilage and connective tissues, such as tendons and ligaments, are also included in this system.

The *muscular system* allows the body to move about and helps internal organs perform various tasks. The human body contains three types of muscles: skeletal, cardiac, and smooth. Skeletal muscles provide mobility, cardiac muscles keep the heart pumping, and smooth muscles aid in various bodily functions, including digestion.

The *endocrine system* contains glands that produce hormones. These hormones send various messages to different parts of the body. The release of certain hormones tells the body to perform certain tasks. Some of the structures involved in hormone production include the hypothalamus, the pituitary gland, and the thyroid gland.

The *renal system*, or urinary system, works to filter impurities from the blood. The organs of the renal system include the kidneys, the bladder, the ureters, and the urethra.

The *cardiovascular system* moves blood throughout the body. The blood provides organs and cells with the nutrients and oxygen they need to function. The structures of the cardiovascular system include the heart, arteries, veins, and capillaries.

The *respiratory system* supplies the entire body with oxygen. The lungs, nose, pharynx, larynx, trachea, bronchi, bronchioles, and alveoli are all part of the respiratory system.

The *integumentary system*, which is made up of the skin and its appendages, protects the body's organs and allows humans to sense pain and changes in temperature or pressure.

The *immune system* is a network of cells and organs that work together to protect the body and help fight off illness. White blood cells are an important part of the immune system. These cells are produced and stored in the thymus, spleen, and bone marrow.

The *reproductive system* allows humans to reproduce. In females, the reproductive system includes the vagina, uterus, fallopian tubes, and ovaries. In males, the reproductive system includes the testicles, epididymis, vas deferens, seminal vesicles, prostate gland, and penis.

The *nervous system* is responsible for maintaining homeostasis in the body by sending messages that coordinate the various systems functions. This system is divided into two parts: the central nervous system and the peripheral nervous system. The central nervous system includes the brain and the spinal cord. The peripheral nervous system links the central nervous system to the rest of the body through a network of nerves.

Anatomy of the Head and Neck

To recognize abnormalities, a dental hygienist must be familiar with the normal structure of the head and neck.

The human head is made up of eight cranial bones and fourteen facial bones. Besides the mandible, most of the bones in the head and face are immovable. The mandible is the only bone in the skull that contains a moveable joint.

The bones of the neck allow for movement of the head. The atlas allows the head to move up and down and the axis allows for back and forth movement. The hyoid bone serves as an anchor for the tongue. The hyoid is unique in that it does not articulate with any other bones.

In addition to the bones of the head and neck, the dental hygienist must also be familiar with the various nerves located throughout the head and neck. Several nerve ailments, including trigeminal neuralgia and Bell's palsy, can affect the human head and neck.

To provide adequate treatment, dental hygienists should also know the locations of the arteries and veins, muscles, and glands in the head and neck.

Dental Anatomy

Dental hygienists must become familiar with the anatomy of the teeth and the structures that support them, including various tissues, muscles, and glands.

> **NOTE**
> The submandibular gland produces 60 to 65 percent of the total saliva volume.

The teeth are made up of four main tissue structures: enamel, dentin, cementum, and pulp. Enamel, which is primarily made of the mineral hydroxyapatite, is the hardest tissue in the body. It is the visible part of the tooth that covers the underlying structure of the crown. The enamel is supported by dentin, which makes up the majority of the tooth structure. Dentin is covered by enamel at the crown and cementum at the root. Cementum covers the root of the tooth. This is the dental tissue that most resembles bone. Underneath the enamel, dentin, and cementum is the pulp. The pulp consists of soft connective tissue, nerves, and blood vessels that supply the tooth with nutrients. The nerves in the pulp can sense pain and extreme changes in temperature or pressure in or around the tooth. Dental hygienists should be familiar with the normal structures of the enamel, dentin, cementum, and pulp so they can recognize abnormalities.

It is also important for dental hygienists to understand the normal size, shape, and location of different teeth. Dental hygienists should also know the eruption dates for various teeth. This will help you recognize developmental abnormalities.

Root Anatomy

Teeth can have one, two, or three roots, which are embedded in the tooth socket of the jaw bone. Incisors, canines, maxillary second premolars, and mandibular premolars have one root. Maxillary first premolars and mandibular premolars have two roots. Maxillary molars have three roots. Single roots are mostly cone shaped. Teeth with more than one root may have fused roots. Dental hygienists should be conscious of variations in root formation, including supernumerary roots, dilacerations, and hypercementosis.

Review these topics related to atomic sciences before taking the NBDHE:

- Relationship of oral structures to other body systems

- Health issues in other body systems that can affect the teeth and gums

- Bones of the head and neck

- Muscles of the head and neck, including the following:

    o Muscles of mastication

    o Facial muscles

    o Muscles of the pharynx

    o Muscles of the tongue

    o Muscles of the palate

- Major and minor salivary glands

- Lymph glands of the head and neck

- Nerves of the head and neck

- Arteries and veins of the head and neck

- Abnormalities of the enamel, dentin, cementum, and pulp

- Shapes, locations, and eruption dates for various teeth

- Developmental abnormalities, including the following:

  o Anodontia

  o Concrescence

  o Dens in dente/dens invaginatus

  o Dentogenesis imperfecta

  o Dilaceration

  o Fusion

  o Gemination

  o Macrodontia/Microdontia

  o Taurodontism

  o Tetracycline staining

- Supporting structures of the teeth, including the following:

  o Bone

  o Periodontal ligament

- Occlusion

- Angle's classification of malocclusion

- Occlusal disturbances

- Mucosal tissues

- Tongue

- Variations in root formation

EXERCISES: ATOMIC SCIENCES

Directions: Choose the option that best answers the question.

1. Which body system controls the skeletal muscles?
   (A) Integumentary system
   (B) Renal system
   (C) Muscular system
   (D) Skeletal system
   (E) Nervous system

   Although skeletal muscles are part of the muscular system, they are controlled by the nervous system. The nervous system sends messages from the brain to the muscles to make them move. **The correct answer is (E).**

2. Which of these is the strongest muscle of mastication?
   (A) Lateral pterygoid
   (B) Medial pterygoid
   (C) Temporalis
   (D) Masseter
   (E) Mentalis

   The masseter is the largest and strongest muscle of mastication. The lateral pterygoid, medial pterygoid, and temporalis are weaker. The mentalis is a facial muscle. **The correct answer is (D).**

3. Which type of dentin is found between the dentinal tubules?
   (A) Primary dentin
   (B) Secondary dentin
   (C) Globular dentin
   (D) Circumpupal dentin
   (E) Intertubular dentin

   Intertubular dentin is found between the dentinal tubules. This is a highly mineralized form of dentin. **The correct answer is (E).**

4. Which of these determines the shape of the root?
   (A) Sharpey's fibers
   (B) Mesenchyme
   (C) Hertwig's root sheath
   (D) Epithelial rest of Malassez
   (E) Acellular cementum

   Hertwig's root sheath determines the shape of the root. It initiates the formation of dentin in the root and eventually disintegrates. **The correct answer is (C).**

BIOCHEMISTRY AND NUTRITION

Nutrition is an important part of oral health. Because all body systems are interconnected, keeping the entire body healthy through proper nutrition is important. Furthermore, nutrition has specific impacts on oral health. For example, eating too many carbohydrates often leads to tooth decay, and eating a diet lacking in certain vitamins and minerals can weaken teeth.

The human body requires six essential nutrients: (1) carbohydrates, (2) fats, (3) proteins, (4) vitamins, (5) minerals, and (6) water. Proper nutrition occurs when people consume the right balance of these six nutrients. If people have too much or too little of these nutrients, they can develop specific health problems. Monitoring a patient's nutrition can help you better understand the person's body and overall health. Counseling patients about their nutrition and ways to improve it can help ensure patients' oral health.

Review these topics related to biochemistry and nutrition before taking the NBDHE:

- Carbohydrates

  o Simple carbohydrates

  o Complex carbohydrates

- o Sugar alcohols
- Fats (Lipids)
  - o Essential fatty acids
  - o Synthetic fats
  - o Lipoproteins
- Proteins
- Vitamins
  - o Water-soluble vitamins
  - o Fat-soluble vitamins
- Minerals
- Water
- Nutrition
  - o Nutritional disorders
  - o Monitoring nutrition
  - o Nutritional counseling
  - o Nutrition for specific medical and dental conditions
  - o Nutrition and weight control

EXERCISES: BIOCHEMISTRY AND NUTRITION

Directions: Choose the option that best answers the question.

1. A deficiency in which of the following vitamins can cause rickets in children?
   (A) Vitamin A
   (B) Vitamin C
   (C) Vitamin D
   (D) Vitamin E
   (E) Vitamin K

   Rickets is normally caused by a vitamin D deficiency. Deficiencies in vitamins A, C, E, and K do not cause rickets. **The correct answer is (C).**

2. Each of the following symptoms is a sign of diabetes mellitus **EXCEPT** one. Which one is the **EXCEPTION**?
   (A) Contracting gingival infections
   (B) Exhibiting little to no appetite
   (C) Being excessively thirsty
   (D) Urinating frequently
   (E) Feeling fatigued and tired

   Symptoms of diabetes mellitus include contracting gingival infections, being excessively thirsty, urinating frequently, feeling fatigued and tired, and exhibiting extreme hunger. Therefore, exhibiting little to no appetite is *not* a symptom of diabetes mellitus. **The correct answer is (B).**

MICROBIOLOGY AND IMMUNOLOGY

Microbiology is a branch of biology that studies microscopic life forms, including bacteria, funguses, and viruses. *Immunology* is the study of the human immune system. Together, the study of microbiology and immunology gives dental hygienists important knowledge about how diseases spread and develop and ways to combat particular diseases.

Microorganisms are found everywhere—including the human body. The oral cavity of an adult human is home to hundreds of microorganisms, and dental hygienists must have a clear understanding of how to prevent the spreading of disease through these microorganisms. Diseases can be easily spread if dental hygienists neglect to use the correct preventive measures. Although only 3 percent of microbes are pathogenic, the bacteria, viruses, fungi, and other microbes that are harmful to humans can cause dangerous, and even life-threatening, diseases.

> **TIP**
>
> Some questions on the NBDHE include the words **NOT** and **EXCEPT**. When the words **NOT** and **EXCEPT** appear on the NBDHE, they are capitalized and bolded so you will more easily notice them. When you see these words, pay close attention to the question, as these words will change a question's meaning.

Microorganisms are also responsible for dental problems, including the formation of caries, the formation of calculus, gingival disease, and periodontal disease. Because microbes are so influential in the human oral cavity, it is important to understand them and the human body's response to them.

Review these topics related to microbiology and immunology before taking the NBDHE:

- Microorganisms
  - Eukaryotes
  - Prokaryotes
  - Viruses
  - Nomenclature
- Microbe cell structure
- Microbe growth and development
- Microbes and disease transmission
  - Common transmissible diseases
  - Modes of disease transmission
- Barriers to disease transmission
- Immunity
  - Acquired immunity
  - Humoral immunity
  - Cell-mediated immunity
  - Immunodeficiency

- Oral microflora

  o Sites of colonization

  o Development of microflora

- Oral infections from microbes

  o Gingival disease

  o Periodontal disease

  o Formation of caries and calculus

EXERCISES: MICROBIOLOGY AND IMMUNOLOGY

Directions: Choose the option that best answers the question.

1. Which of the following microorganisms are classified as prokaryotes?
   (A) Viruses
   (B) Bacteria
   (C) Fungi
   (D) Algae
   (E) Amoeba

   Bacteria are prokaryotes, and like all prokaryotes they have no nuclear membrane. Bacteria, fungi, and amoebas are eukaryotes, and viruses are not classified as either a prokaryote or a eukaryote. **The correct answer is (B).**

2. Bacteria of the *Streptococcus* genus are commonly found in the human oral cavity. Which species of bacteria commonly causes tonsillitis, scarlet fever, strep throat, and rheumatic fever?
   (A) *Streptococcus pneumoniae*
   (B) *Streptococcus mutans*
   (C) *Streptococcus sanguinis*
   (D) *Streptococcus pyogenes*
   (E) *Streptococcus mitis*

   Streptococcus pyogenes is the species in the *Streptococcus* genus that commonly causes diseases such as tonsillitis and rheumatic fever. **The correct answer is (D).**

GENERAL AND ORAL PATHOLOGY

Dental hygienists must have a full understanding of the diseases their patients may suffer from, the causes of those diseases, and the best ways to treat those diseases. Knowledge of general pathology is important because many systemic, developmental, and infectious diseases affect different parts of the body. By understanding the causes, symptoms, and treatments of multiple diseases, dental hygienists can better contribute to the patient-treatment process.

General Pathology

Understanding general pathology helps dental hygienists evaluate their patients' overall health, and it allows them to make informed decisions about their patients' care. Furthermore, many concepts of general pathology relate to oral health. For example, inflammation in the oral cavity can be a sign of an illness that affects other parts of the body. Dental hygienists must also have a sound understanding of wound healing, which is another aspect of general pathology.

Oral Pathology

Understanding oral pathology is vital for dental workers to properly diagnose and treat oral conditions. In emergency situations, a thorough understanding of oral pathology is especially important. By recognizing the signs or symptoms of different pathologies, dental hygienists can help determine which findings are normal and which could be problematic. When dental hygienists understand oral pathology, they can better collaborate with other dental workers.

Review these topics related to general and oral pathology before taking the NBDHE:

- Oral lesions
  - o Ulcerative lesions
  - o Skin lesions
  - o Raised lesions
  - o Lesions designated by color, texture, and size

> **NOTE**
> When pathologic conditions occur, they often change the structure and function of certain body tissues.

- Inflammation
- Wound healing
- Infectious disease
  - o Bacterial infections
  - o Fungal infections
  - o Viral infections
- Diseases of the bone
- Developmental disorders
- Neoplasia
  - o Classifications of tumors
  - o Soft tissue tumors
  - o Bone and cartilage tumors
  - o Other tumors
- Systematic diseases
  - o Endocrine disorders
  - o Blood disorders
  - o Cardiovascular disorders
  - o Respiratory disorders
  - o Skeletal disorders

o Gastrointestinal disorders

o Neurological disorders

EXERCISES: GENERAL AND ORAL PATHOLOGY

Directions: Choose the option that best answers the question.

1. What is the most common symptom of epidermis bullosa?
   (A) Crusty, white or red flat growth
   (B) Nodules on the arms, hands, and legs
   (C) Black and brown filiform papillae
   (D) Blisters on the skin and oral mucosa
   (E) Creamy, white substance on tongue

   The most common symptom of epidermis bullosa is the appearance of blisters on the skin and oral mucosa. **The correct answer is (D).**

2. Benign lesions of the soft tissue usually grow slowly. After they are removed, benign lesions of the soft tissue often recur.
   (A) Both statements are true.
   (B) Both statements are false.
   (C) The first statement is true, and the second statement is false.
   (D) The first statement is false, and the second statement is true.

   Benign lesions of the soft tissue usually grow slowly. After they are removed, however, they usually do not recur. **The correct answer is (C).**

> **TIP**
>
> Certain foods and drinks can affect the absorption and actions of particular drugs. Be sure you know what, if any, foods and drinks can interact with commonly prescribed drugs.

PHARMACOLOGY

To give patients the best quality care, dental hygienists must understand drugs, drugs actions and interactions, and drug uses. Dental hygienists need to understand pharmacology because sometimes patients will have symptoms of diseases or conditions that require the use of drugs. Some patients may already be taking prescriptions for another illness or chronic condition. Dental hygienists need to understand how those drugs work and interact so they can properly treat the patient. Nearly all the drugs used by dental professionals are controlled by different laws and agencies. Dental hygienists should understand the laws and restrictions concerning the handling and use of these drugs.

Review these topics related to pharmacology before taking the NBDHE:

- Drugs

  o Analgesics

  o Antianxiety drugs

  o Anti-infective drugs

  o Autonomic drugs

  o Cardiovascular drugs

  o Local and general anesthetics

o Neuromuscular blocking agents

o Psychotherapeutic agents

o Other drugs

o Nomenclature

- Drug action

- Adverse reactions

- Handling and administering drugs

- Drug interactions

- Substance abuse

- Toxicology

- Administrative agencies and laws governing drugs

EXERCISES: PHARMACOLOGY

Directions: Choose the option that best answers the question.

1. Each of the follow drugs can produce xerostomia **EXCEPT** one. Which one is the **EXCEPTION**?
   (A) Nystatin
   (B) Lorazepam
   (C) Atropine
   (D) Loratadine
   (E) Clozapine

   The drug nystatin, which is an antifungal, does not produce xerostomia, or dry mouth. The other drugs (lorazapam, atropine, loratadine, and clozapine) do cause dry mouth, and patients taking these drugs should be treated for the condition if necessary. **The correct answer is (A).**

2. A patient at a dental facility has been diagnosed with periodontal infection. Which one of the following would best treat the patient?
   (A) Albuterol
   (B) Tetracycline
   (C) Zidovudine
   (D) Fluoxetine
   (E) Cyclizine

   A patient with a periodontal infection should be treated with an anti-infective agent. Tetracycline is an antibiotic that can be used to treat infections such as periodontal infections. **The correct answer is (B).**

FOUR TIPS FOR ANSWERING SCIENTIFIC BASIS QUESTIONS

When you are taking the NBDHE, it may be helpful to remember these hints:

1. **The oral cavity is part of the digestive system.** Relate all of the organ systems in the human body to each other and the oral cavity. Digestion begins in the oral cavity and then proceeds through the other systems.

2. **The head and neck are made up of bones, nerves, arteries, muscles, and glands.** It is important to know the anatomy of the head and neck as well as the names of all of its components. Memorizing acronyms can often help you learn the important body parts.

3. **Have a thorough understanding of different type of microorganisms, such as algae, bacteria, fungi, protozoa, and viruses.** Cells are divided into two groups: eukaryotes and prokaryotes. Eukaryotes are unicellular and contain a nucleus. Algae, protozoa, and fungi fall into this category. Prokaryotes can be unicellular or multicellular and are not so complex as eukaryotes. Bacteria fall into this category.

4. **Oral pathology is the study of the destructive conditions associated with the mouth, head, and neck.** As a dental hygienist, it is important to be able to recognize the different types of cysts and tumors that may be present inside the oral cavity. In addition, it is important to identify their origins and treatment if necessary.

> **NOTE**
>
> Before you take the NBDHE, you need to schedule a date and time to take it. If you need to cancel or reschedule the date of your exam, you must give the testing center at least 24 hours' notice of your change in plans. Otherwise, you will be charged a fee.

PRACTICE QUESTIONS

Directions: Choose the option that best answers the question.

1. Where is stratified squamous located?
   (A) Epidermis, esophagus, oral cavity, vagina
   (B) Stomach, small intestine, colon, gallbladder
   (C) Kidney tubules, ovary surface, small ducts of endocrine glands
   (D) Respiratory tract lining, vascular system, Bowman's capsules
   (E) Heart, liver, large intestine, uterus

2. During the cap stage, the ectoderm becomes the
   (A) dental papilla.
   (B) periodontal ligament.
   (C) alveolar bone.
   (D) enamel organ.
   (E) dental sac.

3. Which of the following is **NOT** part of the respiratory system?
   (A) Trachea
   (B) Cerebellum
   (C) Pharynx
   (D) Alveoli
   (E) Bronchi

4. How many ameloblasts does it take to form one enamel rod?
   (A) 1
   (B) 2
   (C) 3
   (D) 4
   (E) 5

5. Which teeth are characterized as being simplest and the smallest?
   (A) Mandibular first premolar
   (B) Mandibular canine
   (C) Mandibular lateral incisor
   (D) Mandibular central incisor
   (E) Mandibular third molar

6. Which one of the following is a non-mineralized, organized, mixed microbial biofilm made up of 80-percent water and 20-percent solids?
   (A) Enamel
   (B) Plaque
   (C) Dentin
   (D) Saliva
   (E) Pulp

7. A cyst presents itself as asymptomatic and is found in areas of unerupted teeth such as the mandibular third molars, maxillary third molars, and maxillary canines. It is solid and well defined surrounding the crown. Which one of the following best describes the cyst?
   (A) Dentigerous or follicular cyst
   (B) Gingival cyst
   (C) Globulomaxillary cyst
   (D) Lateral periodontal cyst
   (E) Apical periodontal cyst

8. Which one of the following best describes xerostomia?
   (A) A minute collection of tissue
   (B) A flat, discolored patch of skin
   (C) Dry mouth due to a lack of saliva production
   (D) An elevated lesion that contains serous fluid
   (E) Large, red lesions on the tongue

9. Which one of the following best describes therapeutic action?
   (A) A reaction particular to a patient
   (B) The desired effect of a drug
   (C) The desired reaction of a drug
   (D) The study of harmful or toxic effects
   (E) An interaction of certain chemicals

10. Each of the following symptoms is a sign of excess protein **EXCEPT** one. Which one is the **EXCEPTION**?
    (A) Anemia
    (B) Kidney damage
    (C) Dehydration
    (D) Increased calcium excretion
    (E) Weight gain

ANSWER KEY AND EXPLANATIONS

1. A	3. B	5. D	7. A	9. C
2. D	4. D	6. B	8. C	10. A

1. **The correct answer is (A).** There are specialized types of epithelial tissue that are divided into simple and stratified epithelial tissue. Simple epithelial tissue is located in the internal organs. Stratified epithelial tissue is located on the skin, glands, and some linings near entrances and exits of the body. Choice (A) is the only list that includes skin, glands, and places for entrance and exit from the body.

2. **The correct answer is (D).** During the cap stage tissues start to morphodifferentiate into either ectoderm or mesenchyme tissue. The ectoderm then becomes the enamel organ that produces enamel. The mesoderm develops into the dental papilla, pulp and dentin, dental sac, the periodontal ligament, alveolar bone, and cementum.

3. **The correct answer is (B).** The cerebellum is responsible for coordination and muscle movement and is part of the nervous system. The trachea, alveoli, and bronchi are part of the lower respiratory tract. The pharynx is part of the upper respiratory tract.

4. **The correct answer is (D).** Enamel is generated by the ameloblasts. Ameloblasts are hexagonal, tall, columnar cells. Four ameloblasts form one enamel rod during the apposition stage of enamel development.

5. **The correct answer is (D).** The mandibular central incisor is characterized as being the simplest and the smallest teeth. They are symmetrical and appear around age 6 or 7.

6. **The correct answer is (B).** Plaque is a living and highly organized ecosystem composed of more than 300 species of bacteria and is the most common reason for gingivitis.

7. **The correct answer is (A).** The dentigerous or follicular cyst is the most common follicular cyst. It forms around the crown of an unerupted or developing tooth and is usually small; however, it can get larger and spread over other teeth.

8. **The correct answer is (C).** Xerostomia is dry mouth and it can occur for several different reasons. Chemotherapy, aging, salivary gland shrinkage, and medication are all causes of dry mouth. People with xerostomia are at a greater risk for oral candidiasis.

9. **The correct answer is (C).** Therapeutic action is the desired reaction of a drug. Idiosyncrasy is a reaction particular to a specific patient. Efficacy is the desired effect of a drug. Toxicology is the study of toxic effects.

10. **The correct answer is (A).** Anemia is the result of not enough protein. Too much protein can cause liver and kidney damage, dehydration, increased calcium excretion, and weight gain.

SUMMING IT UP

- The scientific basis for dental hygiene practice questions will require an understanding of the human body, its construction, and the ways its systems work together. It is also necessary to know about diseases that affect the human body and the medications that can be used to combat diseases. Knowledge of overall nutrition and its effects on oral well-being is needed too, since the oral cavity is affected by what people eat and the body's overall health.

- When studying questions pertaining to the human body and the oral cavity, focus on how all the systems are interrelated with one another.

- Pay close attention to specific details in the questions. Know the vocabulary and definitions of nomenclature associated with each topic.

- Do not just prepare for questions concerning the oral cavity. As a dental hygienist it is necessary to have an understanding of how the whole human body works and how each system affects the others.

CHAPTER 6

Clinical Dental Hygiene Services Questions

OVERVIEW

- Assessing patient characteristics
- Obtaining and interpreting radiographs
- Planning and managing dental hygiene care
- Handling medical emergencies
- Educating patients
- Controlling pain and anxiety
- Performing periodontal procedures
- Using preventive agents
- Providing supportive treatment services
- Understanding professional responsibilities
- Five tips for answering clinical dental hygiene services questions
- Practice questions
- Answer key and explanations
- Summing it up

The National Board Dental Hygiene Examination (NBDHE) will also require you to answer questions about the provision of clinical dental hygiene services. Because assessing and treating patients is such a central part of your job, this subject matter represents a large number of questions on the test. About 58 percent of the examination questions, or approximately 120 items, test your knowledge on how to most effectively work with and treat patients.

The Provision of Clinical Dental Hygiene Services section consists of multiple-choice questions that deal with all topics relative to dental hygiene services, such as evaluating healthy patients and those with special needs, protecting yourself and the patient when taking radiographs, planning and managing hygienic care, assessing and conducting periodontal work, applying preventive agents, and providing the patient with supportive treatment services such as tooth desensitization. The multiple-choice items are formatted as questions, incomplete statements, and scenarios.

ASSESSING PATIENT CHARACTERISTICS

You should carefully assess all patients when they visit the dental office. Your goal with this assessment is to create a baseline of information about the patient so that you can design and conduct appropriate treatment. Treatment is most effective when it takes the health and medical conditions of the patient into account. Therefore, as part of the screening process, you will be looking to determine the patient's general state of health by taking a complete medical history, which includes any pre-existing conditions or current medications. You will take the patient's vital signs and review and discuss any symptoms the patient may be experiencing. If diagnostic radiographs are available, you can review them in terms of what they may mean for the patient's current (or past) condition. You can complete your evaluation by conducting a careful patient oral examination and recording your clinical findings. Screening examinations include the extraoral examination (head and neck), intraoral examination (mouth), and an assessment of the patient's periodontal and dentition conditions as appropriate.

Besides general information about the patient, such as height, weight, and so on, as well as vital signs such as pulse rate, respiratory rate, and blood pressure, some other useful questions you will want to ask patients include:

- Are you currently ill or experiencing any problems?

- Are you taking any medications? If so, what kinds?

- What medications have you taken in the past?

- Do you have any known diseases or medical conditions?

- What medical procedures have you undergone?

- Do you have allergies? If so, to what?

- Do you smoke or use other tobacco products?

- How much alcohol do you drink in a typical day/week?

- Are you pregnant or trying to get pregnant?

To correctly answer test questions about patient assessment, you will need to identify appropriate assessment procedures for patients who are healthy as well as those with physical conditions or disabilities. You will be required to recognize common abnormalities that may become apparent during head and neck examinations or via radiograph. You will also be required to demonstrate your knowledge of procedure and the steps to follow to complete both the extraoral examination of the patient's head and neck as well as the intraoral examination of the patient's mouth.

Review these topics related to assessing patient characteristics before taking the NBDHE:

- Completing a medical history

- Taking patient vital signs

- Conditions requiring pre-medication

- Recommended pre-medication substances and dosing

- Completing the general assessment—extraoral and intraoral examinations

- Completing the periodontal assessment, including gingival evaluation and pocket probing

- Completing the dentition assessment, including Black's classification of caries, overhang classifications, and plaque scoring

- Working with patients with special needs or medical conditions; for example, ADHD, Alzheimer's, blood disorders, cancer, cardiovascular problems, Down's syndrome, hearing impaired, muscular dystrophy, Parkinson's, visually impaired, wheelchair-bound

EXERCISES: ASSESSING PATIENT CHARACTERISTICS

Directions: Choose the option that best answers the question.

1. Each of the following patients is at high risk for endocarditis **EXCEPT** one. Which one is the **EXCEPTION**?
   (A) A patient with a palliative shunt
   (B) A patient with a prosthetic heart valve
   (C) A patient with a history of endocarditis
   (D) A patient with non-insulin dependent diabetes
   (E) A patient with unrepaired cyanotic congenital heart disease

   A patient with non-insulin dependent diabetes would not be at a higher risk for endocarditis. Endocarditis is an inflammation of the inside lining of the heart chambers that is commonly caused by bacterial infections. Dental procedures can sometimes introduce bacteria into the bloodstream, so patients at higher risk for endocarditis should take antibiotics prior to treatment. **The correct answer is (D).**

2. Which of the following represents an elevated temperature for an adult?
   (A) 97.4°F
   (B) 97.8°F
   (C) 98.9°F
   (D) 99.4°F
   (E) 99.8°F

   A normal temperature range for a healthy adult is 97.0–99.5°F. An elevated temperature would be 99.8°F. Dental hygienists should take the temperature of patients who complain about feeling ill. **The correct answer is (E).**

OBTAINING AND INTERPRETING RADIOGRAPHS

One important diagnostic tool you will be using is the *radiograph*, or X-ray. The radiograph is helpful for detecting conditions affecting the teeth, gums, and bones in the mouth as well as identifying oral abnormalities that might not otherwise be readily apparent. Radiographs are also useful for evaluating the condition of dental implants in patients who have them.

Radiographs pose some level of risk for both the patient and the radiographer, because the photons in radiation can be absorbed by human tissue and cause damage. Thus, radiographs should be taken with care, following the guidelines published by the Occupational Safety and Health Administration (OSHA). Protective equipment is used to mitigate this risk and includes gloves, eyewear, masks, and lead aprons.

Radiographs are produced by passing controlled radiation through the X-ray machine into the patient's mouth. The radiation is absorbed by the patient's hard tissue (teeth and bones) and passed through to film, on which radiographic images develop. The horizontal and vertical angles of the film are important to produce usable images that are not blurry or overlapping and can be used for diagnostic purposes.

Once images are produced, you can evaluate them for conditions:

- Disturbances to hard structures

- Bone levels and degree of bone loss

- Abnormalities such as iatrogenic abnormality and periapical abscess

For the examination, you should be able to answer questions about what radiography is and how it works. You may be asked to describe the techniques used to produce and develop usable images. You may be asked to distinguish different oral conditions that can be detected by radiography. Finally, you should be able to identify the protective equipment that should be worn and demonstrate understanding of how it is used, when it is used, and who uses it.

Review these topics related to obtaining and interpreting radiographs before taking the NBDHE:

- The principles of radiation, including electromagnetic radiation, radiation wavelengths and frequencies, digital radiography, and maximum permissible doses (MPD)

- The principles of radiobiology, including classic scatter radiation, characteristic/photoelectric radiation, the Compton effect, and the behavior of photons and free radicals

- Radiological protection for both the operator and the patient, including the identification and usage of protective equipment

- Radiological techniques, including radiographic quality, horizontal and vertical angulation, and the buccal object rule

- Anatomical landmarks used in radiography, including the condyle, zygomatic arch, eye orbit, maxillary sinus, nasal septum, coronoid process, mandibular notch, mandible angle, inferior mandibular border, mandibular canal, geneial tubercles, mental foramen, and external oblique ridge

- Radiographic interpretation and the detection of abnormalities

EXERCISES: OBTAINING AND INTERPRETING RADIOGRAPHS

Directions: Choose the option that best answers the question.

1. Which of the following tissues is most sensitive to free radicals?
   (A) Liver
   (B) Muscles
   (C) Lymphocytes
   (D) Connective tissue
   (E) Salivary glands

   X-ray photons create free radicals that then intermingle with the water and oxygen found in biological tissues. Some tissues are more sensitive to free radicals than others. Lymphocytes, a type of white blood cell, are more sensitive to free radicals than liver, muscles, connective tissues, and salivary glands are. **The correct answer is (C).**

2. Which film speed is typically used for dental radiographic films?
   (A) A
   (B) B
   (C) C
   (D) E
   (E) F

   Film speeds range from A to F. Most dental radiographic films are speeds D or E. Speed E requires less exposure time than other films. **The correct answer is (D).**

PLANNING AND MANAGING DENTAL HYGIENE CARE

Once you have thoroughly evaluated the patient, you will be able to devise an individualized treatment plan which addresses all of the patient's unique needs. The treatment plan should focus on addressing issues with the patient's dentition and supporting structures; provide for any restorative procedures that may be needed; and address any supporting treatments that may be desired by the patient, such as the desensitization of teeth prior to treatment, or tooth whitening services. And, of course, the treatment plan should make recommendations for ongoing preventive care.

Treatment plans should be thorough and complete so that patients understand what you are planning to do and why. The design and order of treatment will depend upon the patient's overall health, the severity of his or her issues, and the individual's willingness and ability to participate. When you share the treatment plan with the patient, you should identify the procedures to be performed, explain why they are needed, and describe exactly what they involve. You should identify any risk factors associated with either undergoing or refusing to undergo the treatment, and you should address any concerns the patient may have regarding pain or discomfort. In addition, you should outline the general time frame required and indicate the number of appointments needed to complete the schedule of treatment. Depending on the norms in your dental practice, you may also want to let the patient know how much each part of the treatment will cost.

Controlling Infection

Due to the type of work performed, dental personnel and their patients are at high risk for exposure to a variety of contaminants. Dental hygienists in particular can be frequently exposed to infection caused by air- and blood-borne pathogens, such as cytomegalovirus, hepatitis B, influenza, tuberculosis, and others. Because pathogens can be transmitted in a variety of ways, it is important to always exercise caution when working in the dental office. This means following the Centers for Disease Control and Prevention (CDC) recommendations for universal precautions, such as hand-washing, surface cleaning, pre-procedural mouth rinsing, and so on. In addition, you should adhere to Occupational Safety and Health Administration (OSHA) regulations for appropriate protective equipment such as gloves and safety goggles. You should also follow all office procedures for other activities such as sterilization, disinfection, and the management of waste. Also, for your own personal protection, it is critical that you keep your immunizations are up-to-date.

It is important that you understand and follow these procedures carefully with every patient. When studying for your exam, spend time reviewing modes of infection transmission as well as standard procedures for protecting yourself and your patients.

HANDLING MEDICAL EMERGENCIES

Part of the reason for thorough patient screening procedures is to ensure that you have the right information on hand if any type of medical complication or emergency arises during treatment. A sickly, anxious patient might be predisposed to have an anxiety attack, for example, or an otherwise healthy individual might react adversely to a medication or substance used during treatment. You will need to be prepared to recognize when an emergency is taking place and also to follow appropriate procedures when one occurs. The most important advice you can follow in crisis situations is to call 911. Time is frequently of the essence in medical emergencies.

Part of your education involves cardiopulmonary resuscitation (CPR) training as well as medical management training, so you should pay special attention to that material while studying for the examination. You should understand the difference between the primary and secondary assessment as well as the difference between a sign (something you observe) and a symptom (something the patient says about his or her condition). You should know how to monitor a patient's vitals and to perform CPR if it becomes necessary. You should recognize signs and symptoms of particular conditions and understand the procedures to follow to assist the patient while waiting for help (if additional help is required). The following list contains more common conditions you will be expected to know during the examination.

- Allergic reactions
- Cardiovascular emergencies
- Drug-related crises
- Eye injuries
- Locked jaws
- Respiratory distress
- Seizures

EXERCISES: HANDLING MEDICAL EMERGENCIES

Directions: Choose the option that best answers the question.

1. A seemingly healthy 19-year-old boy having his teeth cleaned complains of a quickened heartbeat, shortness of breath, and an odd feeling in his fingertips. The boy is most likely experiencing which of the following?
   (A) Partial seizure
   (B) Hyperventilation
   (C) Adrenal crisis
   (D) Asthma attack
   (E) Septic shock

   Signs of hyperventilation include abnormally fast or deep respiration, causing loss of carbon dioxide from the blood, further causing a fall in blood pressure, tingling of the extremities, and sometimes fainting. Partial seizures cause a change in muscle and sensory activity. Signs of an adrenal crisis include vomiting and abdominal pain. Signs of an asthma attack include the inability to catch one's breath. Signs of septic shock include chills, an abnormally high or low body temperature, rapid breathing, and a drop in blood pressure. **The correct answer is (B).**

2. Cardiovascular pulmonary resuscitation (CPR) is most likely indicated in which of the following circumstances?
   (A) The patient is unresponsive.
   (B) The patient is unconscious.
   (C) The patient is still breathing.
   (D) The patient has no pulse.
   (E) The patient goes in and out of consciousness.

   CPR is indicated for patients who are unresponsive, not breathing, or gasping for breath, because they are most likely in cardiac arrest. If the patient is obviously breathing or regaining consciousness, other interventions are more appropriate. It is sometimes difficult to locate a pulse in an emergency situation, so a better indicator of CPR needs is the patient's breathing/responsive level. **The correct answer is (A).**

EDUCATING PATIENTS

Part of your role as a hygienist involves educating patients on appropriate self-care activities. Surprisingly, many patients do not know how to brush and floss properly or otherwise take effective preventive measures. In addition, patients with specific diagnoses, such as frequent cavities, gingivitis, periodontal disease, bone loss, or other oral conditions, need to know what to do to manage the problem, resolve the problem, or prevent it from recurring.

The most effective patient education involves all three of the patient's learning domains: *cognitive* (increasing the patient's knowledge of the subject matter), *affective* (changing any negative attitudes or beliefs about the subject matter), and *psychomotor* (developing the patient's related skills). In addition, the self-care strategies you devise should not only be understandable to the patient, but should also be strategies to which the patient can reasonably be expected to adhere.

When reviewing the education of patients for the exam, you should consider the following:

- Human motivation theories

- Dental treatment strategies

- Individualized patient instruction

- Learning domains

- Learning theories

- Educating patients on the prevention and management of specific oral diseases, such as dental caries, periodontal disease, and other conditions

- Understanding and applying theories of human motivation

Maslow's Hierarchy of Needs

When you set self-care goals for patients, they need to be motivated to complete them. A tool to help you understand why a patient might or might not be responsive to particular goals is to understand human motivation via *Maslow's Hierarchy of Needs*. In this model, Abraham Maslow classified human needs as a pyramid. He theorized that the more fundamental needs at the bottom of the pyramid must be filled before humans will be motivated by needs higher up the pyramid. The five needs in *descending* order are:

- Self-actualization
  ↓
- Self-esteem/ego
  ↓
- Love and belonging
  ↓
- Safety and security
  ↓
- Physiological needs

In other words, a person is not motivated by goals or activities that help them to, for example, build self-esteem or become self-actualized unless lower-level needs, such as hunger and safety, are fulfilled. For example, your patient might feel better about himself if his teeth were whiter (self-esteem needs) but this will be less important to him if, for example, he has been unemployed for a period of time and is concerned about his financial condition (safety and security needs).

EXERCISES: EDUCATING PATIENTS

Directions: Choose the option that best answers the question.

1. Your patient is a 35-year-old long-time tobacco chewer. He is aware of the risks associated with this habit but has been historically unresponsive to suggestions to change. Which of the following is more likely to elicit a more positive response from this patient?
   (A) Providing the patient with literature describing the health conditions caused by continued tobacco use
   (B) Suggesting the patient try hypnosis, acupressure, or acupuncture to quit the tobacco habit
   (C) Asking the patient to talk about why he chews tobaccos and how this need might otherwise be fulfilled
   (D) Showing the patient photographs of individuals who have undergone surgical treatment for oral cancer
   (E) Calculating how much money the patient spends monthly on cigarettes

Helping the patient to identify the needs that smoking fulfills for him will assist him in understanding why he chews tobacco and may help him find motivation to quite. The patient demonstrates awareness of the risks he is taking, therefore neither choices (A) nor (D) will likely be effective. The patient may be open to alternative health remedies such as hypnosis, but is likely not motivated to follow them at this time. Calculating the financial cost of the habit does not help the patient to identify the root causes of his addiction. **The correct answer is (C).**

2. One of your patients is a 9-year-old elementary student. As part of her ongoing treatment plan, you show her how to use dental floss correctly to remove plaque and debris. During each visit over the course of the year, you ask her to demonstrate this technique for you. What learning domain are you engaging?
   (A) Affective domain
   (B) Cognitive domain
   (C) Ego domain
   (D) Self-esteem domain
   (E) Psychomotor domain

The psychomotor domain involves developing the patient's motor skills. The affective domain involves changes to the patient's attitudes or beliefs. The cognitive domain involves increasing the patient's knowledge of the subject matter. The ego domain and self-esteem domain do not exist. **The correct answer is (E).**

CONTROLLING PAIN AND ANXIETY

Dental work can be uncomfortable and some procedures are downright painful. Patient tolerance for discomfort and pain can vary greatly, so part of your job is not only understanding the amount of pain a procedure might generally produce but also recognizing the variability in a patient's ability to deal with pain. Pain management is an important part of your job duties.

Pain can be controlled in a number of ways:

- Topical anesthetics, used to numb the area to be treated prior to the introduction of a local anesthetic

- Local anesthetics, generally applied via injection prior to the treatment start

- Computer-controlled/electronically administered anesthesia, used as an alternative to local anesthetic, and involving the application of electrical impulses to the treatment area

- Nitrous oxide-oxygen, inhaled with a face mask (also called "laughing gas")

> **NOTE**
>
> Patients with certain health conditions, including pregnancy, should not receive nitrous oxide-oxygen. Before taking the NBDHE, be sure you understand which patients can receive which treatments for pain and anxiety.

More invasive pain-management procedures are also available, such as oral sedation and general anesthesia. However, these are generally performed only in extreme cases and only under the supervision of the dentist and a trained anesthesiologist.

Related to pain management is patient anxiety. Many patients are afraid of the dentist; as a matter of fact, fear is probably the number-one reason many people neglect their oral health. You can and should address this anxiety, especially if the patient seems particularly nervous and anxiety-filled. Some of the techniques you can utilize to address this anxiety include the following:

- **Distraction techniques:** Distracting patients from the procedure can help lower anxiety levels. For example, many dental offices make TV available and visible from the chair. Others play soothing music or make it a habit to speak in a comforting voice during the procedure.

- **Education:** Many patients feel more confident and less anxious if they know exactly what to expect. Walking patients through the treatment beforehand can help them to take a more realistic look at what they are going to experience.

- **Relaxation techniques:** Patients can learn how to relax themselves through deep breathing, guided imagery, and other, similar activities.

- **Therapy:** Patients with extreme dental phobia may need to address this issue with a therapist or support group.

When reviewing pain and anxiety management for the examination, make sure you study the following topics:

- Anesthetic agents, including chemical structures, physiological effects, dosage calculation, and levels of toxicity

- Anesthetic armamentarium, including needles, cartridges, and syringes

- Computer-controlled/electronically controlled anesthesia

- Legal documentation requirements

- Physiology of pain, including nerves, pain pathways, and patient perception of pain

EXERCISES: CONTROLLING PAIN AND ANXIETY

Directions: Choose the option that best answers the question.

1. Gingivitis is the least common periodontal disease.

   Smoking puts adults at great risk for periodontal diseases such as gingivitis.
   (A) Both statements are true.
   (B) Both statements are false.
   (C) The first statement is true, the second is false.
   (D) The first statement is false, the second is true.

   The first statement is false. Gingivitis is one of the most prominent periodontal diseases, affecting nearly 70 percent of adults in all countries. The second statement is true. Smoking is a risk factor for periodontal diseases, including gingivitis. **The correct answer is (D).**

2. Which of the following is **NOT** an indication for nitrous oxide usage?
   (A) Anxiety
   (B) Pregnancy
   (C) Hypertension
   (D) Cerebral palsy
   (E) Stress-induced asthma

   Pregnancy is not an indication for nitrous oxide usage. The use of nitrous oxide on a pregnant patient could have harmful effects on the unborn child. **The correct answer is (B).**

PERFORMING PERIODONTAL PROCEDURES

Due to the prevalence of conditions such as gingivitis, periodontal treatment is one of the primary roles of the dental hygienist. You will need to understand the etiology, histology, and classification of periodontal conditions. You will need to recognize appropriate treatment options for different classifications, such as lavage, debridement, and curettage; surgical and non-surgical options; and the use of chemotherapeutic agents.

Much of your work in periodontics will focus on evaluating patients for signs of periodontal conditions, including identifying specific abnormalities on radiographic images. You will educate your patients on the risks involved in periodontal disease as well as self-care activities designed to prevent periodontal disease from occurring. You will perform treatments on conditions such as gingivitis and early-stage periodontal disease while maintaining the patient's health once the treatment is complete. You will, of course, sometimes work with patients who present more severe periodontal conditions. These patients will require more extensive and invasive interventions and management in order to restore them to health.

Dental Materials

Dental materials can be classified into four categories:

1. Ceramics

2. Composites

3. Metals

4. Polymers

The properties of each of these categories include:

- Biological

- Chemical

- Electrical

- Mechanical

- Physical

- Thermal

Review these topics related to performing periodontal procedures before taking the NBDHE:

- Bacterial plaque biofilm, including supragingival plaque and subgingival plaque, bacterial specificity, and dental calculus

- Classification of periodontal diseases, including gingivitis, chronic periodontitis, aggressive periodontitis, periodontic abscess, and periodontitis associated with systemic disease or endodontic lesions

- Diagnostic tools, including radiographic abnormalities

- Etiology and pathology of periodontal diseases

- Treatment, such as lavage, debridement, and curettage; surgical and non-surgical options; and the use of chemotherapeutic agents

EXERCISES: PERFORMING PERIODONTAL PROCEDURES

Directions: Choose the option that best answers the question.

1. Gingival curettage is a periodontal procedure that
   (A) uses an incision to remove the crevicular epithelium.
   (B) removes soft tissue from the wall of the periodontal pocket.
   (C) adjusts the gingiva contour into a more healthy shape.
   (D) grinds teeth to make them more even.
   (E) removes inflamed tissue in the periodontal pocket.

   Gingival curettage is a periodontal procedure that removes inflamed tissue in the periodontal pocket. An excisional new attachment procedure uses an incision to remove the crevicular epithelium lining. Occlusal adjustment grinds teeth to make them more even. **The correct answer is (E).**

2. Periodontal abscesses usually swell before they become painful.

   Endodontic abscesses usually become painful before they swell.
   (A) Both statements are true.
   (B) Both statements are false.
   (C) The first statement is true, the second is false.
   (D) The first statement is false, the second is true.

   Periodontal abscesses and endodontic abscesses are characterized by different symptoms. Periodontal abscesses usually swell before they become painful, and endodontic abscesses usually become painful before they swell. **The correct answer is (A).**

USING PREVENTIVE AGENTS

Preventive care is an important part of maintaining oral health. Although the treatment of oral conditions such as dental caries is vital to patient health, preventing these conditions is even more important. Along with teaching patients about proper oral hygiene, dental professionals can use preventive agents to prevent oral health problems, including dental caries.

As a dental hygienist, it is important to know what types of preventive agents exist and how they work. Two main types of preventive agents are fluoride and sealants for pits and fissures.

Fluoride

Fluoride is probably the most important preventive agent in dental health. Fluoride acts by remineralizing the tooth enamel. By keeping the tooth enamel hard and intact, the fluoride helps prevent bacteria from entering the teeth. Fluoride treatment is especially important in children whose teeth are still forming, but people of all ages can benefit from fluoride's effects. The following is a list of the benefits of fluoride.

- Remineralizing teeth

- Boosting teeth's resistance to acid

- Fighting germs that cause acid in the mouth

- Speeding up the growth of teeth

Generally, fluoride is administered topically and systematically. Fluoride can be administered systematically through fluoridated water and through fluoride supplements. In the United States, most public water systems put fluoride into the water. Water fluoridation, as it is called, has been a common practice in the country since the 1950s. In areas where fluoridated water is not available, many young children take fluoride supplements and use fluoride rinses to ensure they are getting the proper amount of fluoride. Pregnant and breastfeeding women should not take fluoride supplements.

Fluoride can be administered topically in many different ways. Some of the most common and widely used products containing fluoride include mouth rinse and toothpaste. Fluoride can also be applied topically by dental professionals. Such applications are most often used for children.

Although fluoride has many oral health benefits, it can be dangerous if it is not used carefully. Fluoride can be toxic if it is ingested in large doses. Fluoride's toxicity has made it the target of claims that its use in water and in other items (such as toothpaste) is bad for people's health. Generally, however, fluoride toxicity is only a problem when large doses are consumed. Children 6 years old and younger are at the highest risk of accidental fluoride overdose. For that reason, young children should not use toothpaste with fluoride and when children begin using toothpaste and other products with fluoride, they should be monitored.

NOTE

Patients who receive too much fluoride can experience white streaking or spotting on the teeth. This condition is called fluorosis, and it can be prevented by ensuring patients are not being administered too much fluoride.

Sealants for Pits and Fissures

Just as advancements in fluoride treatments have improved oral health, so have advancements in the use of sealants for pits and fissures. These sealants help to stop tooth decay in areas where the tooth enamel has cracked or worn away. The sealants seep into the fissures and pits and protect these areas from harmful bacteria. For sealants to be effective, they have to stay intact in the mouth and be compatible with teeth.

Sealants are often used on children and teenagers because these age groups are especially prone to dental caries. Sealants are also effective treatments for other patient populations, such as people suffering from xerostomia and people who are otherwise prone to dental caries.

Today, most sealants are resins to which fillers, such as silica and quarts, are added. Some sealants are unfilled, however. Some sealants even include fluoride to help make the teeth more resistant to caries.

Follow these eight steps when applying sealants:

1. Clean all debris from the area of the pit or fissure.

2. Wash and dry the area.

3. Etch the surface with an acid mixture. After etching is complete, the area should look chalky and white. Etching the surface will allow the sealant to better adhere to surface.

4. Wash and dry the etched area.

5. Prepare the sealant. Different sealants need to be prepared in different ways:

   o Self-cured, or autopolymerized, sealants are made up of two different materials that must be mixed together before they can be used. Generally self-cured sealants take 60 to 90 seconds to activate. Because of their makeup, self-cured sealants have time restrictions.

o Light-cured, or photopolymerized, sealants are activated using a curing light. Generally, the sealant must be exposed to the light for 20 to 30 seconds.

6. Apply the sealant according to the manufacturer's instructions.

7. Remove any excess material and examine the area for appropriate coverage and hardness.

8. Instruct patients about how to clean and care for the area.

EXERCISES: USING PREVENTIVE AGENTS

Directions: Choose the option that best answers the question.

1. Which of the following statements is true about using sealants for pits and fissures?
   (A) Photopolymerized sealants should be activated for 60 to 90 seconds.
   (B) After sealants are applied, teeth should be etched.
   (C) Sealants are generally 75-percent effective in preventing dental caries.
   (D) The etching process should make the teeth chalky and white.
   (E) People with xerostomia should not be treated with sealants.

When preparing to apply a sealant to a pit or a fissure, it is important to etch the tooth so that the sealant can properly adhere. The etching process should make the teeth a chalky white color. **The correct answer is (D).**

2. Which of the following is true about self-administered fluoride?
   (A) It generally comes in high doses.
   (B) It is more effective than water fluoridation.
   (C) It can cause fluoride toxicity.
   (D) It is almost always used on adults.
   (E) It prevents all dental caries.

Self-administered fluoride generally comes in low doses, but it can still cause fluoride toxicity if too much of it is ingested. Because of the potential for fluoride toxicity, children using products containing fluoride should be monitored. **The correct answer is (C).**

PROVIDING SUPPORTIVE TREATMENT SERVICES

Although preventive care treatments are often necessary in proper dental care, providing the proper and thorough treatments will help ensure patients' happiness and well-being. To answer the questions on the NBDHE, you will have to understand how to best treat patients and what materials to use during treatment.

The Properties of and Use of Treatment Materials

Many times, the treatments used in dental care require special materials, such as dental fillings, dental ceramics, and dental implants. Understanding how and why these materials are used is vital for excelling on the NBDHE.

All the materials used in dental care have different uses and different properties. Often, the properties of the materials impact how the materials are handled and used. All the materials used in dental treatments have physical properties, thermal properties, electrical properties, mechanical proper ties, and biological properties.

Some of the materials used to treat and prevent dental problems include:

- **Dental amalgams:** Dental amalgams are materials produced by mixing metal powder and mercury. Dental amalgams are often used to fill dental caries, and they are generally strong and long lasting. Despite containing mercury, dental amalgams are generally safe for adults.

- **Sealants:** Sealants are used to fill fissures and fits and are generally made from resin and filler material. These materials are very effective if applied properly.

- **Bonding agents:** Bonding agents are materials that are used to bond items (including bridges, orthodontic brackets, and amalgams) to teeth. Bonding agents are generally applied after teeth have been etched so the agents remain intact.

- **Dental composites and ceramics:** Dental composites and ceramics can be used to produce veneers, bridges, and other devices. Although ceramics tend to be brittle, they have a high tensile strength. Dental composites wear better when they have more filler in them.

- **Dental implants:** Dental implants are generally made from titanium or a titanium alloy. Dental implants are inserted into the bone, so they are sometimes coated with a ceramic material to stop them from corroding.

> **TIP**
> Before taking the NBDHE, review all the materials used to treat and prevent dental problems. Be sure that you understand what the materials are used for and what properties they have.

Maintaining Oral Health by Polishing Surfaces

Reducing plaque and bacteria in the mouth is an important goal of dental care. When surfaces in the mouth, including teeth and other materials, such as dental amalgams, have rough or irregular surfaces, bacteria will thrive. One important way of reducing plaque and bacteria is by making all the surfaces in the oral cavity smooth.

The following is a list of three steps involved in smoothing and polishing the surface of teeth:

1. Remove large amounts of excess material from the surface using a tool with a high hardness.

2. Finish the area by refining the surface and removing the small amounts of remaining excess material.

3. Polish and smooth the area by removing the fine scratches.

Some dental materials, such as metal implants, are polished in a laboratory and do not need to be polished in the dental office.

Making Impressions and Casts

Impressions and casts are important parts of dental care and dental health. These tools help dental professionals perform many important tasks, including creating orthodontic appliances. Impressions are negative models of mouth, and casts are positive models of the mouth.

Because impressions are negative models of the mouth, they are made by molding a material around the teeth and surrounding tissue. The impression can be used to make a cast or it can be used for another purpose. Generally, impressions are made with flexible material, but they can also be made using rigid material. Some materials used to create impressions include the following:

- Alginate hydrocolloid (flexible)

- Silicone (flexible)

- Plaster (rigid)

- Compound (rigid)

- Polysulfide (flexible)

- Polyether (flexible)

- Zinc oxide (rigid)

Casts are usually made from impressions of the mouth. Casts are generally created from plaster, stone, die stone, or other gypsum products. After the products are mixed with water, they are poured into impressions and allowed to set. Usually casts set in 45 to 60 minutes.

Other Types of Patient Care

Patients sometimes need or desire other treatments such as tooth desensitization and tooth bleaching. Hypersensitivity in the teeth is generally caused by the exposure of dentin and dentinal tubules. Patients with hypersensitivity can be treated with a number of different agents. One of the most popular and effective agents for treating hypersensitivity is fluoride. Other agents used to treat hypersensitivity include calcium hydroxide, sodium citrate, and ferric oxalate.

> **NOTE**
>
> Wax is another commonly used material in dental offices. It was one of the earliest materials used to make impressions. Today, it is widely used to create casts, help make impressions, and prepare reproductions.

Some patients choose to have elective treatments such as tooth bleaching. At-home tooth bleaching kits generally use the same chemical, hydrogen peroxide, as the in-office whitening systems; however, the in-office systems use a much higher concentration of the chemical. (In-office systems generally contain 30 to 35 percent hydrogen peroxide, and at-home kits generally contain 10 percent.) Generally, the in-office systems use heat or light to activate the hydrogen peroxide. The effectiveness of the bleaching depends on the amount of hydrogen peroxide and the length of time it is used.

EXERCISES: PROVIDING SUPPORTIVE TREATMENT SERVICES

Directions: Choose the option that best answers the question.

1. Waxes are not appropriate materials to make impressions for molds **BECAUSE** they soften when they are heated.
   (A) Both the statement and the reason are correct and related.
   (B) Both the statement and the reason are correct but NOT related.
   (C) The statement is correct but the reason is NOT.
   (D) The statement is NOT correct, but the reason is correct.
   (E) NEITHER the statement NOR the reason is correct.

   Waxes are often used to create impressions for molds and to help with other laboratory procedures, so the statement is incorrect. The reason is correct, however, because waxes do soften when they are heated and harden when they are cooled. **The correct answer is (D).**

2. Which of these best describes finishing?
   (A) Removing large amounts of excess material from surfaces
   (B) Removing material to refine the surface
   (C) Removing small scratches to smooth the surface
   (D) Removing hard tissue using air
   (E) Removing surface stains with an abrasive

   Finishing occurs when you remove material from the surface to refine the surface. Cutting is the removing of large amounts of excess material from surfaces. Polishing is the removing of small scratches to smooth the surface. Air polishing, or air abrasion, occurs when air is used to remove or polish hard tissue. Removing surface stains with an abrasive is microabrasion. **The correct answer is (B).**

UNDERSTANDING PROFESSIONAL RESPONSIBILITIES

Certain laws and ethical standards exist to protect both patients and dental hygienists. As a dental hygienist, it is important that you understand the various ethical and legal issues that you may encounter while on the job. This will ensure that you act in a professional manner that is always within the confines of the law.

Ethical Principles

Dental hygienists have a responsibility to help prevent disease and encourage healthy oral hygiene practices. When executing these responsibilities, you must always make sure that you are working within the confines of the law. There are two major types of laws: criminal law and civil law. *Criminal law* is an offense against society. *Civil laws* are created to protect individual citizens.

Tort law is a kind of civil law concerned with civil wrongdoings against an individual. Tort law is further broken down into intentional torts and unintentional torts. *Intentional torts* are conscious actions that result in the harm of an individual, including assault and battery. *Unintentional torts* involve negligence and malpractice. A medical professional is guilty of *negligence* when he or she does not provide the patient with prudent care. *Malpractice* is when a medical professional fails to adhere to professional standards, causing injury to the patient. Understanding these concepts will help you protect your patients and yourself.

Dental hygienists should also be aware of the laws that protect patients. Certain state and federal laws, including the Health Insurance Portability and Accountability Act (HIPAA), protect patient confidentiality. This prevents medical professionals from disclosing a patient's personal and health information. Violations of these laws have serious consequences. HIPAA also guarantees patients access to their medical records.

Another ethical principle that dental hygienists should understand is *informed consent*. Before any procedure is undertaken, patients must be informed of their diagnosis, prognosis, treatment plan, treatment options, and treatment risks. This helps patients make informed decisions about their health. Once everything is explained, the dental hygienist should have the patient sign a consent form to show that he or she understands the treatment plan. However, a patient may refuse care. If this is the case, you should document the reasons for the refusal carefully. In some cases, you may need to have the patient sign a form that indicates that the treatment plan was fully explained to the patient, who then made an informed decision to refuse care.

Regulatory Compliance

State legislatures establish dental practice acts, which set forth the rules and regulations that govern dental professionals within the state. Dental practice acts also determine whether dental hygienists can perform various tasks, such as the administration of local anesthesia or nitrous oxide. These rules and regulations are enforced by a state board, sometimes referred to as the State Board of Dental Examiners. This board is also responsible for developing the requirements for licensure and monitoring educational protocols. Some states also have dental hygiene advisory committees, which assist in regulating dental hygiene practices. It is important for dental hygienists to know and understand all the rules and regulations established by their state governing agencies.

Dental Hygiene Advisory Committees

The following states have dental hygiene advisory committees or subcommittees:

- Arizona
- California
- Connecticut
- Delaware
- Florida
- Iowa
- Maine
- Maryland

- Missouri
- Montana
- Nevada
- New Mexico
- Oklahoma
- Oregon
- Texas
- Washington

Patient and Professional Communication

Dental hygienists should always act in a professional manner, whether they are communicating with patients, staff members, or other medical professionals. Clear and effective communication is an important part of every dental hygienist's job. This is especially critical when dealing with patients. Communicating in a professional manner will not only help patients understand any procedures they may need, but may also alleviate any anxiety they may be experiencing. Dental hygienists can ensure that they are communicating effectively by monitoring their body language and verbal behaviors. Communicate all information in a manner that the patient can understand. When the patient asks questions, you should always maintain eye contact and focus on what the patient is saying. This will help you understand any fears or confusion the patient may be experiencing. Actively listening to patients and addressing their concerns in a clear yet empathetic manner establishes a bond of trust between the dental hygienist and his or her patients.

Review these topics related to professional responsibility before taking the NBDHE:

- Invasion of privacy
- Types of contracts
- Breach of contract
- Fraud
- Misrepresentation
- Health Insurance Portability and Accountability Act (HIPAA)

- Standard level of care
- Duties of the State Board of Dental Examiners
- Elements of dental practice acts
- Provisions for licensure across states
- Requirements for practice
- Employment laws
- Effective written communication

EXERCISES: UNDERSTANDING PROFESSIONAL RESPONSIBILITIES

Directions: Choose the option that best answers the question.

1. Each of the following statements is true about informed consent **EXCEPT** one. Which one is the **EXCEPTION**?
   (A) Patients should have adequate time to ask questions.
   (B) Doctors should weigh the risks and benefits of treatments.
   (C) Patients should understand the purpose of treatments.
   (D) Doctors should have the right to immediate patient answers.
   (E) Patients should understand the nature of treatments.

   Doctors do not have the right to immediate patient answers because patients should have adequate time to consider treatments, ask questions, and make decisions. Informed consent helps doctors and patients make well-informed and deliberate decisions. **The correct answer is (D).**

2. Which of these best describes the purpose of the Health Insurance Portability and Accountability Act (HIPAA)?
   (A) To ensure patients have the opportunity to enroll in free or reduced-cost insurance
   (B) To ensure medical professionals are fully licensed and qualified for their positions
   (C) To ensure patients' medical records and health information are properly used and protected
   (D) To ensure medical professionals treat patients with proper therapies and medications
   (E) To ensure medical professionals inform patients about the possible risks related to procedures

   The purpose of HIPAA, which was passed by Congress and signed into law in 1996, is to ensure patients' medical records and health information are properly used and protected. Because of HIPAA, medical professionals must carefully handle and store all patients' medical information. This act also protects the health insurance of workers who lose or change jobs. **The correct answer is (C).**

FIVE TIPS FOR ANSWERING CLINICAL DENTAL HYGIENE SERVICES QUESTIONS

When you are taking the NBDHE, it may be helpful to remember these hints:

1. **Assessing a patient's condition requires attention to detail.** Whether you are asking a patient about his or her health or assessing radiographs, it is important to pay attention to everything you can so you can get a full understanding of the person's condition.

2. **Educating patients is an important part of a dental hygienist's job.** Dental hygienists make important contributions to their patients' health when they educate them. Understanding what information to give patients and when to give it is an important step in becoming a dental hygienist.

3. **Emergencies can arise during dental procedures.** Although most dental procedures will not result in emergency situations, emergencies can happen. Make sure you know the different types of emergencies that can arise and the proper ways to handle them.

4. **Different materials are used for different treatments.** Dental treatments use a number of different materials that have different properties. You should understand the different materials, the ways they are used, and their properties.

5. **As a dental professional, you must keep in mind the law and ethics.** Dental professionals must follow all the laws that apply to dental professions in the areas in which they live. They should also follow all the ethical guidelines set for their profession.

PRACTICE QUESTIONS

Directions: Choose the option that best answers the question.

1. What has the National Institutes of Health deemed as Stage I hypertension?
   (A) <100/60
   (B) <120/<80
   (C) <140/<90
   (D) 140–160/90–100
   (E) 160–180/100–110

2. While assessing the gingiva, you notice that the margins are knife-edged. What does this indicate?
   (A) The dentitions are healthy.
   (B) The dentitions may be diseased.
   (C) The dentitions are diseased.
   (D) The dentitions are also soft.
   (E) The dentitions are spongy.

3. All of the following are radiopaque landmarks **EXCEPT** one. Which one is the **EXCEPTION**?
   (A) Nasal septum
   (B) Inverted Y
   (C) Median palatine suture
   (D) Zygomatic arch
   (E) Hamular process

4. While looking at a radiograph it is clear that overlap occurred and a new X-ray must be taken. How can the problem be corrected?
   (A) The dental hygienist should use fresh film for every exposure.
   (B) The patient must be instructed not to move.
   (C) Make sure all equipment is out of the way of the central beam.
   (D) Direct the central beam in a perpendicular line to the film through the interproximal surfaces.
   (E) The vertical angle must be adjusted on the machine prior to exposure.

5. At what temperature does the steam autoclave sterilize?
   (A) 25°C
   (B) 100°C
   (C) 121°C
   (D) 132°C
   (E) 160°C

6. The main function of the dentoperiosteal primary gingival fiber group is to
   (A) give gingival support.
   (B) attach gingiva to bone.
   (C) anchor teeth.
   (D) support free gingival.
   (E) maintain associations with other teeth.

7. Which of the following is classified as type IV cementum?
   (A) Accellular, afibrullar cementum is coronal cementum
   (B) Acellular, extrinsic fiber cementum
   (C) Cellular, intrinsic fiber cementum
   (D) Cellular, mixed-fiber cementum
   (E) Cellular, collagen fiber cementum

8. Which type of tissue inspection uses only one finger?
   (A) Bidigital
   (B) Digital
   (C) Bilateral
   (D) Bimanual
   (E) Circular

9. Which of these should be done before sealants are applied to teeth?
   (A) Sealants should be evaluated for retention problems.
   (B) A curing light should be placed over teeth for 20 to 30 seconds.
   (C) Phosphoric acid should be applied to generate micropores on teeth.
   (D) Fluoride must be applied to the teeth and teeth should be thoroughly dried.
   (E) Self-curing sealants should rest for 1 to 3 minutes prior to use.

10. Each of the following is a physical property of a material **EXCEPT** one. Which one is the **EXCEPTION**?
    (A) Hardness
    (B) Weight
    (C) Volume
    (D) Mass
    (E) Density

ANSWER KEY AND EXPLANATIONS

1. C	3. C	5. C	7. D	9. C
2. A	4. D	6. C	8. B	10. A

1. **The correct answer is (C).** Stage I hypertension is described as a blood pressure reading of 140–159/90–99. Stage II hypertension is described as >160/>100.

2. **The correct answer is (A).** During a gingival assessment you should notice that the margins are knife-edged. This indicates that the dentitions are healthy. If they are blunted, cratered, rolled, or bulbous, disease may be present. If the tissues are soft and spongy, disease is present.

3. **The correct answer is (C).** Median palatine suture is a maxillary radiolucent landmark. This represents the juncture of the two palatal shelves.

4. **The correct answer is (D).** When overlapping occurs, incorrect horizontal angulation was applied to the camera. The central beam should be perpendicular to the film through the interproximal surfaces.

5. **The correct answer is (C).** The steam autoclave kills all life forms and therefore sterilizes. It sterilizes at 121°C or 250°F at pounds of pressure for 15 to 30 minutes. Other methods of sterilization include statims, flash cycles, dry heat, chemical vapor, and ethylene oxide.

6. **The correct answer is (C).** The function of the dentoperiosteal primary gingival fiber group is to anchor teeth. Other primary fiber groups include: dentogingival which offers gingival support, alveologingival which attaches gingiva to bone, circular fibers which support free gingiva, and transeptal fibers which maintain associations with other teeth.

7. **The correct answer is (D).** There are four classifications of cementum. Type IV is classified as cellular, mixed-fiber cementum, which is located at the apical third and in furcations.

8. **The correct answer is (B).** Digital inspection uses only one finger. Bimanual inspection uses two hands, bidigital inspection uses two fingers, bilateral inspection uses two hands, and circular inspection uses the fingers of one hand for rotation.

9. **The correct answer is (C).** Before applying sealants, the tooth must be cleaned and dried. Next, an acid-etch material is applied to generate micropores on which the sealant can adhere. Acid-etch solutions should be dabbed on and gels should be applied with a syringe or a brush.

10. **The correct answer is (A).** Hardness is considered a mechanical property and is the ability of a material to resist indentation. Knoops hardness is the most commonly used test of hardness. Weight, volume, density, mass, boiling point, melting point, and vapor pressure are all physical properties of materials.

SUMMING IT UP

- Questions related to the provision of dental hygiene services require a working knowledge of how dental hygienists assess and treat patients. This section makes up the largest portion of the NBDHE test.

- When studying questions pertaining to provision of dental hygiene services, you should understand how each procedure affects the patient.

- It is important to understand how radiography works in order to answer the questions on the test.

- Review the types of patients who would most benefit from anxiety and pain-control techniques. You should also understand which patients should not receive certain anxiety-relieving medications.

- You should understand the proper treatments for periodontal diseases, such as gingivitis.

- It is also critical that you review the various preventive agents used in the dental office and understand how they help patients maintain good oral hygiene.

- You should understand the legal and ethical issues involved in dental practice to ensure that you are always working within the confines of the law.

- Preventive agents, such as fluoride and pit-and-fissure sealants, help keep patients' teeth healthy. Be sure you understand how these agents work and how they are administered.

- Despite preventive measures, some patients require treatments for dental problems. Before you take the NBDHE, be sure you understand the materials and procedures used to treat dental problems.

CHAPTER 7

Community Health and Research Questions

OVERVIEW

- **Promoting health and preventing disease within groups**
- **Developing and participating in community programs**
- **Analyzing scientific literature, understanding statistical concepts, and applying research results**
- **Five tips for answering community health and research questions**
- **Practice questions**
- **Answer key and explanations**
- **Summing it up**

The first part of the National Board Dental Hygiene Examination (NBDHE) contains 200 questions about these three subject areas: (1) Scientific Basics for Dental Hygiene Practice, (2) Provision of Clinical Dental Hygiene Services, and (3) Community Health and Research Principles. In this chapter, you will learn about the third subject area: Community Health and Research Principles.

About 24 test questions, or 12 percent, are about Community Health and Research Principles. These questions cover the following topics:

- Promoting health and preventing disease in groups

- Developing and participating in community programs

- Analyzing scientific literature, understanding statistical concepts, and applying research results

While this chapter does not review every detail of the subjects you learned in school, it highlights some very important information and provides you with practice questions to test your knowledge in these areas. If you have trouble remembering the information in this chapter or answering the practice questions, review your textbooks and notes from school.

PROMOTING HEALTH AND PREVENTING DISEASE WITHIN GROUPS

The World Health Organization (WHO) defines wellness as "...the optimal state of health of individuals and groups." The promotion of health and wellness in the local community is an important part of a dental practice. Due to their proximity to patients and their focus on preventive care, dental hygienists are in a unique position to educate patients on how to prevent oral diseases or keep them from spreading.

As a dental hygienist, you can encourage healthy behavior by taking the following actions:

- Sharing appropriate oral self-care techniques with your patients

- Explaining how poor lifestyle choices, such as smoking, affect oral health

- Teaching your patients how to identify and remove potential health hazards that may exist in their living or working environments

As a dental hygienist, you can also educate your community about these issues as well as the prevention of disease.

Health Promotion

The World Health Organization defines health promotion as the practice of helping people gain more control over their physical and emotional well-being by motivating them to adopt healthier behaviors. Health promotion is a comprehensive model of health care that focuses on educating both the individual and the community. Health promotion facilitates wellness by strengthening the skills of individuals and by identifying and changing conditions in the community that might impact individual or public health. To be most effective, health promotion requires both caregivers and citizens to play an active role.

The health promotion model of care differs from other health-care models that are more focused on either disease treatment or prevention. Although both disease treatment and prevention play important roles in a model of health care that focuses on health, they are not the primary focus. Rather, in a health-promoting model of care, the focus is on changing behaviors through education and the sharing of health-related information.

Effective health promotion can really make a difference in changing attitudes and behaviors by raising awareness of the dangers associated with self-destructive behaviors. For example, in 1955, smoking was considered the norm, with almost 57 percent of men and 28 percent of women classifying themselves as smokers. However, as the consequences of tobacco use and the dangers of secondhand smoke became more widely known through a variety of education and awareness campaigns, the incidence of smoking has steadily declined. In 2007, less than 24 percent of men and 18 percent of women classified themselves as smokers.

Taken from U.S. Centers for Disease Control and Prevention

Preventing the Spread of Disease

As a dental hygienist, you play a key role in helping patients improve their health by teaching them how diseases are spread through both direct and indirect contact. For example, you can help your patients to prevent the spread of the flu by showing them how to properly cover their mouths and noses when they sneeze or cough. You can also promote public health by providing this kind of education at the community level; for example, by hosting workshops for caregivers at local daycare centers.

At the individual level, you can use the process-of-care model to assess, diagnose, implement, and evaluate a plan of oral care. This model presents a sequence of events that you can follow to build and reinforce a patient's ability to engage in appropriate self-care practices. This model also helps you identify risky patient behaviors, such as smoking, and find ways to diplomatically suggest self-care techniques to minimize problems associated with such behaviors. To be most effective in your ability to change or modify patient behaviors and attitudes, you should understand and be able to apply theories of human behavior, teaching, and learning.

Review the following topics related to the promotion of health and the prevention of the spreading of diseases before you take the NBDHE:

- Health-care models (disease treatment, disease prevention, and prevention-oriented)

- Strategies and interventions that support preventive oral health care

- Process-of-care model

- Theories and strategies that can help facilitate change in a population's behaviors and attitudes

  o Principles of teaching and learning

  o Principles of human behavior

  o Learning ladder

  o Maslow's Hierarchy of Needs

> **TIP**
>
> Before taking the NBDHE, you should have completed course work in psychology and sociology. Reviewing information from these courses can help you answer the community health questions that appear on the NBDHE.

EXERCISES: PROMOTING HEALTH AND PREVENTING DISEASE WITHIN GROUPS

Directions: Choose the option that best answers the question.

1. In the second week in December, a number of students in a local school district are out sick with the flu. When a number of individuals suffer from the same condition at the same time, this is called a(an)
   (A) prevalence.
   (B) epidemic.
   (C) pandemic.
   (D) endemic.
   (E) epidemiological.

   Prevalence is defined as the number of all persons with a condition in a given population at a given time. An epidemic refers to an outbreak of a contagious disease that spreads rapidly and widely. A pandemic is an outbreak of contagious disease that spreads over a wide geographic area and affects a large proportion of the population, such as an entire country or continent. Endemic refers to a condition that is peculiar to a particular locality, region, or people. Epidemiological refers to the study and distribution of disease and disability in a population. **The correct answer is (A).**

2. Your patient is a long-time tobacco chewer who has historically resisted changing this habit even though he is aware of the potential problems associated with it. How might you be more effective in approaching him?
   (A) Provide the patient with literature that outlines the consequences of long-term tobacco use.
   (B) Make sure the patient understands the quality-of-life issues he may experience as he ages.
   (C) Help the client to understand that his oral health and general wellness are his responsibility.
   (D) Show the client dramatic pictures of patients with oral cancer.
   (E) Do nothing; the patient will quit the habit if he develops cancer.

   It is important to emphasize personal responsibility for health and wellness, because only the patient himself has the capability of changing his own behavior. Providing the patient with literature or even dramatic film probably won't help since he is already aware of the consequences of this behavior. Choice (E) supports a disease-treatment model of health. **The correct answer is (C).**

DEVELOPING AND PARTICIPATING IN COMMUNITY PROGRAMS

Most modern dental practices are concerned not only with the health of their individual patients but also with the health of the general public—the lifestyle, behavior, culture, and health of the surrounding community. As a dental hygienist, you will be part of such an organization, so you should understand the systematic process of defining and assessing a population as well as building and revising suitable educational programs for that population.

This section of the NBDHE assesses your understanding of the following topics:

- Identification and analysis of a population to determine that population's issues or challenges

- Based on this analysis, definition of objectives or goals for an educational program designed to resolve the issue or raise awareness

- Design and implementation of an educationally sound program that is appropriate for the issues, objectives, and population

- Evaluation and ongoing revision of the program to ensure maximal success

During the assessment phase, the individuals conducting the research identify and define the population in question. This population might be as big as a city or state or as small as a school or assisted-living center. The assessment focuses on a variety of factors related to the population, such as age, gender, geographical location, cultural background, the type and quality of available health care, and cultural norms associated with healthful living. Other considerations might include the availability of government or private funding and the general political climate in the area.

Once a population has been defined, researchers can collect data about this population. This information can be collected in a number of ways, including the following:

- Epidemiological surveys
- Interviews/focus groups
- Observations

- Physical examinations
- Questionnaires
- Review of medical records

Epidemiological surveys are studies of the health of specific populations and are used to determine the amount and distribution of diseases, disabilities, or other health conditions among the population. These surveys analyze issues such as lifestyle, geographic location, access to health care, and the environment. Epidemiological surveys frequently focus on the comparison between certain groups or defined populations.

A commonly utilized epidemiological device is the dental index (plural: indices), which is used to measure a defined condition or disease in a selected population. The measurement is presented along a defined numerical scale that allows researchers to easily compare conditions between or among groups. Indices are classified as reversible when they measure conditions that can be reversed or irreversible when they measure conditions that cannot be reversed. Indices should be valid, reliable, clear, and quantifiable. They should also be reasonable to the population in question. For example, the collection of information should not put anyone in harm's way.

Commonly used dental indices include oral hygiene indices, dental fluorosis indices, and dental caries indices. As part of the NBDHE, you will be asked to analyze whether a particular index is appropriate for measuring a condition in a particular population.

Collected data can be analyzed to determine the condition or problem to be addressed. Next, the researchers will define set specific, measurable objectives for the program. Objectives represent the end goal of the educational program and answer the question, "What do you want participants to think or know or do differently after they have completed the program?"

The program is designed following an educational approach appropriate to the population and situation. Instructional activities, such as lectures, demonstrations, panel discussions, and online learning, are selected. The program is created, promoted, conducted, evaluated, and adjusted as necessary to achieve optimal success.

Review the following topics related to the development and implementation of community programs before you take the NBDHE:

- Definition of private versus community/public health
- Population identification and analysis
- Data-collection techniques

- Conditions measured by common dental indices, including the following:

  o Dental caries indices

  o Fluorisis indices

  o Gingivitis indices

  o Oral hygiene indices

  o Periodontal indices

  o Root caries indices

  o Sulcular bleeding indices (SBI)

- Principles of systematic instructional design, including the following:

  o Crafting of specific, measurable objectives

  o Selecting suitable educational strategies and activities

  o Appropriately conducting the program

  o Evaluating and revising the approach/materials

EXERCISES: DEVELOPING AND PARTICIPATING IN COMMUNITY PROGRAMS

Directions: Choose the option that best answers the question.

1. The OHI-S is used to study which of the following?
   (A) Advanced decay as evidenced by inflammation along the gum line
   (B) Oral cleanliness as evidenced by the amount of debris or calculus on 6 specific teeth
   (C) Oral hygiene regimen as self-reported by the patient
   (D) Degree of fluorosis as evidenced by opaque areas on all teeth
   (E) Periodontal needs as evidenced by inflammation and pain

   The OHI-S is a simplified oral hygiene index in which 6 teeth are evaluated for debris. Choice (A) does not make sense as decay would be present in teeth and not in the gum line. Choice (C) would be measured by PHP, the patient hygiene performance index. Choice (D) would be measured with a fluorosis index. Choice (E) would be measured by a periodontal disease index. **The correct answer is (B).**

2. You recently designed an educational program on the importance of regular dental checkups for low-income families in your community. You want to design a text-based brochure that is delivered via the Internet. Which of the following outlines the primary issues you should consider before moving forward?
   (A) Should you include items of visual interest, such as pictures and diagrams, along with the text-based information?
   (B) Are the families in your target population primarily English speakers or is their primary dialect some other language?
   (C) Does your population have access to the Internet?
   (D) All of the above
   (E) None of the above

   When designing educational programs, carefully evaluate your target population to make sure the program you develop is appropriate and reachable. The questions outlined here are just a few of the areas you should take into consideration as you move forward. In addition, one tenet of good design is to include items of visual interest, as these can grab a person's attention and enhance the text. **The correct answer is (D).**

ANALYZING SCIENTIFIC LITERATURE, UNDERSTANDING STATISTICAL CONCEPTS, AND APPLYING RESEARCH RESULTS

As part of your program development, you will want to ensure that the information you are providing is accurate and current. Thus, you will have many opportunities to review published research. For example, you might be interested in the existing incidence of periodontal disease among the local population, or you might want to read current opinions on fluoride in drinking water. It is important that you be able to understand the information presented in scientific literature so you can review it with a critical eye. Having the ability to analyze the validity (or lack thereof) of the data being presented or the conclusions being drawn is an important part of reviewing research.

Much of the research you review will likely be statistical in nature, so it is important that you have a working knowledge of statistics. You should know how to read and analyze statistical content. You should be able to understand common statistical concepts such as sample size, variables, data sets, and correlations. In addition, you should understand more basic scientific concepts such as the scientific method, hypotheses, and data-presentation techniques.

Review the following topics related to scientific research and statistics before you take the NBDHE:

- Common statistical concepts and techniques
- Data selection and statistical reporting methods
- Drawing conclusions from collected data
- Evaluating the validity of published literature

EXERCISES: ANALYZING SCIENTIFIC LITERATURE, UNDERSTANDING STATISTICAL CONCEPTS, AND APPLYING RESEARCH RESULTS

Directions: Use the following scenario to answer questions 1–2.

A recent research study published by the American Dental Association considered the relationship between the use of methamphetamines and an increase in dental disease. As part of this study, participating physicians provided comprehensive medical and oral assessments for adults dependent on this substance, and trained interviewers collected self-reports from patients on their oral health and substance use. The authors used propensity score matching (PSM) to create a matched comparison group of nonusers from participants in NHANES III.

1. In this study, who is the control group?
   - (A) The methamphetamine users
   - (B) The trained interviewers
   - (C) The NHANES III group
   - (D) All of the above
   - (E) None of the above

   A control group is a group of people who share many characteristics with the subjects under study except for the primary factor being studied (in this case, methamphetamine use). The control groups serve as a comparison group. **The correct answer is (C).**

2. Which of the following best describes propensity score matching, the research methodology used?
   - (A) PSM attempts to provide an unbiased estimation of treatment-effects
   - (B) PSM attempts to match all variables of the control group to the treatment group
   - (C) PSM relies on observational methodology to determine treatment effects
   - (D) PSM prevents participants from reporting on the placebo effect
   - (E) PSM is a single blind trial that removes observational bias

   Propensity score matching is a common research technique in which characteristics of the group under study (the treatment group) are compared with characteristics of the control group. **The correct answer is (A).**

FIVE TIPS FOR ANSWERING COMMUNITY HEALTH AND RESEARCH QUESTIONS

When you are taking the NBDHE, it may be helpful to remember these hints:

1. **Public health and individual health are different but interrelated concepts.** Public health is concerned with issues and conditions in the larger community, while individual health is concerned with issues of a specific person.

2. **Promoting health is a specific health-care model.** While the health-promoting model includes disease treatment and prevention, its primary focus is on education. This type of model teaches the community at large to facilitate superior public health and prevent the origination or spread of disease.

> **TIP**
>
> When answering questions on the NBDHE that are based on cases, be sure to carefully read each case. You may want to reread a case after you reviewed the questions that follow it, so you can pick out specific information that you need to answer the questions. Use specific details listed in the case to help you determine the correct answers.

3. **Development of community programs follows a systematic process.** You need to understand the objectives of your program before you begin devising educational strategies and instructional activities. Remember the SMART acronym: objectives should be Specific, Measurable, Achievable, Realistic, and Timed. The educational activities you select should be appropriate for the population and the community. After it has been conducted, the program should be carefully evaluated and continually revised to ensure maximal success.

4. **Different indices measure different conditions.** Being able to recognize the specific condition being measured by an index is an important skill. During your review, try to make mental associations between the names of each common index and its purpose.

5. **Understanding statistics can make or break your program.** Being able to review statistical and other scientific information published in professional literature and possessing the ability to analyze it with a critical eye are key skills. They will help ensure that your programs always include the most current, accurate information available.

NOTE

Applicants taking the NBDHE who have a disability covered by the Americans with Disabilities Act may have certain accommodations made for them. Contact the Joint Commission on National Dental Examinations for more information about testing accommodations for people with disabilities.

PRACTICE QUESTIONS

Directions: Use the following scenario to answer questions 1–10.

As part of an elementary school's campaign to promote healthy eating among students, the administration has asked you to present a workshop on cavity prevention.

1. While researching your program, you review a popular published index to get a read on current incidences of cavities among the elementary school population. The index you selected was the DMFT index. What type of index is this?
   (A) Root caries index
   (B) Simplified oral hygiene index
   (C) Dental caries index
   (D) Fluorosis index
   (E) Periodontal index

2. The DMFT index is used to measure which of the following?
   (A) Past and present caries experience of a population
   (B) Likelihood of participants to develop root caries
   (C) Past and present oral hygiene practices
   (D) Past and present periodontal disease rates
   (E) Current oral cleanliness of participants

3. One of the most accurate ways you could collect data on this population is to
   (A) ask the children to self-report the number of cavities they have.
   (B) observe lunchroom food choices and draw appropriate correlations.
   (C) review the children's past and present dental records.
   (D) conduct focus groups with parents and care-givers of the children.
   (E) survey the teachers for their opinion on student behaviors.

4. Which of the following represents a good objective for this workshop?
   (A) Eliminate the number of cavities among the student population for the next 5 years as evidenced by self-reporting by creating awareness of the relationship between poor eating habits and cavities.
   (B) Lower the number of cavities among the student population over the next year as evidenced by dental examination by creating awareness of the relationship between poor eating habits and cavities.
   (C) Prevent cavities among the school population for the next several years by identifying sugar-rich foods and relating them to the incidence of cavities.
   (D) Lower the number of cavities among the student population over the next year by asking the students to identify and group foods that promote tooth decay.
   (E) Eliminate the number of cavities as reported via survey by asking students to analyze their eating habits and determine ways in which these can be improved.

5. As part of your research, you come across a local statistical study that ranks nearby communities according to the incidence of cavities in the under-12 population. In this published document, each community is ranked in descending order, with the community featuring the highest incidence of cavities listed first, followed by the next highest community, and so on. What type of scale is this?
   (A) Interval scale
   (B) Nominal scale
   (C) Ordinal scale
   (D) Ratio scale
   (E) Variable scale

6. Indices are a form of epidemiological study. How can indices be best described?
   (A) Indices are used to measure the controlled incidence of disease among a random population.
   (B) Indices are used to measure the incidence of disease or disability among a defined population.
   (C) Indices are set up as double-blind studies of a defined group measured over a long period of time.
   (D) Indices measure the incidence of irreversible disease or disability among a group or population.
   (E) Indices measure the incidence of reversible disease or disability among a group or population.

7. This index identifies the population at risk for developing a particular caries condition. This index evaluates the four surfaces of the tooth root: (1) mesial, (2) distal, (3) facial, and (4) lingual. It scores the patient based on the most severely affected surface(s). Which of the following indices is this?
   (A) Dental caries index
   (B) Gingival index
   (C) Periodontal index
   (D) Root caries index
   (E) Sulcular bleeding index

8. This index is a device used to identify the population at risk for developing a particular oral condition. This index assigns a score to each of four gingival surfaces: mesial, distal, facial, and lingual. It scores the patient based on the presence and amount of inflammation. Which of the following indices is this?
   (A) Dental caries index
   (B) Gingival index
   (C) Periodontal index
   (D) Root caries index
   (E) Sulcular bleeding index

9. A dental caries index measures past and present cavity experience of a particular population. If this type of index is carried out on individuals aged 12 and older, how many teeth are evaluated?
   (A) 12
   (B) 16
   (C) 20
   (D) 24
   (E) 28

10. A dental caries index measures past and present caries experience of a particular population. If this type of index is carried out on individuals aged 11 and younger, how many teeth are evaluated?
   (A) 12
   (B) 16
   (C) 20
   (D) 24
   (E) 28

ANSWER KEY AND EXPLANATIONS

1. C	3. C	5. C	7. D	9. E
2. A	4. B	6. B	8. B	10. C

1. **The correct answer is (C).** The DMFT—Decayed, Missing, Filled Teeth—index is an irreversible index used to measure the past and present caries experience of a defined population. It evaluates the percentage of decayed, missing, and filled teeth. A root caries index measures the extent of a population's root caries experience. A simplified oral hygiene index measures the cleanliness and plaque of a population's teeth. A fluorosis index measures the degree of fluorosis (intake of fluoride) in a population. A periodontal index measures the incidence of periodontal disease.

2. **The correct answer is (A).** As indicated above, the DMFT considers both the past and present experiences of the population in question. The other options do not apply to this type of index.

3. **The correct answer is (C).** The best, most objective way to collect data about caries incidence in this population is to review their dental records, if available. Self-reporting does not necessarily produce accurate results due to the age of the population in question, which might not know or understand what a cavity is or whether he or she has experienced one or more. Observation in the lunchroom or surveying teachers may not be an accurate representation of the population's behaviors outside of the school, which might be quite different under other circumstances (i.e., parental supervision, availability of healthy/ unhealthy food choices). Conducting a focus group with parents and caregivers might be problematic due to the desire to represent their children in the most positive light.

4. **The correct answer is (B).** The best educational objectives meet the SMART criteria—specific, measurable, achievable, realistic, and timely. In the answer options, only choice (B) meets all of these. Choice (A) is unrealistic (eliminate cavities) and the measurement device selected (self-reporting) is unreliable due to reporting bias. Choice (C) does

not provide a specific time frame in which results will be measured, nor does it indicate how results will be measured. Choice (D) does not provide a measurement device; in addition, the suggested activity does not complete the correlation between unhealthy choices and tooth decay. Choice (E) has an unrealistic goal (eliminate) and relies on a survey device for self-reported results, which may be subject to reporting bias.

5. **The correct answer is (C).** In statistical documentation, an ordinal scale is used to rank characteristics in an empirical order. An interval scale displays characteristics along a timeline or continuum. A nominal scale presents information by category. A ratio scale presents information within an absolute zero value such as weight or height. A variable scale does not exist.

6. **The correct answer is (B).** Indices are used to measure the incidence of disease or disability among a defined population. The keywords here are "measure," "disease or disability," and "defined population." Choice (A) refers to a random population. Choice (C) is an example of an index that might be used, but does not provide an actual definition of an index. Choices (D) and (E) limit an index to either reversible or irreversible conditions. An index might measure one or the other, but the definition is not exclusive.

7. **The correct answer is (D).** The type of condition being measured is indicated in the phrase "evaluates four surfaces of the tooth root" as well as in the description of the specific evaluation method. A dental caries index measures the incidence of tooth decay; the tooth surface is evaluated. A gingival index measures the presence and severity of gingivitis. Evaluation is conducted on gingival surfaces. A periodontal index measures the presence and severity of periodontal disease. All teeth are evaluated for inflammation. A sulcular bleeding index also

measures the presence and severity of gingivitis as evidenced by bleeding upon sulcus probing.

8. **The correct answer is (B).** The type of condition being measured is indicated in the phrase "assigns a score to four gingival surfaces" and refers to inflammation as the indicator. A dental caries index measures the incidence of tooth decay; the tooth surface is evaluated. A periodontal index measures the presence and severity of periodontal disease. All teeth are evaluated for inflammation. A root caries index measures the risk for the development of root caries and is evaluated at the roots. A sulcular bleeding index also measures for the presence and severity of gingivitis as evidenced by bleeding upon sulcus probing.

9. **The correct answer is (E).** As you will recall from your studies, in populations age 12 and older, it is standard practice to evaluate 28 teeth.

10. **The correct answer is (C).** As you will recall from your studies, in populations age 11 and younger, it is standard practice to evaluate 20 teeth.

SUMMING IT UP

- Health-promoting models of health care focus on facilitating both individual and public health. It is important to understand the difference between these two concepts, as well as to be able to identify other models of health care, such as disease treatment and disease-prevention models.

- One key way to influence the attitudes and behaviors of the larger community is to develop and/or participate in community educational programs. You can design programs for specific populations using available research materials. The process you follow, however, should be systematic, to ensure that the approach is sound, that the audience can meet the objectives, and that you can measure your results to know if you were successful or not.

- As part of your involvement in educational programs, you will spend time reviewing published scientific literature. You will benefit from being able to recognize sound research from that which is less valid. You will also need to understand basic statistical concepts and data representation so that you can apply results appropriately.

PART IV

NBDHE COMPONENT B QUESTIONS

CHAPTER 8

Case-Based Questions

OVERVIEW

- **Patient categories**
- **Case components**
- **Practice questions**
- **Answer key and explanations**
- **Summing it up**

As you learned earlier in this book, the National Board Dental Hygiene Exam (NBDHE) is administered in two sessions, called components. Component A of the test contains 200 discipline-based multiple-choice questions. Component B of the NBDHE contains 150 case-based multiple-choice items. In this chapter, you will learn about the questions in Component B. According to the Joint Commission on National Dental Examinations (JCNDE), the test items in this component address the following procedures of dental hygiene care delivery:

- Assessing patient characteristics
- Obtaining and interpreting radiographs
- Planning and managing dental hygiene care
- Performing periodontal procedures
- Using preventive agents
- Providing supporting treatment services
- Professional responsibility

PATIENT CATEGORIES

The questions in Component B are about patients in two categories: adults and children. Eighty percent of the test questions are about adults, and 20 percent are about children. At least two cases address how to manage a compromised patient, a patient whose health requires modified care. Each exam contains at least one case for each of the following types of patients:

- Geriatric
- Adult-periodontal

- Pediatric

- Special-needs

- Medically-compromised

CASE COMPONENTS

Dental hygienists must be able to apply their knowledge to solve patient problems. Component B of the NBDHE assesses your ability to do this. The questions in this session are groups of questions about a particular patient's case. Expect to see about 12 to 15 cases on the test, each with 8 to 15 test items. The patient cases in Component B contain the following information:

> **TIP**
> Refer back to the case components as you answer the items. This is not cheating and will help you choose the correct answer option.

- Patient history

- Dental chart

- Radiographs

- Clinical photographs

- Photographs of casts (when appropriate)

Patient History

The patient history contains patient information such as age, gender, relevant physical characteristics, vital signs, medical and dental histories, relevant social history, and the chief complaint. A patient history on the NBDHE might look like this:

SYNOPSIS OF PATIENT HISTORY　　　　　CASE ___1___

Age ___58___

Sex ___Male___

Height _6'2"_

Weight _250_ lbs

_113.6_ kgs

Vital Signs
Blood pressure ___136/80___

Pulse rate ___63___

Respiration rate ___14___

---

1. Under Care of Physician
   Yes ☑ No ☐

   Condition: _____ *Osteoarthritis* _____

2. Hospitalized within the last 5 years
   Yes ☑ No ☐

   Reason: _____ *Appendicitis* _____

3. Has or had the following conditions:

   Received steroid injections for acute pain.
   _____

4. Current medications:

   Ketorolac for inflammation and acetaminophen
   for pain.
   _____

5. Smokes or uses tobacco products
   Yes ☐ No ☑

6. Is pregnant
   Yes ☐ No ☐ N/A ☑

MEDICAL HISTORY:
The takes medication occasionally for pain flare-ups. He has had many X-rays of his neck and back during the last five years.

DENTAL HISTORY:
He has not seen a dentist in nearly seven years.

SOCIAL HISTORY:
He is married with three children.

CHIEF COMPLAINT:
He says his gums bleed sometimes when he brushes.

TIP

Some dental charts include supplemental oral examine findings. Do not confuse this with the key on the chart and be sure to read these findings carefully. They will help you answer the questions following the chart.

Dental Chart

A dental chart is also included in each scenario. Note the information included in the following chart and the key to the right of the chart.

ADULT CLINICAL EXAMINATION

Case 1

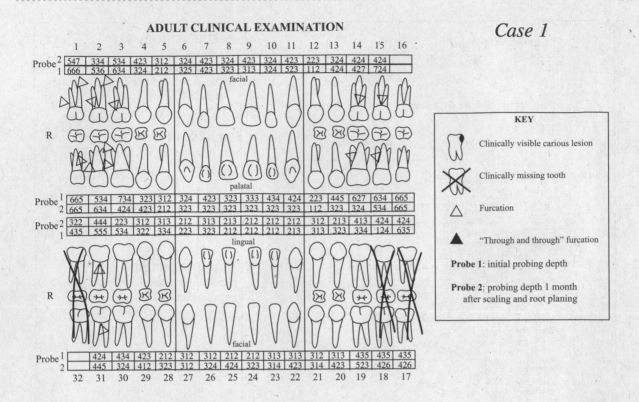

	1	2	3	4	5	6	7	8	9	10	11	12	13	14	15	16
Probe 2	547	334	534	423	312	324	423	324	423	324	423	223	324	424	424	
Probe 1	666	536	634	324	212	325	423	323	313	324	523	112	424	427	724	

facial

KEY

Clinically visible carious lesion

Clinically missing tooth

Furcation

"Through and through" furcation

Probe 1: initial probing depth

Probe 2: probing depth 1 month after scaling and root planing

palatal

	1	2	3	4	5	6	7	8	9	10	11	12	13	14	15	16
Probe 1	665	534	734	323	312	324	423	323	333	434	424	223	445	627	634	665
Probe 2	665	634	424	423	212	323	323	323	323	323	323	112	323	324	534	665

	32	31	30	29	28	27	26	25	24	23	22	21	20	19	18	17
Probe 2	322	444	223	312	313	212	313	213	212	212	212	312	213	413	424	424
Probe 1	435	555	534	322	334	223	212	212	212	212	213	313	323	334	124	635

lingual

facial

	32	31	30	29	28	27	26	25	24	23	22	21	20	19	18	17
Probe 1		424	434	423	212	312	312	212	212	313	313	312	313	435	435	435
Probe 2		445	324	412	323	312	324	424	323	314	423	314	423	523	426	426

Radiographs and Photographs

The NBDHE contains radiographs and photographs. Bitewing radiographs and/or a panoramic view may be included. Color photographs, slides, or digital images may also be included to help you better understand a patient's condition. Note that you may also be asked about technical errors in radiographs. For example, a test question might ask you if a radiograph has had the film overlapped during processing or has too little angulation. Review your textbook and notes to refresh your memory on the following radiographic errors:

- **Elongation:** Vertical angulation caused by too little angulation.

- **Distortion:** Bent or curbed film on the palate and cuspid area of the mandible.

- **Overlapping:** Incorrect horizontal angulation caused by an incorrectly angled cone.

- **Foreshortening:** Vertical angulation error caused by too much angulation.

- **Cone cutting:** Film is only partially exposed because the X-ray beam missed part of the film.

- **Underexposed film:** Film appears light.

- **Overexposed film:** Film appears dark.

- **Double exposure:** Film is exposed twice, which causes images to look indistinct.

PRACTICE QUESTIONS

Directions: Study the case components and answer questions 1–10.

SYNOPSIS OF PATIENT HISTORY   CASE ___2___

Age ___28___

Sex ___Female___

Height ___5'4"___

Weight ___145___ lbs

___65.77___ kgs

Vital Signs

Blood pressure ___122/78___

Pulse rate ___76___

Respiration rate ___14___

---

1. Under Care of Physician
   Yes ☑ No ☐

   Condition: ___Pregnancy___

2. Hospitalized within the last 5 years
   Yes ☐ No ☑

   Reason: _____

3. Has or had the following conditions:

   _____
   _____

4. Current medications:

   Pregnancy vitamins
   _____
   _____

5. Smokes or uses tobacco products
   Yes ☐ No ☑

6. Is pregnant
   Yes ☑ No ☐ N/A ☐

MEDICAL HISTORY:
The patient is 16 weeks' pregnant and is currently taking pregnancy vitamins. She experienced morning sickness during her first trimester, which has subsided. The patient is not allergic to any medications.

DENTAL HISTORY:
The patient's last visit to the dentist was for a cleaning and exam one year prior. The patient brushes her teeth once/day with a manual toothbrush and flosses only when she gets a food impaction.

SOCIAL HISTORY:
Patient is employed as a full-time teller at a bank.

CHIEF COMPLAINT:
Patient states, "My gums are bleeding almost every time I brush, and I have a large swelling on the gums between my right front tooth and the one next to it. I have bad breath."

ADULT CLINICAL EXAMINATION

Case 2

	1	2	3	4	5	6	7	8	9	10	11	12	13	14	15	16
Probe 2 / 1		434	434	424	432	333	323	333	333	334	334	434	424	434	434	

facial

R

palatal

	1 / 2															
Probe		424	434	424	432	333	323	323	333	333	334	424	424	434	434	

	2 / 1															
Probe		424	434	424	432	333	323	323	333	333	334	424	424	434	434	

lingual

R

facial

	1 / 2															
Probe		434	434	424	432	333	323	333	333	334	334	434	424	434	434	

| 32 | 31 | 30 | 29 | 28 | 27 | 26 | 25 | 24 | 23 | 22 | 21 | 20 | 19 | 18 | 17 |

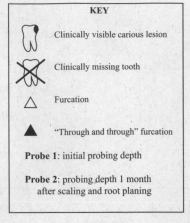

KEY

Clinically visible carious lesion

Clinically missing tooth

Furcation

"Through and through" furcation

Probe 1: initial probing depth

Probe 2: probing depth 1 month
after scaling and root planing

SUPPLEMENTAL ORAL EXAMINATION FINDINGS

1. Fair oral hygiene.
2. Localized areas of moderate plaque. Slight calculus mandibular anterior linuals.
3. Minimal light stain maxillary anterior linguals.
4. Generalized gingival bleeding upon upon probing.
5. Area of localized swelling on facial interdental papillae between #7 and #8, red, 6mm, not painful.

1. Which of the following is the AAP classification for this patient's periodontal condition?
   (A) Type 1
   (B) Type 2
   (C) Type 3
   (D) Type 4

2. Which of the following is the best diagnosis for this patient's periodontal disease?
   (A) Localized moderate periodontitis
   (B) Generalized severe periodontitis
   (C) Gingivitis
   (D) Generalized moderate periodontitis

3. The swollen, deep red, 6mm area on the interproximal tissue between #7 and #8 is most likely which of the following?
   (A) Localized hormonal gingival cyst
   (B) Periodontal abscess
   (C) Pregnancy tumor or pyogenic granuloma
   (D) Pyrogenic Granulitis

4. Which of the following is true about the pocketing in the posterior teeth?
   (A) It is due to attachment loss.
   (B) It is pseudopocketing due to hormonally exaggerated tissue response to plaque biofilm.
   (C) It is indicative of moderate periodontitis.
   (D) It is irreversible.

5. Patient's home-care regimen should include all of the following **EXCEPT**
   (A) brush 2–3 times daily with an automatic toothbrush.
   (B) dental floss once a day in the evening prior to brushing.
   (C) use toothpicks on a daily basis to massage the swollen tissue.
   (D) use a tongue scraper daily.

6. Which position is contraindicated for the patient during dental hygiene treatment?
   (A) Sits upright
   (B) Lies supine with legs gently elevated
   (C) Lies on left side
   (D) Head and back moderately raised

7. Which trimester of pregnancy is optimum for dental treatment?
   (A) Throughout
   (B) First trimester
   (C) Second trimester
   (D) Third trimester

8. The patient states that she is too tired at night to brush her teeth before bedtime. Which of the following is the best response from the dental hygienist?
   (A) "Once a day is better than not at all."
   (B) "If you continue with this attitude, you will probably lose your teeth."
   (C) "Skip the brushing, but use an alcohol-free antimicrobial mouth rinse."
   (D) "Why not try to get a second brushing in immediately after dinner?"

9. The patient is due for bitewing X-rays. Which of the following is most appropriate?
   (A) Use two lead shields, one with a thyroid collar and the other without.
   (B) Use a lead shield on the back as well as the front of the patient.
   (C) Take only two bitewings rather than the usual four.
   (D) Do not take X-rays on this patient.

10. What is the best treatment for this patient's periodontal condition?
   (A) Quadrant debridement with local anesthesia
   (B) Debridement; placement of local antibiotic tetracycline delivery system
   (C) Full mouth light scaling and selective polishing
   (D) Gross scaling

ANSWER KEY AND EXPLANATIONS

1. A	3. C	5. C	7. C	9. D
2. C	4. B	6. B	8. D	10. A

1. **The correct answer is (A).** Type 1 periodontal disease is gingivitis that is reversible with no attachment loss.

2. **The correct answer is (C).** The patient's periodontal disease is gingivitis because there is no loss of attachment. Swollen tissues create pseudopocketing and are a result of hormonal exaggeration to plaque biofilm.

3. **The correct answer is (C).** Gingivitis is a condition occasionally found in pregnant women on the interproximal facial surfaces of the gingiva due to hormonal factors. Gingivitis often requires no treatment and typically disappears after pregnancy.

4. **The correct answer is (B).** Pocketing is due to swollen tissues exacerbated by hormonal factors, not a loss of attachment. Pocketing is completely reversible.

5. **The correct answer is (C).** Toothpicks would not be as beneficial in this regiment as other home-care devices and could potentially damage tissues.

6. **The correct answer is (B).** Lying supine with legs gently elevated could place undue pressure on the fetus from the mother.

7. **The correct answer is (C).** During the second trimester, there is less risk to the developing fetus and the mother is less apt to be fatigued or to go into preterm delivery.

8. **The correct answer is (D).** The hygienist is proposing a win-win situation to maintain optimal oral health as well as to cope with the patient's fatigue.

9. **The correct answer is (D).** The bitewing X-rays can most likely be put off until after the patient has her baby, thus minimizing risk.

10. **The correct answer is (A).** The patient does not require extensive deep scaling. The treatment can be completed in one visit.

SUMMING IT UP

- Component B of the National Board Dental Hygiene Examination (NBDHE) contains 150 case-based multiple-choice items. These items address the following procedures of dental hygiene care delivery: assessing patient characteristics, obtaining and interpreting radiographs, planning and managing dental hygiene care, performing periodontal procedures, using preventive agents, providing supporting treatment services, and professional responsibility.

- Eighty percent of the cases in Component B are about adults and 20 percent of the questions are about children.

- Each NBDHE exam contains at least one case for geriatric, adult-periodontal, pediatric, special-needs, and medically-compromised patients.

- Each case on the NBDHE contains a patient history, a dental chart, radiographs, and clinical photographs.

PART V

TWO PRACTICE TESTS

ANSWER SHEET PRACTICE TEST 2

Component A

1. Ⓐ Ⓑ Ⓒ Ⓓ Ⓔ	41. Ⓐ Ⓑ Ⓒ Ⓓ Ⓔ	81. Ⓐ Ⓑ Ⓒ Ⓓ Ⓔ	121. Ⓐ Ⓑ Ⓒ Ⓓ Ⓔ	161. Ⓐ Ⓑ Ⓒ Ⓓ Ⓔ
2. Ⓐ Ⓑ Ⓒ Ⓓ Ⓔ	42. Ⓐ Ⓑ Ⓒ Ⓓ Ⓔ	82. Ⓐ Ⓑ Ⓒ Ⓓ Ⓔ	122. Ⓐ Ⓑ Ⓒ Ⓓ Ⓔ	162. Ⓐ Ⓑ Ⓒ Ⓓ Ⓔ
3. Ⓐ Ⓑ Ⓒ Ⓓ Ⓔ	43. Ⓐ Ⓑ Ⓒ Ⓓ Ⓔ	83. Ⓐ Ⓑ Ⓒ Ⓓ Ⓔ	123. Ⓐ Ⓑ Ⓒ Ⓓ Ⓔ	163. Ⓐ Ⓑ Ⓒ Ⓓ Ⓔ
4. Ⓐ Ⓑ Ⓒ Ⓓ Ⓔ	44. Ⓐ Ⓑ Ⓒ Ⓓ Ⓔ	84. Ⓐ Ⓑ Ⓒ Ⓓ Ⓔ	124. Ⓐ Ⓑ Ⓒ Ⓓ Ⓔ	164. Ⓐ Ⓑ Ⓒ Ⓓ Ⓔ
5. Ⓐ Ⓑ Ⓒ Ⓓ Ⓔ	45. Ⓐ Ⓑ Ⓒ Ⓓ Ⓔ	85. Ⓐ Ⓑ Ⓒ Ⓓ Ⓔ	125. Ⓐ Ⓑ Ⓒ Ⓓ Ⓔ	165. Ⓐ Ⓑ Ⓒ Ⓓ Ⓔ
6. Ⓐ Ⓑ Ⓒ Ⓓ Ⓔ	46. Ⓐ Ⓑ Ⓒ Ⓓ Ⓔ	86. Ⓐ Ⓑ Ⓒ Ⓓ Ⓔ	126. Ⓐ Ⓑ Ⓒ Ⓓ Ⓔ	166. Ⓐ Ⓑ Ⓒ Ⓓ Ⓔ
7. Ⓐ Ⓑ Ⓒ Ⓓ Ⓔ	47. Ⓐ Ⓑ Ⓒ Ⓓ Ⓔ	87. Ⓐ Ⓑ Ⓒ Ⓓ Ⓔ	127. Ⓐ Ⓑ Ⓒ Ⓓ Ⓔ	167. Ⓐ Ⓑ Ⓒ Ⓓ Ⓔ
8. Ⓐ Ⓑ Ⓒ Ⓓ Ⓔ	48. Ⓐ Ⓑ Ⓒ Ⓓ Ⓔ	88. Ⓐ Ⓑ Ⓒ Ⓓ Ⓔ	128. Ⓐ Ⓑ Ⓒ Ⓓ Ⓔ	168. Ⓐ Ⓑ Ⓒ Ⓓ Ⓔ
9. Ⓐ Ⓑ Ⓒ Ⓓ Ⓔ	49. Ⓐ Ⓑ Ⓒ Ⓓ Ⓔ	89. Ⓐ Ⓑ Ⓒ Ⓓ Ⓔ	129. Ⓐ Ⓑ Ⓒ Ⓓ Ⓔ	169. Ⓐ Ⓑ Ⓒ Ⓓ Ⓔ
10. Ⓐ Ⓑ Ⓒ Ⓓ Ⓔ	50. Ⓐ Ⓑ Ⓒ Ⓓ Ⓔ	90. Ⓐ Ⓑ Ⓒ Ⓓ Ⓔ	130. Ⓐ Ⓑ Ⓒ Ⓓ Ⓔ	170. Ⓐ Ⓑ Ⓒ Ⓓ Ⓔ
11. Ⓐ Ⓑ Ⓒ Ⓓ Ⓔ	51. Ⓐ Ⓑ Ⓒ Ⓓ Ⓔ	91. Ⓐ Ⓑ Ⓒ Ⓓ Ⓔ	131. Ⓐ Ⓑ Ⓒ Ⓓ Ⓔ	171. Ⓐ Ⓑ Ⓒ Ⓓ Ⓔ
12. Ⓐ Ⓑ Ⓒ Ⓓ Ⓔ	52. Ⓐ Ⓑ Ⓒ Ⓓ Ⓔ	92. Ⓐ Ⓑ Ⓒ Ⓓ Ⓔ	132. Ⓐ Ⓑ Ⓒ Ⓓ Ⓔ	172. Ⓐ Ⓑ Ⓒ Ⓓ Ⓔ
13. Ⓐ Ⓑ Ⓒ Ⓓ Ⓔ	53. Ⓐ Ⓑ Ⓒ Ⓓ Ⓔ	93. Ⓐ Ⓑ Ⓒ Ⓓ Ⓔ	133. Ⓐ Ⓑ Ⓒ Ⓓ Ⓔ	173. Ⓐ Ⓑ Ⓒ Ⓓ Ⓔ
14. Ⓐ Ⓑ Ⓒ Ⓓ Ⓔ	54. Ⓐ Ⓑ Ⓒ Ⓓ Ⓔ	94. Ⓐ Ⓑ Ⓒ Ⓓ Ⓔ	134. Ⓐ Ⓑ Ⓒ Ⓓ Ⓔ	174. Ⓐ Ⓑ Ⓒ Ⓓ Ⓔ
15. Ⓐ Ⓑ Ⓒ Ⓓ Ⓔ	55. Ⓐ Ⓑ Ⓒ Ⓓ Ⓔ	95. Ⓐ Ⓑ Ⓒ Ⓓ Ⓔ	135. Ⓐ Ⓑ Ⓒ Ⓓ Ⓔ	175. Ⓐ Ⓑ Ⓒ Ⓓ Ⓔ
16. Ⓐ Ⓑ Ⓒ Ⓓ Ⓔ	56. Ⓐ Ⓑ Ⓒ Ⓓ Ⓔ	96. Ⓐ Ⓑ Ⓒ Ⓓ Ⓔ	136. Ⓐ Ⓑ Ⓒ Ⓓ Ⓔ	176. Ⓐ Ⓑ Ⓒ Ⓓ Ⓔ
17. Ⓐ Ⓑ Ⓒ Ⓓ Ⓔ	57. Ⓐ Ⓑ Ⓒ Ⓓ Ⓔ	97. Ⓐ Ⓑ Ⓒ Ⓓ Ⓔ	137. Ⓐ Ⓑ Ⓒ Ⓓ Ⓔ	177. Ⓐ Ⓑ Ⓒ Ⓓ Ⓔ
18. Ⓐ Ⓑ Ⓒ Ⓓ Ⓔ	58. Ⓐ Ⓑ Ⓒ Ⓓ Ⓔ	98. Ⓐ Ⓑ Ⓒ Ⓓ Ⓔ	138. Ⓐ Ⓑ Ⓒ Ⓓ Ⓔ	178. Ⓐ Ⓑ Ⓒ Ⓓ Ⓔ
19. Ⓐ Ⓑ Ⓒ Ⓓ Ⓔ	59. Ⓐ Ⓑ Ⓒ Ⓓ Ⓔ	99. Ⓐ Ⓑ Ⓒ Ⓓ Ⓔ	139. Ⓐ Ⓑ Ⓒ Ⓓ Ⓔ	179. Ⓐ Ⓑ Ⓒ Ⓓ Ⓔ
20. Ⓐ Ⓑ Ⓒ Ⓓ Ⓔ	60. Ⓐ Ⓑ Ⓒ Ⓓ Ⓔ	100. Ⓐ Ⓑ Ⓒ Ⓓ Ⓔ	140. Ⓐ Ⓑ Ⓒ Ⓓ Ⓔ	180. Ⓐ Ⓑ Ⓒ Ⓓ Ⓔ
21. Ⓐ Ⓑ Ⓒ Ⓓ Ⓔ	61. Ⓐ Ⓑ Ⓒ Ⓓ Ⓔ	101. Ⓐ Ⓑ Ⓒ Ⓓ Ⓔ	141. Ⓐ Ⓑ Ⓒ Ⓓ Ⓔ	181. Ⓐ Ⓑ Ⓒ Ⓓ Ⓔ
22. Ⓐ Ⓑ Ⓒ Ⓓ Ⓔ	62. Ⓐ Ⓑ Ⓒ Ⓓ Ⓔ	102. Ⓐ Ⓑ Ⓒ Ⓓ Ⓔ	142. Ⓐ Ⓑ Ⓒ Ⓓ Ⓔ	182. Ⓐ Ⓑ Ⓒ Ⓓ Ⓔ
23. Ⓐ Ⓑ Ⓒ Ⓓ Ⓔ	63. Ⓐ Ⓑ Ⓒ Ⓓ Ⓔ	103. Ⓐ Ⓑ Ⓒ Ⓓ Ⓔ	143. Ⓐ Ⓑ Ⓒ Ⓓ Ⓔ	183. Ⓐ Ⓑ Ⓒ Ⓓ Ⓔ
24. Ⓐ Ⓑ Ⓒ Ⓓ Ⓔ	64. Ⓐ Ⓑ Ⓒ Ⓓ Ⓔ	104. Ⓐ Ⓑ Ⓒ Ⓓ Ⓔ	144. Ⓐ Ⓑ Ⓒ Ⓓ Ⓔ	184. Ⓐ Ⓑ Ⓒ Ⓓ Ⓔ
25. Ⓐ Ⓑ Ⓒ Ⓓ Ⓔ	65. Ⓐ Ⓑ Ⓒ Ⓓ Ⓔ	105. Ⓐ Ⓑ Ⓒ Ⓓ Ⓔ	145. Ⓐ Ⓑ Ⓒ Ⓓ Ⓔ	185. Ⓐ Ⓑ Ⓒ Ⓓ Ⓔ
26. Ⓐ Ⓑ Ⓒ Ⓓ Ⓔ	66. Ⓐ Ⓑ Ⓒ Ⓓ Ⓔ	106. Ⓐ Ⓑ Ⓒ Ⓓ Ⓔ	146. Ⓐ Ⓑ Ⓒ Ⓓ Ⓔ	186. Ⓐ Ⓑ Ⓒ Ⓓ Ⓔ
27. Ⓐ Ⓑ Ⓒ Ⓓ Ⓔ	67. Ⓐ Ⓑ Ⓒ Ⓓ Ⓔ	107. Ⓐ Ⓑ Ⓒ Ⓓ Ⓔ	147. Ⓐ Ⓑ Ⓒ Ⓓ Ⓔ	187. Ⓐ Ⓑ Ⓒ Ⓓ Ⓔ
28. Ⓐ Ⓑ Ⓒ Ⓓ Ⓔ	68. Ⓐ Ⓑ Ⓒ Ⓓ Ⓔ	108. Ⓐ Ⓑ Ⓒ Ⓓ Ⓔ	148. Ⓐ Ⓑ Ⓒ Ⓓ Ⓔ	188. Ⓐ Ⓑ Ⓒ Ⓓ Ⓔ
29. Ⓐ Ⓑ Ⓒ Ⓓ Ⓔ	69. Ⓐ Ⓑ Ⓒ Ⓓ Ⓔ	109. Ⓐ Ⓑ Ⓒ Ⓓ Ⓔ	149. Ⓐ Ⓑ Ⓒ Ⓓ Ⓔ	189. Ⓐ Ⓑ Ⓒ Ⓓ Ⓔ
30. Ⓐ Ⓑ Ⓒ Ⓓ Ⓔ	70. Ⓐ Ⓑ Ⓒ Ⓓ Ⓔ	110. Ⓐ Ⓑ Ⓒ Ⓓ Ⓔ	150. Ⓐ Ⓑ Ⓒ Ⓓ Ⓔ	190. Ⓐ Ⓑ Ⓒ Ⓓ Ⓔ
31. Ⓐ Ⓑ Ⓒ Ⓓ Ⓔ	71. Ⓐ Ⓑ Ⓒ Ⓓ Ⓔ	111. Ⓐ Ⓑ Ⓒ Ⓓ Ⓔ	151. Ⓐ Ⓑ Ⓒ Ⓓ Ⓔ	191. Ⓐ Ⓑ Ⓒ Ⓓ Ⓔ
32. Ⓐ Ⓑ Ⓒ Ⓓ Ⓔ	72. Ⓐ Ⓑ Ⓒ Ⓓ Ⓔ	112. Ⓐ Ⓑ Ⓒ Ⓓ Ⓔ	152. Ⓐ Ⓑ Ⓒ Ⓓ Ⓔ	192. Ⓐ Ⓑ Ⓒ Ⓓ Ⓔ
33. Ⓐ Ⓑ Ⓒ Ⓓ Ⓔ	73. Ⓐ Ⓑ Ⓒ Ⓓ Ⓔ	113. Ⓐ Ⓑ Ⓒ Ⓓ Ⓔ	153. Ⓐ Ⓑ Ⓒ Ⓓ Ⓔ	193. Ⓐ Ⓑ Ⓒ Ⓓ Ⓔ
34. Ⓐ Ⓑ Ⓒ Ⓓ Ⓔ	74. Ⓐ Ⓑ Ⓒ Ⓓ Ⓔ	114. Ⓐ Ⓑ Ⓒ Ⓓ Ⓔ	154. Ⓐ Ⓑ Ⓒ Ⓓ Ⓔ	194. Ⓐ Ⓑ Ⓒ Ⓓ Ⓔ
35. Ⓐ Ⓑ Ⓒ Ⓓ Ⓔ	75. Ⓐ Ⓑ Ⓒ Ⓓ Ⓔ	115. Ⓐ Ⓑ Ⓒ Ⓓ Ⓔ	155. Ⓐ Ⓑ Ⓒ Ⓓ Ⓔ	195. Ⓐ Ⓑ Ⓒ Ⓓ Ⓔ
36. Ⓐ Ⓑ Ⓒ Ⓓ Ⓔ	76. Ⓐ Ⓑ Ⓒ Ⓓ Ⓔ	116. Ⓐ Ⓑ Ⓒ Ⓓ Ⓔ	156. Ⓐ Ⓑ Ⓒ Ⓓ Ⓔ	196. Ⓐ Ⓑ Ⓒ Ⓓ Ⓔ
37. Ⓐ Ⓑ Ⓒ Ⓓ Ⓔ	77. Ⓐ Ⓑ Ⓒ Ⓓ Ⓔ	117. Ⓐ Ⓑ Ⓒ Ⓓ Ⓔ	157. Ⓐ Ⓑ Ⓒ Ⓓ Ⓔ	197. Ⓐ Ⓑ Ⓒ Ⓓ Ⓔ
38. Ⓐ Ⓑ Ⓒ Ⓓ Ⓔ	78. Ⓐ Ⓑ Ⓒ Ⓓ Ⓔ	118. Ⓐ Ⓑ Ⓒ Ⓓ Ⓔ	158. Ⓐ Ⓑ Ⓒ Ⓓ Ⓔ	198. Ⓐ Ⓑ Ⓒ Ⓓ Ⓔ
39. Ⓐ Ⓑ Ⓒ Ⓓ Ⓔ	79. Ⓐ Ⓑ Ⓒ Ⓓ Ⓔ	119. Ⓐ Ⓑ Ⓒ Ⓓ Ⓔ	159. Ⓐ Ⓑ Ⓒ Ⓓ Ⓔ	199. Ⓐ Ⓑ Ⓒ Ⓓ Ⓔ
40. Ⓐ Ⓑ Ⓒ Ⓓ Ⓔ	80. Ⓐ Ⓑ Ⓒ Ⓓ Ⓔ	120. Ⓐ Ⓑ Ⓒ Ⓓ Ⓔ	160. Ⓐ Ⓑ Ⓒ Ⓓ Ⓔ	200. Ⓐ Ⓑ Ⓒ Ⓓ Ⓔ

Component B

1. Ⓐ Ⓑ Ⓒ Ⓓ	31. Ⓐ Ⓑ Ⓒ Ⓓ	61. Ⓐ Ⓑ Ⓒ Ⓓ	91. Ⓐ Ⓑ Ⓒ Ⓓ	121. Ⓐ Ⓑ Ⓒ Ⓓ
2. Ⓐ Ⓑ Ⓒ Ⓓ	32. Ⓐ Ⓑ Ⓒ Ⓓ	62. Ⓐ Ⓑ Ⓒ Ⓓ	92. Ⓐ Ⓑ Ⓒ Ⓓ	122. Ⓐ Ⓑ Ⓒ Ⓓ
3. Ⓐ Ⓑ Ⓒ Ⓓ	33. Ⓐ Ⓑ Ⓒ Ⓓ	63. Ⓐ Ⓑ Ⓒ Ⓓ	93. Ⓐ Ⓑ Ⓒ Ⓓ	123. Ⓐ Ⓑ Ⓒ Ⓓ
4. Ⓐ Ⓑ Ⓒ Ⓓ	34. Ⓐ Ⓑ Ⓒ Ⓓ	64. Ⓐ Ⓑ Ⓒ Ⓓ	94. Ⓐ Ⓑ Ⓒ Ⓓ	124. Ⓐ Ⓑ Ⓒ Ⓓ
5. Ⓐ Ⓑ Ⓒ Ⓓ	35. Ⓐ Ⓑ Ⓒ Ⓓ	65. Ⓐ Ⓑ Ⓒ Ⓓ	95. Ⓐ Ⓑ Ⓒ Ⓓ	125. Ⓐ Ⓑ Ⓒ Ⓓ
6. Ⓐ Ⓑ Ⓒ Ⓓ	36. Ⓐ Ⓑ Ⓒ Ⓓ	66. Ⓐ Ⓑ Ⓒ Ⓓ	96. Ⓐ Ⓑ Ⓒ Ⓓ	126. Ⓐ Ⓑ Ⓒ Ⓓ
7. Ⓐ Ⓑ Ⓒ Ⓓ	37. Ⓐ Ⓑ Ⓒ Ⓓ	67. Ⓐ Ⓑ Ⓒ Ⓓ	97. Ⓐ Ⓑ Ⓒ Ⓓ	127. Ⓐ Ⓑ Ⓒ Ⓓ
8. Ⓐ Ⓑ Ⓒ Ⓓ	38. Ⓐ Ⓑ Ⓒ Ⓓ	68. Ⓐ Ⓑ Ⓒ Ⓓ	98. Ⓐ Ⓑ Ⓒ Ⓓ	128. Ⓐ Ⓑ Ⓒ Ⓓ
9. Ⓐ Ⓑ Ⓒ Ⓓ	39. Ⓐ Ⓑ Ⓒ Ⓓ	69. Ⓐ Ⓑ Ⓒ Ⓓ	99. Ⓐ Ⓑ Ⓒ Ⓓ	129. Ⓐ Ⓑ Ⓒ Ⓓ
10. Ⓐ Ⓑ Ⓒ Ⓓ	40. Ⓐ Ⓑ Ⓒ Ⓓ	70. Ⓐ Ⓑ Ⓒ Ⓓ	100. Ⓐ Ⓑ Ⓒ Ⓓ	130. Ⓐ Ⓑ Ⓒ Ⓓ
11. Ⓐ Ⓑ Ⓒ Ⓓ	41. Ⓐ Ⓑ Ⓒ Ⓓ	71. Ⓐ Ⓑ Ⓒ Ⓓ	101. Ⓐ Ⓑ Ⓒ Ⓓ	131. Ⓐ Ⓑ Ⓒ Ⓓ
12. Ⓐ Ⓑ Ⓒ Ⓓ	42. Ⓐ Ⓑ Ⓒ Ⓓ	72. Ⓐ Ⓑ Ⓒ Ⓓ	102. Ⓐ Ⓑ Ⓒ Ⓓ	132. Ⓐ Ⓑ Ⓒ Ⓓ
13. Ⓐ Ⓑ Ⓒ Ⓓ	43. Ⓐ Ⓑ Ⓒ Ⓓ	73. Ⓐ Ⓑ Ⓒ Ⓓ	103. Ⓐ Ⓑ Ⓒ Ⓓ	133. Ⓐ Ⓑ Ⓒ Ⓓ
14. Ⓐ Ⓑ Ⓒ Ⓓ	44. Ⓐ Ⓑ Ⓒ Ⓓ	74. Ⓐ Ⓑ Ⓒ Ⓓ	104. Ⓐ Ⓑ Ⓒ Ⓓ	134. Ⓐ Ⓑ Ⓒ Ⓓ
15. Ⓐ Ⓑ Ⓒ Ⓓ	45. Ⓐ Ⓑ Ⓒ Ⓓ	75. Ⓐ Ⓑ Ⓒ Ⓓ	105. Ⓐ Ⓑ Ⓒ Ⓓ	135. Ⓐ Ⓑ Ⓒ Ⓓ
16. Ⓐ Ⓑ Ⓒ Ⓓ	46. Ⓐ Ⓑ Ⓒ Ⓓ	76. Ⓐ Ⓑ Ⓒ Ⓓ	106. Ⓐ Ⓑ Ⓒ Ⓓ	136. Ⓐ Ⓑ Ⓒ Ⓓ
17. Ⓐ Ⓑ Ⓒ Ⓓ	47. Ⓐ Ⓑ Ⓒ Ⓓ	77. Ⓐ Ⓑ Ⓒ Ⓓ	107. Ⓐ Ⓑ Ⓒ Ⓓ	137. Ⓐ Ⓑ Ⓒ Ⓓ
18. Ⓐ Ⓑ Ⓒ Ⓓ	48. Ⓐ Ⓑ Ⓒ Ⓓ	78. Ⓐ Ⓑ Ⓒ Ⓓ	108. Ⓐ Ⓑ Ⓒ Ⓓ	138. Ⓐ Ⓑ Ⓒ Ⓓ
19. Ⓐ Ⓑ Ⓒ Ⓓ	49. Ⓐ Ⓑ Ⓒ Ⓓ	79. Ⓐ Ⓑ Ⓒ Ⓓ	109. Ⓐ Ⓑ Ⓒ Ⓓ	139. Ⓐ Ⓑ Ⓒ Ⓓ
20. Ⓐ Ⓑ Ⓒ Ⓓ	50. Ⓐ Ⓑ Ⓒ Ⓓ	80. Ⓐ Ⓑ Ⓒ Ⓓ	110. Ⓐ Ⓑ Ⓒ Ⓓ	140. Ⓐ Ⓑ Ⓒ Ⓓ
21. Ⓐ Ⓑ Ⓒ Ⓓ	51. Ⓐ Ⓑ Ⓒ Ⓓ	81. Ⓐ Ⓑ Ⓒ Ⓓ	111. Ⓐ Ⓑ Ⓒ Ⓓ	141. Ⓐ Ⓑ Ⓒ Ⓓ
22. Ⓐ Ⓑ Ⓒ Ⓓ	52. Ⓐ Ⓑ Ⓒ Ⓓ	82. Ⓐ Ⓑ Ⓒ Ⓓ	112. Ⓐ Ⓑ Ⓒ Ⓓ	142. Ⓐ Ⓑ Ⓒ Ⓓ
23. Ⓐ Ⓑ Ⓒ Ⓓ	53. Ⓐ Ⓑ Ⓒ Ⓓ	83. Ⓐ Ⓑ Ⓒ Ⓓ	113. Ⓐ Ⓑ Ⓒ Ⓓ	143. Ⓐ Ⓑ Ⓒ Ⓓ
24. Ⓐ Ⓑ Ⓒ Ⓓ	54. Ⓐ Ⓑ Ⓒ Ⓓ	84. Ⓐ Ⓑ Ⓒ Ⓓ	114. Ⓐ Ⓑ Ⓒ Ⓓ	144. Ⓐ Ⓑ Ⓒ Ⓓ
25. Ⓐ Ⓑ Ⓒ Ⓓ	55. Ⓐ Ⓑ Ⓒ Ⓓ	85. Ⓐ Ⓑ Ⓒ Ⓓ	115. Ⓐ Ⓑ Ⓒ Ⓓ	145. Ⓐ Ⓑ Ⓒ Ⓓ
26. Ⓐ Ⓑ Ⓒ Ⓓ	56. Ⓐ Ⓑ Ⓒ Ⓓ	86. Ⓐ Ⓑ Ⓒ Ⓓ	116. Ⓐ Ⓑ Ⓒ Ⓓ	146. Ⓐ Ⓑ Ⓒ Ⓓ
27. Ⓐ Ⓑ Ⓒ Ⓓ	57. Ⓐ Ⓑ Ⓒ Ⓓ	87. Ⓐ Ⓑ Ⓒ Ⓓ	117. Ⓐ Ⓑ Ⓒ Ⓓ	147. Ⓐ Ⓑ Ⓒ Ⓓ
28. Ⓐ Ⓑ Ⓒ Ⓓ	58. Ⓐ Ⓑ Ⓒ Ⓓ	88. Ⓐ Ⓑ Ⓒ Ⓓ	118. Ⓐ Ⓑ Ⓒ Ⓓ	148. Ⓐ Ⓑ Ⓒ Ⓓ
29. Ⓐ Ⓑ Ⓒ Ⓓ	59. Ⓐ Ⓑ Ⓒ Ⓓ	89. Ⓐ Ⓑ Ⓒ Ⓓ	119. Ⓐ Ⓑ Ⓒ Ⓓ	149. Ⓐ Ⓑ Ⓒ Ⓓ
30. Ⓐ Ⓑ Ⓒ Ⓓ	60. Ⓐ Ⓑ Ⓒ Ⓓ	90. Ⓐ Ⓑ Ⓒ Ⓓ	120. Ⓐ Ⓑ Ⓒ Ⓓ	150. Ⓐ Ⓑ Ⓒ Ⓓ

Practice Test 2

COMPONENT A

Directions: Choose the option that best answers the questions.

1. Pain intensity is primarily determined by the
   (A) type of stimulation.
   (B) severity of stimulation.
   (C) number of fibers stimulated.
   (D) body area that is stimulated.
   (E) nerve cells' degree of stimulation.

2. Penumbra refers to
   (A) magnification.
   (B) distance.
   (C) exposure time.
   (D) a partial shadow.
   (E) the number of photons.

3. Which of the following illnesses has an incubation period of approximately 2 to 3 weeks?
   (A) Common cold
   (B) Tuberculosis
   (C) Scarlet fever
   (D) Chicken pox
   (E) Strep throat

4. Dental hygiene professionals should regularly review relevant professional literature. Each of the following is a criterion that can help dental health professionals determine the overall quality of professional literature **EXCEPT** one. Which one is the **EXCEPTION**?
   (A) The quality of article references
   (B) Whether an article is current
   (C) Whether the author is qualified
   (D) The cost of the journal or article
   (E) Whether the journal is peer reviewed

5. Which of the following cautions should be provided to a patient taking acetaminophen?
   (A) Avoid if taking Warfarin
   (B) Avoid physical activity
   (C) Avoid hot foods and drinks
   (D) Avoid operating machinery
   (E) Avoid taking with alcohol

6. Which of the following is a characteristic of enamel hypoplasia?
   (A) Pitted enamel
   (B) Mottled enamel
   (C) Brown bands on enamel
   (D) Green staining on enamel
   (E) Demineralization of enamel

7. During which of the following mitosis phases do the chromosomes line up along the midplane?
   (A) Interphase
   (B) Prophase
   (C) Metaphase
   (D) Anaphase
   (E) Telophase

8. The tonsils drain into the
   (A) lacrimal ducts.
   (B) nasal conchae.
   (C) nasal meatuses.
   (D) ethmoid air cells.
   (E) superior deep cervical nodes.

9. To control the spread of infection, dental hygiene professionals should change gloves every 2 hours **BECAUSE** defects usually begin to occur at about this time.
   (A) Both the statement and reason are correct and related.
   (B) Both the statement and reason are correct but NOT related.
   (C) The statement is correct, but the reason is NOT.
   (D) The statement is NOT correct, but the reason is correct.
   (E) NEITHER the statement NOR the reason is correct.

10. Which of the following **BEST** describes gingivoplasty?
    (A) A procedure to remove enlarged tissue
    (B) A procedure to regenerate lost tissue
    (C) A procedure to eliminate periodontal pockets
    (D) A surgery to improve the facial image of the client
    (E) An excisional surgery that reshapes gingival tissues

11. Panoramic radiographs should be used in conjunction with
    (A) E-speed film.
    (B) periapical X-rays.
    (C) extraoral film.
    (D) less exposure time.
    (E) film emulsion.

12. According to the teleological theory of ethics, whether an action can be considered ethical depends on its consequences.

    According to deontologic ethics, the ethicality of an action depends on the intention behind it.
    (A) Both statements are true.
    (B) Both statements are false.
    (C) The first statement is true, the second is false.
    (D) The first statement is false, the second is true.

13. How many chromosomes are found in the human nucleus?
    (A) 12
    (B) 22
    (C) 34
    (D) 46
    (E) 58

14. Tetracyclines often cause suprainfections **BECAUSE** this class of antibiotics binds to the 30S ribosome and impedes the synthesis of proteins.
    (A) Both the statement and reason are correct and related.
    (B) Both the statement and reason are correct but NOT related.
    (C) The statement is correct, but the reason is NOT.
    (D) The statement is NOT correct, but the reason is correct.
    (E) NEITHER the statement NOR the reason is correct.

15. After telling Mark about the importance of flossing to prevent dental caries, Mark shares with Beth that he suffered an injury at the workplace that adversely affected his dexterity. Based on this information, Beth should discuss the use of which of the following ideas during the educational session?
    (A) Floss threaders
    (B) Knitting yarn
    (C) Pipe cleaners
    (D) Wooden toothpicks
    (E) Floss holders

16. Which of the following microorganisms forms protective cysts to survive harsh environments?
    (A) Yeast
    (B) Bacteria
    (C) Viruses
    (D) Protozoa
    (E) Mold

17. Which of the following chemotherapeutic agents is an antimetabolite?
    (A) Melphalan
    (B) Thiotepa
    (C) Busulfan
    (D) Methotraxate
    (E) Cyclophosphamide

18. When populations are assessed, certain groups are often found to be at a high risk of developing oral health issues. Which of the following individuals would **MOST LIKELY** be part of a high-risk group?
    (A) A woman who has a 2-year-old and a 4-year-old
    (B) A 20-year-old currently enrolled in a college program
    (C) A chiropractor who earns more than $100,000 a year
    (D) A 75-year-old man who still resides in his own home
    (E) A man who lives in a house in an urban community

19. During interactions in the dental setting, a dental hygiene professional should avoid entering a patient's second zone of personal space.

    The third zone of personal space extends from approximately 18 inches away from an individual to about 4 feet.
    (A) Both statements are true.
    (B) Both statements are false.
    (C) The first statement is true, the second is false.
    (D) The first statement is false, the second is true

20. Each of the following techniques relies on the sense of touch to assess a patient during the head and neck examination **EXCEPT** one. Which one is the **EXCEPTION**?
    (A) Digital palpation
    (B) Circular compression
    (C) Bilateral palpation
    (D) Auscultation
    (E) Bimanual palpation

21. The mandibular second deciduous molar erupts at
    (A) 6 months.
    (B) 9 months.
    (C) 16 months.
    (D) 20 months.
    (E) 34 months.

22. Which of the following best describes periodontal flap surgery?
    (A) An excisional surgery that removes diseases gingival tissue
    (B) A surgery that corrects diseased pocket beyond the mucogingival junction
    (C) An incisional surgery that exposes underlying bone and root surface for removal of diseased tissue
    (D) A surgery that corrects bone defects by resculpting the bone
    (E) An excisional surgery that reshapes gingival tissues

23. Each of the following is a risk factor for people suffering with metabolic syndrome **EXCEPT** one. Which one is the **EXCEPTION**?
    (A) Chronic obstructive pulmonary disease
    (B) Coronary heart disease
    (C) Type 2 diabetes
    (D) Peripheral vascular disease
    (E) Stroke

24. Dental diagnosis identifies human-needs deficits.

    Dental hygiene diagnosis identifies specific oral diseases.
    (A) Both statements are true.
    (B) Both statements are false.
    (C) The first statement is true, but the second is false.
    (D) The first statement is false, but the second is true.

25. The first step in applying a sealant is to clean debris from the pits and fissures.

    The second step is to apply the sealant.
    (A) Both statements are true.
    (B) Both statements are false.
    (C) The first statement is true, the second is false.
    (D) The first statement is false, the second is true.

26. A patient with orthodontics will benefit most from fluoride
    (A) varnish.
    (B) gel.
    (C) foam.
    (D) tablets.
    (E) sealants.

Use the following scenario to answer questions 27–29.

Beth, a dental hygiene professional, is planning an informal meeting with a patient named Mark. Over the last two years, Mark has had a higher than average number of carious lesions. During his last two visits, Beth noticed that he had significant plaque accumulation both on the surfaces of his teeth and in between his teeth. She also noticed dark brown staining on the lingual surfaces of his teeth. She is hoping a short session of individual instruction can help address these issues.

27. While instructing Mark on how to prevent carious lesions, Beth is planning to demonstrate proper brushing technique. Based on the information above about Mark's oral health issues, which of the following techniques should Beth plan to demonstrate for Mark?
    (A) Bass
    (B) Fones
    (C) Charters
    (D) Leonard
    (E) Stillman

28. Based on the types of stains Beth noticed on Mark's teeth, which of the following should she include in her educational session aside from a demonstration of proper brushing technique?
    (A) Major symptoms of pulp necrosis
    (B) Effects of bacteria on tooth color
    (C) How food pigments can stain teeth
    (D) Removal techniques for coffee stains
    (E) Effects of tobacco on oral health

29. Beth plans to educate Mark about the role of brushing and flossing in dental caries prevention during her individualized education session. Which of the these pieces of information would **MOST LIKELY** also be useful?
    (A) Cariogenic bacteria demineralize tooth surfaces.
    (B) *S. sanguis* is connected to low sugar intake.
    (C) Drinking sugary sodas can increase caries risk.
    (D) *Lactobacilli* can form caries-causing acid.
    (E) A high-carbohydrate diet can lead to teeth staining.

30. If an image is blurred, what is the corrective measure to ensure that the next image is clear?
    (A) Clear all equipment out of the way of the beam.
    (B) Use fresh film.
    (C) Ask the patient to remain still.
    (D) Adjust the vertical angluation.
    (E) Monitor temperature in the dark room.

31. Patients with a history of bulimia are likely to present with each of the following oral manifestations **EXCEPT** one. Which one is the **EXCEPTION**?
    (A) Parotid gland swelling
    (B) Severe caries
    (C) Burning tongue
    (D) Perimyolysis
    (E) Adenoidal hyperplasia

32. Dental hygiene professionals may need to communicate with hearing-impaired individuals in their line of work. One way to improve the quality of communications with these individuals is to
    (A) stand a few inches away from the patient.
    (B) employ affective learning techniques.
    (C) repeat information without being asked.
    (D) speak with the help of another hygienist.
    (E) reduce or eliminate background noise.

33. A benign soft tissue lesion composed of a circumscribed mass of mature fat cells is known as a
    (A) papilloma.
    (B) fibroma.
    (C) hemangioma.
    (D) lipoma.
    (E) granuloma.

34. Recurrent aphthous stomatitis is commonly caused by exposure to *Bacillus fusiformis* or *Borreliavincentii*.

    Patients with this condition usually present with oval or round ulcerations with a yellow-white fibrous surface encircled by a red halo.
    (A) Both statements are true.
    (B) Both statements are false.
    (C) The first statement is true, the second is false.
    (D) The first statement is false, the second is true.

35. A patient suffering from what condition would be particularly likely to develop a brown tumor?
    (A) Hypoparathyroidism
    (B) Hypertension
    (C) Hyperparathyroidism
    (D) Hyperthyroidism
    (E) Hypotension

36. Heartbeats become stronger and slower after taking
    (A) antianginal agents.
    (B) digitalis glycosides.
    (C) antihypertensives.
    (D) angiotensin II blockers.
    (E) vasodilators.

37. Each of the following should be avoided by dental hygiene professionals when communicating oral health information to patients **EXCEPT** one. Which one is the **EXCEPTION**?
    (A) Providing information while sitting alongside a patient
    (B) Providing information while polishing a patient's teeth
    (C) Providing information while standing and facing a patient
    (D) Providing information while filling out a patient's chart
    (E) Providing information while sitting and facing a patient

38. A dental hygiene worker wants to prevent the spread of infection from patient to patient. Which of the following strategies would be most effective in terms of accomplishing this?
    (A) The dental hygiene worker wears a mask while scraping a patient's teeth.
    (B) The dental hygiene worker provides protective eyewear for all patients.
    (C) The dental hygiene worker sterilizes cleaning instruments used on patients.
    (D) The dental hygiene worker uses a rubber dam for certain patient procedures.
    (E) The dental hygiene worker stores instruments in cassettes during cleaning.

39. A child has just gotten his 6-year-old molars. The **BEST** way to prevent dental caries in the molars is to
    (A) use a rotating head toothbrush.
    (B) floss twice a day.
    (C) apply pit-and-fissure sealants.
    (D) take fluoride supplements.
    (E) drink fluoridated water.

40. During a severe bacterial infection, septic shock can occur **BECAUSE** the infection can trigger high levels of different types of leukocytes.
    (A) Both the statement and the reason are correct and related.
    (B) Both the statement and the reason are correct but NOT related.
    (C) The statement is correct but the reason is NOT.
    (D) The statement is NOT correct, but the reason is correct.
    (E) NEITHER the statement NOR the reason is correct.

41. Iodine solutions are disclosing agents that are commonly used as educational tools by dental hygienists **BECAUSE** they can help make bacterial plaque visible.
    (A) Both the statement and reason are correct and related.
    (B) Both the statement and reason are correct but NOT related.
    (C) The statement is correct, but the reason is NOT.
    (D) The statement is NOT correct, but the reason is correct.
    (E) NEITHER the statement NOR the reason is correct.

42. The primary purpose of polishing a restoration is to
    (A) clean the restoration.
    (B) remove surface irregularities.
    (C) improve aesthetic appearance.
    (D) clear plaque buildup.
    (E) extract harmful materials.

43. Fluoridation added to drinking water reduces tooth decay by
    (A) 10–15 percent.
    (B) 15–20 percent.
    (C) 20–25 percent.
    (D) 20–40 percent.
    (E) 25–50 percent.

44. Which of the following essential nutrients is made up of thousands of amino acids?
    (A) Fats
    (B) Proteins
    (C) Carbohydrates
    (D) Vitamins
    (E) Minerals

45. Which of the following is a Gram-negative microorganism?
    (A) *Listeria*
    (B) *Actinomyces*
    (C) *Strepococcus*
    (D) *Staphlococcus*
    (E) *Campylobacter*

46. A lecture is one method that can be used to present instructional units that are part of a community program. Which of the following is a disadvantage usually associated with lectures, or informative talks?
    (A) They stifle the creativity of learners.
    (B) They do not work well with large groups.
    (C) They require the use of technology.
    (D) They must be prepared carefully.
    (E) They may require special facilities.

47. Each of the following is true about the body's clotting system **EXCEPT** one. Which one is the **EXCEPTION**?
    (A) It helps form thrombin.
    (B) It produces kininogens and kallikreins.
    (C) It can be activated by collagen and protease.
    (D) It prevents the spread of infection.
    (E) It localizes microorganisms.

48. Which of the following would a dentist **MOST LIKELY** administer to a patient to reduce anxiety before an operation?
    (A) Lidocaine
    (B) Salicylates
    (C) Benocaine
    (D) Barbiturates
    (E) Ketamine

49. Smoking is a major cause of oral cancer. Which of the following is an educational approach that may be useful in terms of convincing youths not to start smoking?
    (A) Demonstrate how to refuse offers of cigarettes from peers.
    (B) Ban smoking on school property and at school functions.
    (C) Enforce strict consequences for those caught smoking.
    (D) Prohibit all forms of tobacco, including chewing tobacco.
    (E) Offer nicotine replacement therapies such as patches at no cost.

50. While conducting a study, researchers created and compiled a list of oral health scores for members of a community. Five of these scores were 9, 9, 5, 8, and 4. What is the mean oral health score of these five individuals?
    (A) 5
    (B) 6
    (C) 7
    (D) 8
    (E) 9

51. A patient who is allergic to one ester will have an allergic reaction to all other anesthetics derived from ester **BECAUSE** all anesthetics are cross-reactive.
    (A) Both the statement and the reason are correct and related.
    (B) The statement and the reason are correct but NOT related.
    (C) The statement is correct, but the reason is NOT.
    (D) The statement is NOT correct, but the reason is correct.
    (E) NEITHER the statement NOR the reason is correct.

52. What is the normal heart rate range for a healthy adult?
    (A) 60–100 beats per minute
    (B) 70–110 beats per minute
    (C) 80–130 beats per minute
    (D) 100–140 beats per minute
    (E) 120–160 beats per minute

53. Additional quadrant debridement should be accomplished at 2-week intervals.

    Six weeks after the last appointment, another reevaluation of pockets is made.
    (A) Both statements are true.
    (B) Both statements are false.
    (C) The first statement is true, but the second statement is false.
    (D) The first statement is false, but the second statement is true.

54. What percentage of enamel is inorganic?
    (A) 40
    (B) 55
    (C) 60
    (D) 75
    (E) 95

55. Patients taking which type of medication may have a limited ability to metabolize vasoconstrictors?
    (A) MAO inhibitors
    (B) Anticoagulants
    (C) NSAIDs
    (D) ACE inhibitors
    (E) Corticosteroids

56. Systemic fluoride provides topical protection to teeth **BECAUSE** low levels of fluoride in saliva continuously bathe teeth.
    (A) Both the statement and the reason are correct and related.
    (B) Both the statement and the reason are correct but NOT related.
    (C) The statement is correct, but the reason is NOT.
    (D) The statement is NOT correct, but the reason is correct.
    (E) Neither the statement NOR the reason is correct.

57. Acidulated phosphate fluoride should not be used on patients with crowns, bridges, veneers, or composite restorations **BECAUSE** its acidity may lead to the corrosion of metalwork or other surfaces.
    (A) Both the statement and the reason are correct and related.
    (B) Both the statement and reason are correct but NOT related.
    (C) The statement is correct, but the reason is NOT.
    (D) The statement is NOT correct, but the reason is correct.
    (E) Neither the statement NOR the reason is correct.

58. Dental sealant programs should be introduced only in communities where drinking water is not fluoridated.

    Sealants are not covered by insurance so parents will have to pay for them out of pocket.
    (A) Both statements are true.
    (B) Both statements are false.
    (C) The first statement is true, the second is false.
    (D) The first statement is false, the second is true.

59. Which of the following is an example of an injury or illness that would **MOST LIKELY** cause fibrosis?
    (A) Myocardial infarction
    (B) Skin wound
    (C) Partial hepatectomy
    (D) Cirrhosis
    (E) Lobar pneumonia

60. The Internet is one educational aid that may be used in community programs. The main issue with using the Internet as a source of information is
    (A) the Internet contains information that is too complex for the public.
    (B) many community members will not know how to use the Internet.
    (C) the Internet contains inaccurate information about dental health.
    (D) many community members will not have access to the Internet.
    (E) the Internet does not contain much information on dental health.

61. Which of the following is the pH level at which carious enamel lesions occur?
    (A) 4.5–5.5
    (B) 5.5–6.5
    (C) 6.5–7.5
    (D) 7.5–8.5
    (E) 8.5–9.5

62. Which artery supplies the brain with blood?
    (A) Internal carotid artery
    (B) External carotid artery
    (C) Greater palatine artery
    (D) Inferior alveolar artery
    (E) Temporal artery

63. Each of the following vitamins is water soluble **EXCEPT** one. Which one is the **EXCEPTION**?
    (A) Folate
    (B) Vitamin C
    (C) Vitamin E
    (D) Thiamin
    (E) Biotin

64. Nursing-bottle decay does not typically affect the mandibular anterior teeth **BECAUSE** it tends to affect the maxillary anterior teeth first.
    (A) Both the statement and reason are correct and related.
    (B) Both the statement and reason are correct but NOT related.
    (C) The statement is correct, but the reason is NOT.
    (D) The statement is NOT correct, but the reason is correct.
    (E) NEITHER the statement NOR the reason is correct.

65. Patients at risk for endocarditis must be treated with an antibiotic before dental procedures **BECAUSE** some dental procedures can cut up the gums, allowing bacteria into the bloodstream.
    (A) Both the statement and reason are correct and related.
    (B) Both the statement and reason are correct but NOT related.
    (C) The statement is correct, but the reason is NOT.
    (D) The statement is NOT correct, but the reason is correct.
    (E) NEITHER the statement NOR the reason is correct.

66. Which of the following describes the process of incidental curettage as a therapy for periodontitis?
    (A) Removal of calculus deposits
    (B) Removal of bacterial irritants
    (C) Removal of a thin layer of diseased pocket epithelium
    (D) Regrowth of bone that was destroyed by bacteria
    (E) Soft tissue grafting to replace damaged tissue

67. When implementing community health programs, it is important to keep in mind that educational strategies can include both formal and informal activities. Which of the following is an example of an informal activity?
    (A) An educational seminar conducted by several dental health professionals
    (B) A conversation between a dental hygiene professional and a member of the public
    (C) An elementary school program designed to encourage students to floss daily
    (D) A health fair at a local community center designed to promote dental health
    (E) A presentation by a dental hygiene professional on gingivitis to a high school class

68. What is one action of β-1 receptors in the sympathetic autonomic nervous system (SANS)?
    (A) Constricting smooth muscles
    (B) Relaxing smooth muscles
    (C) Increasing heart rate
    (D) Decreasing heart rate
    (E) Stimulating bronchodilation

69. Which of the chemical mediators of acute inflammation causes vasodilatation and pain?
    (A) Histamine
    (B) Bradykinin
    (C) Nitric oxide
    (D) Chemokines
    (E) Prostaglandins

70. What is the name of the sweetener used in some foods and beverages that can help prevent dental health problems by reducing the risk of caries and limiting plaque formation?
    (A) Aspartame
    (B) Saccharin
    (C) Xylitol
    (D) Sucralose
    (E) Neotame

71. Each of the following is a piece of information that should be recorded when administering injected anesthetic **EXCEPT** one. Which one is the **EXCEPTION**?
    (A) The amount of drug administered
    (B) The patient's reactions to the drug
    (C) The ratio of vasoconstrictor
    (D) The percentage of drug administered
    (E) The type of syringe used

72. Each of the following statements is true about viruses **EXCEPT** one. Which one is the **EXCEPTION**?
    (A) Viruses are eukaryotic.
    (B) Viruses are symmetrical.
    (C) Viruses feed off other cells.
    (D) Viruses cannot reproduce outside a host.
    (E) Viruses contain small amounts of DNA.

73. During digestion, the bodily secretion that breaks down fat is
    (A) trypsin.
    (B) pepsin.
    (C) saliva.
    (D) bile.
    (E) mucus.

74. Each of the following should be indicated in a patient's medical history **EXCEPT** one. Which one is the **EXCEPTION**?
    (A) Allergic reaction to a medication
    (B) Tobacco use
    (C) Daily medications
    (D) Dependency on alcohol
    (E) Oral habits such as grinding teeth

75. Bell's palsy is a form of facial paralysis.

    It affects the trigeminal nerve.
    (A) Both statements are true.
    (B) Both statements are false.
    (C) The first statement is true, the second is false.
    (D) The first statement is false, the second is true.

76. Each of the following is an example of a genetic disorder associated with periodontitis **EXCEPT** one. Which one is the **EXCEPTION**?
    (A) HIV-associated periodontitis
    (B) Cohen's syndrome
    (C) Papillon-Lefevre syndrome
    (D) Down syndrome
    (E) Neutropenia

77. What is the normal respiration rate for healthy adults?
    (A) 5 to 10 breaths per minute
    (B) 10 to 15 breaths per minute
    (C) 14 to 20 breaths per minute
    (D) 20 to 25 breaths per minute
    (E) 18 to 30 breaths per minute

78. A dental hygiene professional is reading a scientific study on the incidence of dental caries in African American men. Which of the following parts of the study would represent the second step of the scientific method?
    (A) A discussion of the adverse effects of dental caries in the general population and the prevalence of the problem
    (B) The conclusion that the incidence of dental caries in African American men was lower than expected
    (C) The suggestion that the original hypothesis about African American men and dental caries be rejected
    (D) The hypothesis that African American men are more susceptible to dental caries than Caucasian men
    (E) The section containing charts and tables of the data collected about the study's target population

79. Which branchial arch gives rise to the sphenoid bone?
    (A) First
    (B) Second
    (C) Third
    (D) Fourth
    (E) Fifth

80. Which part of the endocrine system regulates the body's homeostasis?
    (A) Spleen
    (B) Thymus
    (C) Thyroid
    (D) Medulla
    (E) Hypothalamus

81. A male dental hygiene professional is working in a state where he is permitted to take dental X-rays under indirect or close supervision. This means that the dentist
    (A) must be present in the facility while the X-rays are taken.
    (B) must be with the hygienist while the X-rays are taken.
    (C) must be available by phone while the X-rays are taken.
    (D) doesn't need to provide authorization before the X-rays are taken.
    (E) doesn't need to be present or available while the X-rays are taken.

82. Drugs that are more ionized will be absorbed more readily by the body.

    Drugs that are more lipid soluble will be absorbed less readily by the body.
    (A) Both statements are true.
    (B) Both statements are false.
    (C) The first statement is true, the second is false.
    (D) The first statement is false, the second is true.

83. The main purpose of a case presentation is to
    (A) meet legal and ethical requirements, reach a treatment agreement, and obtain informed consent.
    (B) educate clients about the dental hygiene procedures they will need to undergo in order to meet their personal goals.
    (C) provide clients with an overview of their dental health and hygiene needs.
    (D) outline the various commitments clients will have to make in order to reach their personal goals.
    (E) impress upon clients the need for proper dental hygiene care and encourage them to accept your plan.

84. Which of the following is true about walking strokes?
    (A) They are used with all instruments for assessment purposes.
    (B) They are the most difficult type of stroke to learn.
    (C) They act as a scaling stroke and are used with treatment instruments.
    (D) They require tight controlled grasp with heavy pressure.
    (E) They are used with probes since EA varies in depth and contour.

85. A dental hygiene professional is educating a patient on how to manage tooth hypersensitivity. The dental hygienist recommends desensitizing toothpaste and gives the patients a list of ingredients to look for when shopping for toothpaste for sensitive teeth. Each of these ingredients will likely be on the list **EXCEPT** one. Which one is the **EXCEPTION**?
    (A) Potassium nitrate
    (B) Calcium hydroxide
    (C) Chlorine oxalate
    (D) Strontium chloride
    (E) Sodium citrate

86. The main goal of providing individualized patient education is to
    (A) diagnose oral health problems.
    (B) cure oral health problems.
    (C) predict oral health problems.
    (D) prevent oral health problems.
    (E) explain oral health problems.

87. An optimal fluoride level in drinking water as recommended by the U.S. Public Health Service is
    (A) 0.25–.50 parts per million.
    (B) 0.7–1.2 parts per million.
    (C) 0.5–2.0 parts per million.
    (D) 1.0–1.5 parts per million.
    (E) 2.0–3.0 parts per million.

88. Which of the following tests is designed to determine the hardness of a dental material using a square-based diamond point?
    (A) Knoops
    (B) Brinell
    (C) Rockwell
    (D) Vickers
    (E) Mohs

89. Air polishers and ultrasonic scalers should **NOT** be used on patients with
(A) bulimia.
(B) cerebral palsy.
(C) hepatitis.
(D) celiac disease.
(E) diabetes.

90. Which of the following tooth-brushing techniques is **NOT** recommended due to its up and down vertical motion from maxillary to mandibular teeth?
(A) Fones
(B) Bass
(C) Scrub
(D) Leonard
(E) Charter's

91. Corticosteroids are usually prescribed for the treatment of
(A) white sponge nevus.
(B) linea alba.
(C) leukoedema.
(D) nicotine stomatitis.
(E) lichen planus.

92. A program plan should include a section that identifies the resources required for a community program. Each of the following should be considered when determining the resources required for a program **EXCEPT** one. Which one is the **EXCEPTION**?
(A) Whether the resources are appropriate
(B) Whether the resources are adequate
(C) Whether the resources are locally made
(D) Whether the resources will be efficient
(E) Whether the resources will be effective

93. Which of the following word parts indicates a type of bacteria is arranged in chains?
(A) *Diplo*
(B) *Spirillum*
(C) *Strepto*
(D) *Coccus*
(E) *Staphylo*

94. A patient in a dental office has just received a dental prosthesis. The patient should be told to change her diet by eating only
(A) food without fats for 24 hours.
(B) liquid foods for 24 hours.
(C) food without carbohydrates for 24 hours.
(D) soft foods for 24 hours.
(E) food without protein for 24 hours.

95. A periodontal screening of a patient reveals that calculus deposits are present. This patient's periodontal screening and report (PSR) score will most likely be
(A) 0.
(B) 1.
(C) 2.
(D) 3.
(E) 4.

96. Which cranial nerve is the largest nerve in the body?
(A) Optic
(B) Olfactory
(C) Trochlear
(D) Trigeminal
(E) Oculomotor

97. Which of the following describes the characteristics of a Grade IV furcation involvement?
(A) Severe involvement, through-and-through visible furcation, complete loss of interradicular bone
(B) Severe involvement, probe enters root to opposite side, complete loss of interradicular bone
(C) Moderate involvement, probe just enters into furcation, some loss of interradicular bone
(D) Early involvement, probe just into the notch, no interradicular bone loss
(E) No involvement or bone loss present

98. A study is being conducted to assess how effective a new mouthwash is at preventing dental caries. The makers of the mouthwash recommend swishing 15 mL of the mouthwash for 30 seconds for optimal results. The control group would **MOST LIKELY** be given
(A) 5 mL of the mouthwash and told to swish for 30 seconds.
(B) 30 mL of the mouthwash and told to swish for 30 seconds.
(C) 15 mL of another new mouthwash and told to swish for 30 seconds.
(D) 15 mL of the mouthwash and told to swish for 30 seconds.
(E) 15 mL of water and told to swish for 30 seconds.

Use this scenario to answer questions 99–102.

A mother brings her child in for his first routine visit. The child is 5 years old and has already gotten his 6-year-old molars. The dentist likes to have radiographs taken on children at their first dental visits to get close-up readings of their teeth and gums to help diagnose any problems early in their development. The mother does not like the idea of exposing her child to radiation at such a young age, but she agrees with the condition that she must be in the room. The child is situated in the chair, and the backrest and headrest are adjusted to make the patient as comfortable as possible to minimize movement during exposure. The radiographs show darkening between the molar and cuspid on the right side of the mouth.

99. How far away from the child should the mother be when the radiographs are administered?
(A) 60–100 degrees
(B) 75–125 degrees
(C) 85–140 degrees
(D) 90–135 degrees
(E) 100–150 degrees

100. What type of radiograph should be taken of this 5-year-old?
(A) Panoramic radiograph
(B) Bitewing radiograph
(C) Periapical radiograph
(D) Occlusal radiograph
(E) Full-mouth series

101. In order to get an accurate image of the 6-year-old molars, to what degree should the average angulation of the tube be adjusted?
(A) +2 degrees
(B) +5 degrees
(C) +8 degrees
(D) +11 degrees
(E) +12 degrees

102. The FDA recommends radiographs be taken on young children at the first dental visit when the
(A) proximal surfaces cannot be explored with a dental instrument.
(B) parents are in agreement that radiographs are needed.
(C) child is experiencing pain in a certain area of the mouth.
(D) doctor believes that radiographs are warranted.
(E) patient has a strong gag reflex.

103. Each of the following is an example of a type of surgical intervention for periodontitis **EXCEPT** one. Which one is the **EXCEPTION**?
(A) Cortical plate surgery
(B) Excisional surgery
(C) Periodontal flap surgery
(D) Mucogingival surgery
(E) Osseous surgery

104. One of the main symptoms of *staphylococcal* food poisoning is a high fever.

Staphylococcal food poisoning usually occurs from unrefrigerated dairy products.
(A) Both statements are true.
(B) Both statements are false.
(C) The first statement is true, the second is false.
(D) The first statement is false, the second is true.

105. A patient wants to review the information on file about her dental care. The patient
(A) is not permitted to review confidential information.
(B) must submit a formal request for the dentist to review.
(C) may view the information in the office but not remove it.
(D) can both review the information and make copies to remove.
(E) is allowed to dictate which information will remain in the file.

106. A 50-year-old woman has been a dental hygienist for 10 years. The maximum permissible dose per year for this hygienist is
(A) 0.25 rem.
(B) 2.5 rem.
(C) 5 rem.
(D) 100 rem.
(E) 150 rem.

107. Each of the following is a benefit associated with the fluoridation of drinking water **EXCEPT** one. Which one is the **EXCEPTION**?
    (A) Prevention of dental caries
    (B) Fewer incidences of missing teeth
    (C) A decreased incidence of malocclusion
    (D) Decreased need for dental cleanings
    (E) Less need for complex restoration procedures

108. There are several standards of professional responsibility specific to the dental hygiene profession. Which of the following is a responsibility a dental hygienist has to his or her community or to society in general?
    (A) Make an effort to avoid conflicts of interest related to work that may arise.
    (B) Show respect for those employed in professions other than dental hygiene.
    (C) Make an effort to establish a positive image of the dental hygiene profession.
    (D) Report illegal actions by any health-care provider to the proper authorities.
    (E) Try to increase public awareness of oral health practices whenever possible.

109. For how long does a varnish impregnate a tooth with fluoride after it has been applied topically?
    (A) 1–2 hours
    (B) 2–3 hours
    (C) 3–4 hours
    (D) 4–5 hours
    (E) 5–6 hours

110. Which of the following digestive system components produce pepsinogen?
    (A) Parietal cells
    (B) Goblet cells
    (C) Chief cells
    (D) Intrinsic factor
    (E) Gastric lipase

111. Each of the following is true of schedule II drugs **EXCEPT** one. Which one is the **EXCEPTION**?
    (A) The prescriber must sign prescriptions for schedule II drugs.
    (B) Emergency prescriptions for schedule II drugs can be phoned in.
    (C) Morphine and Oxycodone are two examples of schedule II drugs.
    (D) Schedule II drugs are considered to have a great potential for abuse.
    (E) Prescriptions for schedule II drugs can be refilled up to five times.

112. After a quadrant root debridement procedure, each pocket should be reevaluated for
    (A) scaling.
    (B) antibiotic therapy.
    (C) additional root debridement.
    (D) periodontal prophylaxis.
    (E) incidental curettage.

113. Each of the following is a classic sign of inflammation **EXCEPT** one. Which one is the **EXCEPTION**?
    (A) Heat
    (B) Pain
    (C) Redness
    (D) Bleeding
    (E) Swelling

114. A program plan should have clear, yet somewhat flexible, deadlines.

    A strengths, weaknesses, opportunities, and threats (SWOT) analysis is an important element of a program plan.
    (A) Both statements are true.
    (B) Both statements are false.
    (C) The first statement is true, the second is false.
    (D) The first statement is false, the second is true.

115. Fungi are microorganisms classified as eukaryotes.

    Fungi are classified as photosynthetic organisms.
    (A) Both statements are true.
    (B) Both statements are false.
    (C) The first statement is true, the second is false.
    (D) The first statement is false, the second is true.

116. Each of the following is a monosaccharide **EXCEPT** one. Which one is the **EXCEPTION**?
(A) Glucose
(B) Fructose
(C) Lactose
(D) Dextrose
(E) Galactose

117. Which of the following should **NOT** be listed on a dental hygiene treatment plan?
(A) Alternative treatments
(B) Required number of appointments
(C) Specialist referrals
(D) Cost of treatment
(E) Risk factors

118. A dental hygiene professional is reading a scientific study. To collect data for the study, the authors used a list of members residing in a specific community. Names were arranged randomly. The authors compiled data by looking at specific characteristics of every tenth person on the list. The sampling technique the study authors used is called
(A) stratified sampling.
(B) systematic sampling.
(C) purposive sampling.
(D) convenience sampling.
(E) nonrandom sampling.

119. Which facial bone has no muscle attachments?
(A) Occipital bone
(B) Temporal bone
(C) Condyle bone
(D) Vomer bone
(E) Zygoma bone

Use the following scenario to answer questions 120–123.

A mother brings her 2-year-old toddler to your dental practice. The child has never been to the dentist before and is experiencing a high level of anxiety about the appointment. The mother is unaware of any allergies or underlying medical conditions, and the child appears to be in good health with vital signs in the normal range. During the oral evaluation, you assign the patient a plaque index score of 0.4. You also detect no signs of fremitus.

120. Which of the following would be a normal respiratory rate for this patient?
(A) 10–20 breaths per minute
(B) 12–20 breaths per minute
(C) 15–25 breaths per minute
(D) 20–35 breaths per minute
(E) 25–40 breaths per minute

121. Using the physical status classification of the American Society of Anesthesiology (ASA), you should classify this patient as
(A) Category I.
(B) Category II.
(C) Category III.
(D) Category IV.
(E) Category V.

122. Which of the following would be an appropriate rating for this patient's home care?
(A) Inconclusive
(B) Poor
(C) Fair
(D) Good
(E) Excellent

123. Which of the following is the correct fremitus classification for this patient?
(A) 0
(B) N
(C) +
(D) ++
(E) +++

124. A female dental hygienist is conducting a patient education session with an individual who has HIV-associated periodontitis. When the dental hygiene professional discusses managing the disease, which of the following types of medications should she mention?
(A) Analgesics
(B) ACE inhibitors
(C) Anti-inflammatories
(D) Antiviral drugs
(E) Antibiotics

125. Traumatic occlusion can cause periodontal disease **BECAUSE** it can contribute to a more rapid spread of inflammation and cause teeth to become mobile from widening of the periodontal ligament.
(A) Both the statement and reason are correct and related.
(B) Both the statement and reason are correct but NOT related.
(C) The statement is correct, but the reason is NOT.
(D) The statement is NOT correct, but the reason is correct.
(E) NEITHER the statement NOR the reason is correct.

126. Viruses are usually larger than bacteria.

Viruses have more complex structures than bacteria.
(A) Both statements are true.
(B) Both statements are false.
(C) The first statement is true, the second is false.
(D) The first statement is false, the second is true.

127. The research results of one study led the authors to conclude that there is a negative correlation between average brushing time and the number of fillings required before adulthood. This means that
(A) as brushing time increases, the number of fillings decreases.
(B) as brushing time increases, the number of fillings increases.
(C) as brushing time decreases, the number of fillings decreases.
(D) brushing time has a negative effect on dental fillings.
(E) brushing time does not affect dental filling numbers.

128. Into which phase of dental care planning would the placement of implants fall?
(A) Preliminary phase
(B) Phase I
(C) Phase II
(D) Phase III
(E) Phase IV

129. Which of the following describes the process of scaling and root debridement?
(A) Removal of all hard and soft deposits from root and coronal surfaces of teeth
(B) Removal of a thin layer of diseased cementum
(C) Removal of a thin layer of diseased pocket epithelium
(D) Application of antibiotics to area of inflammation
(E) Complete removal of infected teeth

130. Ultrasonic inserts for periodontal debridement have either internal or external water conduits.

Ultrasonic inserts for periodontal debridement come in a number of shapes and sizes.
(A) Both statements are true.
(B) Both statements are false.
(C) The first statement is true, the second is false.
(D) The first statement is false, the second is true.

131. At which week in utero do the tooth buds develop?
(A) 5
(B) 6
(C) 7
(D) 8
(E) 9

132. Fat from foods can coat the teeth and prevent food particles from sticking to the teeth.

Periodontal disease is unrelated to consuming a high-fat diet.
(A) Both statements are true.
(B) Both statements are false.
(C) The first statement is true, the second is false.
(D) The first statement is false, the second is true.

133. Each of the following is used to measure the clinical health of periodontal tissues during reevaluation procedures **EXCEPT** one. Which one is the **EXCEPTION?**
(A) Amount of bacterial plaque present
(B) Amount of inflammation and bleeding
(C) Severity of pocket depth
(D) Amount of neutrophils
(E) Amount of calculus deposits

134. What radiolucent landmark is located between the maxillary incisors?
(A) Median palatine suture
(B) Inverted Y
(C) Incisive foramen
(D) Mandibular canal
(E) Mental foramen

135. Excluding the pharynx, the majority of oral carcinomas occur on the
(A) lips.
(B) tongue.
(C) soft palate.
(D) buccal mucosa.
(E) gingiva.

136. The use of anticholinergic agents should be avoided in patients who have
(A) asthma.
(B) diabetes.
(C) prostatic hypertrophy.
(D) multiple sclerosis.
(E) endometriosis.

137. Which of the following describes the intended use of Chlorhexidine gluconate?
(A) It is used as site-specific therapy during reevaluation of root debridements.
(B) It is the strongest antibiotic used to treat remaining bacteria deposits.
(C) It is the most effective antimicrobial agent for maintenance of periodontal tissues.
(D) It is used as pretreatment before dental implant surgery.
(E) It is used in combination with doxycycline to reduce side effects.

138. Which hormone produces the fight-or-flight response in humans?
(A) Acetylcholine
(B) Norepinephrine
(C) Thyroxine
(D) Calcitonin
(E) Oxytocin

Use the following scenario to answer questions 139–141.

A dental hygienist is treating an elderly female patient. While treating the patient, the hygienist notices a large bruise on the patient's neck. The hygienist asks the patient where the bruise came from, but the patient does not give a clear answer. Then the hygienist asks the patient whether she would like to have a fluoride treatment and explains the benefits. The hygienist is an advocate of fluoride treatments for patients of all ages. The patient refuses and leaves soon after.

139. The hygienist suspects the patient may be a victim of abuse. The hygienist must
(A) provide basic medical care to the patient.
(B) make efforts to confirm her suspicions.
(C) report her suspicions to the authorities.
(D) keep all client communications private.
(E) approach the caregiver with her concerns.

140. If the hygienist decides to break confidentiality rules and tell somebody about the suspected abuse of the patient, this action can be classified as
(A) legal and ethical.
(B) legal and unethical.
(C) illegal and ethical.
(D) illegal and unethical.
(E) illegal only.

141. Ethically, the dental hygienist must respect the client's wish not to have a fluoride treatment. This is related to which of the following principles?
(A) Veracity
(B) Autonomy
(C) Beneficence
(D) Nonmaleficence
(E) Fidelity

142. The hygienist outlined the benefits of fluoride treatment for the patient. For that patient to give informed consent or refusal, what other information must the hygienist provide?
(A) The risks associated with the treatment
(B) Other client experiences with the treatment
(C) Personal views about the treatment
(D) Scientific literature about the treatment
(E) Numbers of patients who have had the treatment

143. A dental hygienist who performs a filling is violating the ethical principle of fidelity **BECAUSE** the dental hygienist is acting outside of his or her scope of practice.
    (A) Both the statement and reason are correct and related.
    (B) Both the statement and reason are correct but NOT related.
    (C) The statement is correct, but the reason is NOT.
    (D) The statement is NOT correct, but the reason is correct.
    (E) NEITHER the statement NOR the reason is correct.

144. Patients with some form of thyroid disease commonly present with
    (A) spontaneous hemorrhaging.
    (B) hypoplastic enamel.
    (C) increased incidence of caries.
    (D) deterioration of the alveolar bone.
    (E) enlarged salivary glands.

145. How does external resorption appear on a radiograph?
    (A) As radiopaque areas with varying degrees of osseous integration opacity
    (B) As bone loss that appears angular
    (C) As a blunted or flat appearance of the apices
    (D) As a fuzzy presentation of the alveolar crest bone
    (E) As a conical appearance of the apices

146. Pulse rate frequency is measured in beats per minute (BPM). If an adult patient is conscious, BPMs are taken from the common carotid artery.

    If a patient is unconscious, BPMs are taken from the radial artery.
    (A) Both statements are true.
    (B) Both statements are false.
    (C) The first statement is true, the second is false.
    (D) The first statement is false, the second is true.

147. The statement "Above all, do no harm" is closely associated with
    (A) virtue ethics.
    (B) principalism ethics.
    (C) Dental Hygienists' Code of Ethics.
    (D) the Oath of Hippocrates.
    (E) AMA's Principles of Medical Ethics.

148. A dental hygienist is conducting an oral health education session with a patient who has a learning disability. The hygienist knows that the patient's dominant learning style is affective. Which of the following techniques would **MOST LIKELY** be effective in terms of convincing this patient to floss more regularly?
    (A) Show a diagram indicating how floss should be held and used.
    (B) Physically guide the patient's hands to demonstrate good technique.
    (C) Praise the patient's efforts to establish a good oral health routine.
    (D) Play an educational video on flossing and why it is important.
    (E) Have the patient complete a reading and worksheet on flossing.

149 To prevent distortion when making an impression using an alginate hydrocolloid, the mold should be removed
    (A) with a direct pull.
    (B) by applying a constant force.
    (C) with a slow, cautious pull.
    (D) with a quick pulling motion.
    (E) by breaking the seal and snapping the mold out.

150. On a periodontal exam chart, a zigzag red arrow in the interproximal space between two teeth indicates
    (A) food impaction.
    (B) deficient contacts.
    (C) a missing tooth.
    (D) an impacted tooth.
    (E) decalcification.

151. Orthostatic hypotension will most likely occur in a dental office when a patient
(A) is nervous about a pending dental procedure.
(B) sits up too quickly after being in the supine position.
(C) loses consciousness during a dental procedure.
(D) is elderly, pregnant, or has Addison's disease.
(E) looks into the overhead dental light for an extended period.

Use the following scenario to answer questions 152–155.

A dental hygienist is helping to organize a community program to reduce the incidence of periodontal disease. The oral health of the community is assessed using questionnaires that are mailed out to community residents. After analyzing the data collected through the survey, the dental hygienist and the rest of the team determine that males between the ages of 40 and 58 are most at risk for periodontal disease; therefore, they decide that their program should be designed to focus specifically on this group.

152. Before the dental hygienist and the team start planning their periodontal disease prevention program, they should create a community profile. Each of the following is a topic the team should research **EXCEPT** one. Which one is the **EXCEPTION**?
(A) The number of people who live in the area
(B) The various languages spoken in the area
(C) The location of schools and clinics in the area
(D) The number of survey responses in the area
(E) The number of dental professionals in the area

153. In the above scenario, questionnaires were used to assess the community's overall oral health. What is one disadvantage of this method?
(A) Results may not be quantifiable.
(B) Results are often difficult to record.
(C) It is a very expensive form of research.
(D) Administering questionnaires is time-consuming.
(E) Respondents could misunderstand the questions.

154. Each of the following is a benefit of fit data collection for dental hygiene teams **EXCEPT** one. Which one is the **EXCEPTION**?
(A) Obtaining information about attitudes and beliefs
(B) Obtaining information to assist with planning
(C) Obtaining information about the status quo
(D) Obtaining information to study behavior
(E) Obtaining information about current conditions

155. In the above scenario, males between the ages of 40 and 58 make up the
(A) dominant group.
(B) target group.
(C) mean group.
(D) victim group.
(E) end group.

156. The earliest manifestations of which skin disease usually appear in the oral cavity?
(A) Pemphigus vulgaris
(B) Behcet syndrome
(C) Erythema multiforme
(D) Stevens-Johnson syndrome
(E) Hyperkeratosis

157. A dental hygiene professional is involved in a school program that is administering fluoride mouth rinses to elementary students. The dental hygiene professional should instruct the students to swish the fluoride solution for
(A) 10 seconds and spit it out.
(B) 30 seconds and spit it out.
(C) 1 minute and spit it out.
(D) 90 seconds and spit it out.
(E) 2 minutes and spit it out.

158. In a medical emergency, it is mandatory that all dental personnel know emergency procedures and have the ability to provide basic life support (BLS) **BECAUSE** the main way to manage emergencies involves BLS.
(A) Both the statement and reason are correct and related.
(B) Both the statement and reason are correct but NOT related.
(C) The statement is correct, but the reason is NOT.
(D) The statement is NOT correct, but the reason is correct.
(E) NEITHER the statement NOR the reason is correct.

159. Bacteria tend to die when humans have high fevers **BECAUSE** bacteria thrive at roughly the same temperature as a normal human body.
(A) Both the statement and the reason are correct and related.
(B) Both the statement and the reason are correct but NOT related.
(C) The statement is correct but the reason is NOT.
(D) The statement is NOT correct, but the reason is correct.
(E) NEITHER the statement NOR the reason is correct.

160. Which type of cement is considered ideal for use on patients with a high rate of caries?
(A) Glass ionomer
(B) Resin cement
(C) Zinc phosphate
(D) Calcium hydroxide
(E) Zinc polycarboxylate

161. Which of the following is the first bone lost in periodontal disease?
(A) Compact bone
(B) Cancellous bone
(C) Alveolar crest bone
(D) Bundle bone
(E) Lamina dura

162. Conducting statistical studies may involve considering independent variables, dependent variables, and extraneous variables. A study is analyzing whether free dental clinics for children under 10 reduces the number of dental surgeries in this age group. Some children who attend these clinics have a family dentist, and they come from various socioeconomic backgrounds and types of neighborhoods. The dependent variable in this study is
(A) the presence of dental clinics in the community.
(B) the number of children who have a family dentist.
(C) the family income of children in the study.
(D) the number of children who live in inner-city areas.
(E) the number of dental surgeries done on children.

163. All the radiographs you just developed are very light and the tooth images are hardly defined. What processing error has occurred?
(A) Fixer splash
(B) Overlap
(C) Film fog
(D) Wrong exposure
(E) A too cool temperature

164. Which of the following errors would result in a black streak?
(A) Bent film
(B) Double exposure
(C) Static electricity
(D) Cone cut
(E) Scratch

165. A female dental hygienist has only five minutes before her next patient arrives and is explaining the causes and symptoms of gingivitis to an at-risk patient. To adequately explain everything to the patient, the hygienist will need at least 10 minutes. What should the hygienist do?
(A) Not present any of the information
(B) Only present some of the information
(C) Speak faster while presenting the information
(D) Ask for patient input when presenting the information
(E) Use visual aids to speed up the presentation of the information

166. Each of the following is a source of systemic fluoride **EXCEPT** one. Which one is the **EXCEPTION**?
    (A) Fluoridated water
    (B) Fluoride supplements
    (C) Fluoridated lozenges
    (D) Fluoridated toothpaste
    (E) Fluoridated food sources

167. Iontophoresis is a procedure most often used in the treatment of
    (A) pyogenic granuloma.
    (B) hypersensitivity.
    (C) gingivitis.
    (D) necrotizing periodontitis.
    (E) caries.

168. Symptoms of sublethal fluoride poisoning are
    (A) cardiac and respiratory distress.
    (B) fever, chills, and vomiting.
    (C) salivation, nausea, and vomiting.
    (D) fever and abdominal distress.
    (E) pulmonary and breathing distress.

169. A dental hygienist is planning an education session on tooth brushing. When educating the patient on how to select a toothbrush, the most important piece of advice the dental hygienist can give the patient is to look for a brush with
    (A) firm, large bristles.
    (B) soft, rounded bristles.
    (C) soft, flat bristles.
    (D) firm, flat bristles.
    (E) firm, rounded bristles.

170. During a periodontal exam, you determine that tooth 19 on the mandibular left has through-and-through furcation involvement and complete bone loss between roots. How would you record this information on a periodontal exam chart?
    (A) Draw an N over the affected area in red ink.
    (B) Draw a partial triangle on the affected area in blue ink.
    (C) Outline the affected area in blue ink.
    (D) Write the Roman numeral III below the affected area in red ink.
    (E) Write the Roman numeral IV on the affected area in red ink.

171. What is the most common current theory regarding root debridement therapy for moderate or severe periodontitis?
    (A) No debridement on first visit after consultation from oral surgeon
    (B) Debride deep pockets first, followed by series of root debridement sessions
    (C) Complete debridement, followed by reevaluation in six weeks
    (D) One to four sessions of root debridement divided by quadrant
    (E) Antibiotics administered on first visit

172. Hypercementosis is characterized by
    (A) calculus deposits on the mandibular anterior teeth.
    (B) cemental spurs found near the cemento-enamel junction.
    (C) a defect in the mineralization of formed enamel matrix.
    (D) calcified masses found in the periodontal ligament.
    (E) an excessive formation of cementum on the root surface.

173. Resins used in pit-and-fissure sealants are formulated from a mixture of monomers that are commonly based on
    (A) titanium dioxide.
    (B) phosphoric acid.
    (C) benzoyl peroxide.
    (D) tertiary zinc phosphate.
    (E) bisphenol A glycidyl methacrylate.

174. Periodontal probing reveals information about the health of subgingival areas.

    Periodontal probing depths should be measured on four tooth sites.
    (A) Both statements are true.
    (B) Both statements are false
    (C) The first statement is true, the second is false.
    (D) The first statement is false, the second is true.

175. A patient is experiencing xerostomia as a side effect of a particular drug. Which of the following recommendations is **MOST LIKELY** to result in relief from the associated symptoms?
    (A) Drink fruit juice.
    (B) Increase caffeine intake.
    (C) Suck on ice chips.
    (D) Take acetaminophen.
    (E) Restrict water intake.

176. A dental hygiene professional is getting vaccinations as part of an overall strategy to protect against the spread of infection in the workplace. Each of the following is an illness for which the worker should get a vaccine **EXCEPT** one. Which one is the **EXCEPTION**?
    (A) Hepatitis B
    (B) HPV
    (C) Influenza
    (D) Polio
    (E) Rubella

177. A patient who complains that her lips are constantly cracking may suffer from a lack of
    (A) potassium.
    (B) vitamin B.
    (C) vitamin C.
    (D) calcium.
    (E) vitamin E.

178. Healthy gingival tissue should follow the contour of the teeth.

    Gingival margins that appear knife-edged indicate the presence of periodontal disease.
    (A) Both statements are true.
    (B) Both statements are false.
    (C) The first statement is true, the second is false.
    (D) The first statement is false, the second is true.

179. Each of the following is an example of an antibiotic designed to suppress the multiplication of bacterial growth in periodontitis **EXCEPT** one. Which one is the **EXCEPTION**?
    (A) Minocycline (Arestin)
    (B) Doxycycline (Periostat)
    (C) Chlorhexidine (Periochip)
    (D) Tetracycline (Actisite)
    (E) Doxycycline (Atridox)

180. Each of the following is a characteristic of trigeminal neuralgia **EXCEPT** one. Which one is the **EXCEPTION**?
    (A) Sudden, debilitating pain
    (B) Permanent paralysis of the face
    (C) Pain may last for days, weeks, or months
    (D) Triggered by mild stimulation of the face
    (E) Irritation of the trigeminal nerve that is usually unilateral

181. Which blood pressure reading from a patient's medical history indicates that the patient has Stage I hypertension?
    (A) 115/75
    (B) 121/88
    (C) 151/97
    (D) 175/102
    (E) 205/120

182. If a dental hygienist violates only the ethics of the dental hygiene profession, sanctions will typically be imposed by
    (A) the employer.
    (B) a judicial body.
    (C) an administrative body.
    (D) a criminal court.
    (E) a civil court.

183. The most common dental setting emergency is
    (A) syncope.
    (B) orthostatic hypotension.
    (C) hyperventilation.
    (D) airway obstruction.
    (E) cardiac arrest.

184. Professionals assess the oral health of individuals or populations using several types of examinations and inspections. Which one is rarely used in public health?
    (A) Type 1
    (B) Type 2
    (C) Type 3
    (D) Type 4
    (E) Type 5

185. The Tagoviride family of viruses is responsible for causing
    (A) rubella.
    (B) mumps.
    (C) pertussis.
    (D) influenza.
    (E) mononucleosis.

186. Each of the following is an example of reassessment procedures for chronic periodontal disease or aggressive periodontitis **EXCEPT** one. Which one is the **EXCEPTION**?
    (A) Periodontal flap surgery
    (B) Occlusal equilibration
    (C) Bacterial culturing
    (D) Systemic antibiotics
    (E) Treatment with doxycycline (Periostat)

187. A patient has an infection that is caused by the bacteria *Legionella pneumophila*. Which of the following medications would **MOST LIKELY** be prescribed to treat this infection?
    (A) Cefuroxime
    (B) Cloxacillin
    (C) Nafcillin
    (D) Erythromycin
    (E) Clindamycin

188. Which type of developmental abnormality is characterized by a sharp bend of a root?
    (A) Fusion
    (B) Concrescence
    (C) Dilaceration
    (D) Dens in dente
    (E) Dentinogenesis imperfecta

189. According to situational ethics, each of the following is something a dental hygienist should consider while deciding a course of action **EXCEPT** one. Which one is the **EXCEPTION**?
    (A) The age of the patient
    (B) The relationship with the patient
    (C) The most humanistic action for the patient
    (D) The health status of the patient
    (E) The virtues of the patient

190. A darkened area of a tooth on a radiograph indicates
    (A) a filling.
    (B) decay.
    (C) enamel.
    (D) dentin.
    (E) plaque.

191. Ultrasonic tools are preferable to handheld tools for periodontal debridement **BECAUSE** they do not require a specific angle to be maintained between the tool and the tooth.
    (A) Both the statement and reason are correct and related.
    (B) Both the statement and reason are correct but NOT related.
    (C) The statement is correct, but the reason is NOT.
    (D) The statement is NOT correct, but the reason is correct.
    (E) NEITHER the statement NOR the reason is correct.

192. Pericoronitis usually occurs with the eruption of the
    (A) maxillary first molar.
    (B) maxillary second molar.
    (C) mandibular central incisor.
    (D) mandibular third molar.
    (E) mandibular lateral incisor.

193. A dental hygienist using hand washing as a means of infection control should lather hands with soap for at least 45 seconds.

    If a dental hygiene professional has visible soil on his hands, alcohol-based hand sanitizers will often remove the soil better than plain or antimicrobial soap.
    (A) Both statements are true.
    (B) Both statements are false.
    (C) The first statement is true, the second is false.
    (D) The first statement is false, the second is true.

194. In statistics, a type I error means that a researcher incorrectly accepted a null hypothesis.

    In the data set 1, 1, 1, 5, 9, 5, the mode is 1.
    (A) Both statements are true.
    (B) Both statements are false.
    (C) The first statement is true, the second is false.
    (D) The first statement is false, the second is true.

195. The human body can survive without water for approximately
    (A) 1 day.
    (B) 2 days.
    (C) 3 days.
    (D) 4 days.
    (E) 5 days.

196. Cells in which part of the adult body are most sensitive to radiation exposure?
    (A) Kidneys
    (B) Muscles
    (C) Connective tissue
    (D) Salivary glands
    (E) Lymphocytes

197. A condition referred to as pink tooth is often observed in patients diagnosed with which of the following?
    (A) Internal resorption
    (B) Periapical granuloma
    (C) Hyperplastic pulpitis
    (D) Chondroma
    (E) Osteoma

198. During education sessions on polishing, dental hygiene professionals should plan to inform patients that they should not have their teeth polished if they have implants or hypersensitive teeth.

    A dental hygiene professional should plan to conduct individual education sessions on tooth polishing whenever clients are found to be at risk for caries formation or periodontal disease.
    (A) Both statements are true.
    (B) Both statements are false.
    (C) The first statement is true, the second is false.
    (D) The first statement is false, the second is true.

199. A dental hygiene professional is educating a patient who has a high risk of developing oral health problems about how to recognize the signs of periodontal disease. Which of the following statements about diseased gingiva would be accurate information to give to the patient?
    (A) The gingiva will be pink or pink-brown in color.
    (B) The gingiva will have contours that are pointed.
    (C) The gingiva will have a firm feel and be resilient.
    (D) The gingiva will be red or blue-red in color.
    (E) The gingiva will have margins that are smooth.

200. Which body system specifically creates the "fight or flight" response?
    (A) Sympathetic nervous system
    (B) Enteric nervous system
    (C) Autonomic nervous system
    (D) Visceral nervous system
    (E) Parasympathetic nervous system

COMPONENT B

Directions: Study the case components and answer questions 1–10.

SYNOPSIS OF PATIENT HISTORY

CASE *PT1-1*

Age _____ *60* _____

Sex _____ *Male* _____

Height *5'9"*

Weight _*180*_ lbs

_*81.65*_ kgs

Vital Signs

Blood pressure _____ *130/85* _____

Pulse rate _____ *100* _____

Respiration rate _____ *16* _____

---

1. Under Care of Physician
   Yes ☐   No ☑
   Condition: _____

2. Hospitalized within the last 5 years
   Yes ☑   No ☐
   Reason: *Broken ankle three years ago* _____

3. Has or had the following conditions:
   _____
   _____

4. Current medications:
   One aspirin a day (preventive) _____
   _____
   _____

5. Smokes or uses tobacco products
   Yes ☑   No ☐   *Cigar once a year on his birthday*

6. Is pregnant
   Yes ☐   No ☐   N/A ☑

MEDICAL HISTORY:
Patient is in good health, and takes one aspirin every day because his physician directed him to. He fractured his ankle skiing three years ago.

DENTAL HISTORY:
He comes in regularly for cleanings and checkups. He has 4 implants on the maxillary arch as a consequence of losing his 4 maxillary anteriors in a fight six years prior.

SOCIAL HISTORY:
He is married and lives with his wife. He is employed as a probation officer for the state.

CHIEF COMPLAINT:
Checkup and cleaning.

ADULT CLINICAL EXAMINATION

Case PT1-1

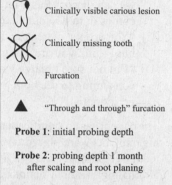

| | | | | | | | | | | | | | | | |
|1|2|3|4|5|6|7|8|9|10|11|12|13|14|15|16|

Probe 2
1: 323 323 323 323 222 | 222 323 323 323 323

R

Probe 1
2: 323 323 323 233 222 | 222 323 323 323 323

Probe 2
1: 323 323 323 222 212 212 212 212 212 212 222 323 323 323

R

Probe 1
2: 323 323 323 222 222 222 212 212 222 222 222 222 323 323

|32|31|30|29|28|27|26|25|24|23|22|21|20|19|18|17|

facial
palatal
lingual
facial

KEY

Clinically visible carious lesion

Clinically missing tooth

Furcation

"Through and through" furcation

Probe 1: initial probing depth

Probe 2: probing depth 1 month after scaling and root planing

---

SUPPLEMENTAL ORAL EXAMINATION FINDINGS

1. All probings < 3 mm.
2. Current Oral Hygiene Status: Good.
3. Light to moderate calculus lower anteriors.

4. Generalized recession 1mm.
5. Patient has minimal bone loss.

---

1. How often should periapical X-rays of this patient's implants be taken?
   (A) Every 6 months
   (B) At every maintenance visit
   (C) Once a year for 3 years, then every other year
   (D) At least once per year

2. What is the **BEST** indicator for diagnosis of implant failure in this patient?
   (A) No bleeding upon probing around the implant
   (B) No tissue inflammation around the implant
   (C) No mobility around the implant
   (D) No deep pocket depths around the implant

3. All of the following are characteristic of a healthy implant site **EXCEPT** one. Which one is the **EXCEPTION**?
   (A) Firm pink tissue that does not bleed when probed

   (B) Only small amounts of purulence when tissue around implant is compressed
   (C) Radiographic evidence of bone in close contact with implant
   (D) Radiographic bone levels with minimal change from previous

4. When taking radiographs of the implant site, which of the following allows for optimum evaluation?
   (A) A vertical bitewing taken in duplicate to be sent to the periodontist
   (B) A periapical taken utilizing a long-cone paralleling technique
   (C) A periapical that is foreshortened so that we can be assured of seeing the apex
   (D) A panograph in order to get a visual of the entire mouth

5. The patient tells you that he no longer wishes to alternate maintenance visits with the periodontist. How do you respond?
   (A) "You have no choice in the matter. You are legally obligated to follow the treatment plan."
   (B) "I'd like to hear your concerns, and then we can discuss this with the doctor when he comes in to do your exam."
   (C) "You are the patient, and it is your decision, but I think you are making a big mistake."
   (D) "I'm not sure I blame you! It is time-consuming to see both the dentist and the periodontist."

6. The patient has no significant periodontal findings; his implants were placed 6 years ago because his teeth were knocked out in a fight. Does he require alternating 3-month maintenance visits with the periodontist?
   (A) Yes, the periodontist placed the implants and needs to monitor them.
   (B) Yes, the patient has generalized recession of less than 2 mm in addition to 4 surgical implants.
   (C) Most likely not; the general practitioner and the hygienist have monitored the patient's implants for 6 years and have provided effective maintenance.
   (D) No, the patient could have stopped seeing the periodontist after the first 6 months following implant surgery.

7. All of the following are reasons why traditional metal curets are contraindicated around implant components **EXCEPT** one. Which one is the **EXCEPTION**?
   (A) If the titanium is scratched, there will be an increase in plaque retention.
   (B) If the titanium is scratched, there is an increased likelihood of periimplantitis.
   (C) There are other instruments that are more versatile and better promote tissue safety.
   (D) Metal can disturb the surface coating of the implant resulting in biocompatibility with periimplant tissues.

8. Should the hygienist polish the implant during the maintenance visit?
   (A) No, only the dentist should polish implants.
   (B) No, unless surface alterations are noted.
   (C) Yes, but a prophy jet should be used.
   (D) Yes, only if the patient requests it.

9. All of the following statements are true regarding probing the periimplant site **EXCEPT** one. Which one is the **EXCEPTION**?
   (A) Routine probing should never be done on implants.
   (B) Routine probing of dental implants is controversial, but is still performed.
   (C) Probing can damage the weak epithelial attachment allowing entry of periodontal pathogens.
   (D) Probing is necessary only in implants where signs of infection are present.

10. What is the **BEST** vehicle for cleaning the interproximal areas between the patient's 4 maxillary anterior implant crowns? He has very limited interdental spacing.
    (A) Round or flat toothpick
    (B) Regular or tufted dental floss
    (C) Wire interdental proxy brush
    (D) Best not to use anything interproximally

Directions: Study the case components and answer questions 11–20.

SYNOPSIS OF PATIENT HISTORY

CASE *PT1-2*

Age ___*32*___

Sex ___*Female*___

Height *5'8"*

Weight *140* lbs

63.5 kgs

Vital Signs

Blood pressure ___*119/78*___

Pulse rate ___*85*___

Respiration rate ___*15*___

1. Under Care of Physician
   Yes ☐ No ☑
                    Condition: _____

2. Hospitalized within the last 5 years
   Yes ☐ No ☑
                    Reason: _____
                    _____

3. Has or had the following conditions:
   _____
   _____

4. Current medications:
   _____
   _____
   _____

5. Smokes or uses tobacco products
   Yes ☐ No ☑

6. Is pregnant
   Yes ☐ No ☑ N/A ☐

MEDICAL HISTORY:
Patient is in excellent health and in excellent physical shape. Exercises on a regular basis. Runs short- and long-distance races.

DENTAL HISTORY:
Patient comes in routinely for dental checkups and cleanings. Last visit was six months ago. No dental caries in four years.

SOCIAL HISTORY:
Patient lives alone and is employed as a psychologist for a hospital. She has never had decay or restorative treatment.

CHIEF COMPLAINT:
"I need my teeth cleaned and would like them to be whiter."

ADULT CLINICAL EXAMINATION

Case PT1-2

| Tooth numbers | 1 | 2 | 3 | 4 | 5 | 6 | 7 | 8 | 9 | 10 | 11 | 12 | 13 | 14 | 15 | 16 |

Probe 2/1 facial: 323 323 323 | 212 212 212 212 212 212 | 323 323 323

R

Probe 1/2 palatal: 323 323 322 | 212 212 212 212 212 212 | 323 323 323

Probe 2/1 lingual: 323 323 323 | 212 212 212 212 212 212 | 323 323 323

R

Probe 1/2 facial: 323 323 322 | 222 222 222 222 222 222 | 323 323 323

| Tooth numbers | 32 | 31 | 30 | 29 | 28 | 27 | 26 | 25 | 24 | 23 | 22 | 21 | 20 | 19 | 18 | 17 |

KEY

Clinically visible carious lesion

Clinically missing tooth

△ Furcation

▲ "Through and through" furcation

Probe 1: initial probing depth

Probe 2: probing depth 1 month after scaling and root planing

---

SUPPLEMENTAL ORAL EXAMINATION FINDINGS

1. Tissue is healthy and probes within 3 mm.
2. Current Oral Hygiene Status: Excellent.
3. Patient has light stain maxillary anterior and mandibular anterior linguals. No calculus evident.
4. X-rays show no bone loss.

---

11. What is the appropriate recall frequency for this patient?
    (A) Once a year
    (B) 6 months
    (C) 4 months
    (D) 3 months

12. How often should this patient have bitewing X-rays taken?
    (A) Every 6 months
    (B) Once a year
    (C) Once each 18 months
    (D) Hygienist discretion

13. The patient is interested in purchasing a power toothbrush. How should the hygienist respond?
    (A) "You don't need a power toothbrush. You are getting good results with a manual brush."
    (B) "Get one tomorrow. You will not be disappointed that you did."

    (C) "Evidence-based research tells us automatic toothbrushes offer many advantages. It is a good idea."
    (D) "Let's ask the dentist if he or she thinks it is necessary before you make your decision."

14. What would be the **MOST** effective way to scale this patient's teeth?
    (A) An ultrasonic scaler with a fine tip
    (B) Select hand instruments
    (C) A combination of ultrasonic and hand instrumentation
    (D) Any of the above instrumentation is acceptable

15. The patient flosses her teeth three times a week. What should be the hygienist's recommendation?
   (A) "Even though you are having excellent results, flossing daily is recommended."
   (B) "You are supposed to be flossing daily. Three days is not enough."
   (C) "You can continue flossing three times a week only if you use a power brush."
   (D) "You should be flossing more. Try 5 days a week."

16. The patient has not requested that her teeth be polished. What action should the dental hygienist take?
   (A) The hygienist can use selective polishing to remove any remaining stain.
   (B) The hygienist should polish the patient's teeth as part of the examination.
   (C) The hygienist should have the dentist speak to the patient about the importance of tooth polishing.
   (D) No action is necessary since polishing should have already been done to remove loose debris.

17. You are about to begin examination of the patient's maxillary arch. All of the following are true of positioning **EXCEPT** one. Which one is the **EXCEPTION**?
   (A) The chair back is parallel to the floor.
   (B) The light is positioned directly over the patient's mouth.
   (C) The arch should be positioned so the occlusal plane is perpendicular to the floor.
   (D) The patient's head is at the top of the chair.

18. The patient has asked you to recommend a mouth rinse that she can use daily. Which do you recommend?
   (A) Any cosmetic breath rinse
   (B) An antimicrobial with fluoride
   (C) Warm salt water rinses
   (D) None. Mouth rinses are not necessary.

19. What is the MOST LIKELY cause of the stain on her anterior linguals?
   (A) Cigarettes
   (B) Tetracycline staining
   (C) Tea
   (D) Age

20. Your patient asks what the **BEST** dentifrice is for her to use. What should be your response?
   (A) "Any highly abrasive toothpaste will remove tarter and soft deposits."
   (B) "Any ADA-approved toothpaste is fine. It is the mechanical action that effectively removes deposits."
   (C) "Choose either a tartar control, antiplaque, desensitizing, or whitening toothpaste based on your personal preference."
   (D) "A mixture of baking soda and hydrogen peroxide have proven to be the most effective in fighting cavities."

Directions: Study the case components and answer questions 21–30.

SYNOPSIS OF PATIENT HISTORY

CASE *PT1-3*

Age   *58*

Sex   *Female*

Height *5'3"*

Weight *150* lbs

68.04 kgs

Vital Signs

Blood pressure   *140/85*

Pulse rate   *110*

Respiration rate   *19*

---

1. Under Care of Physician
   Yes ☑ No ☐

   Condition: *Hypertension*

2. Hospitalized within the last 5 years
   Yes ☐ No ☑

   Reason: _____

3. Has or had the following conditions:

   Hypertension

4. Current medications:

   Cardizen for high blood pressure

5. Smokes or uses tobacco products
   Yes ☑ No ☐

6. Is pregnant
   Yes ☐ No ☑ N/A ☐

MEDICAL HISTORY:
Patient has high blood pressure and takes medication. She has smoked one pack of cigarettes daily since age 30. She does not exercise and is overweight. She has tried to quit smoking without success.

DENTAL HISTORY:
New patient in the practice. She states she has not had regular care, and only goes in for extractions.

SOCIAL HISTORY:
The patient is divorced and lives alone.

CHIEF COMPLAINT:
"I have lost a few teeth and do not wish to lose any more. I need my teeth cleaned, and a couple of them are loose."

ADULT CLINICAL EXAMINATION

Case PT1-3

	1	2	3	4	5	6	7	8	9	10	11	12	13	14	15	16
Probe 2		646		646	646	444	444	444	444	444	444	646		656	656	
Probe 1		646		646	646	444	444	444	444	444	444	646		656	656	

facial

R

palatal

Probe 1		656		656	646	444	444	444	444	444	444	646		666	666	
Probe 2		656		656	545	444	444	444	444	444	444	646		656	656	

Probe 2		666	666		646											
Probe 1		666	666		646											

lingual

R

facial

Probe 1		656	656		646	444	444	444	444	444	444	666	646		646	
Probe 2		656	666		646	444	444	444	444	444	444	646	646		646	

| | 32 | 31 | 30 | 29 | 28 | 27 | 26 | 25 | 24 | 23 | 22 | 21 | 20 | 19 | 18 | 17 |

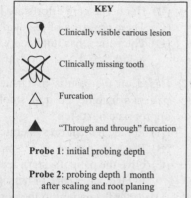

KEY

Clinically visible carious lesion

Clinically missing tooth

Furcation

"Through and through" furcation

Probe 1: initial probing depth

Probe 2: probing depth 1 month after scaling and root planing

SUPPLEMENTAL ORAL EXAMINATION FINDINGS

1. Current Oral Hygiene Status: Fair, with moderate calculus and heavy stain.
2. X-rays reveal moderate horizontal bone loss.
3. Generalized pocketing 4–6 mm with no bleeding.
4. Tissues appear fibrotic and leathery.
5. #2 and #14 have class 1 mobility.
6. Generalized recession 2 mm, greater in mandibular anterior.
7. #18 and #30 have early furcation involvement.
8. Teeth show evidence of severe bruxism.

21. What diagnosis is **MOST LIKELY** to be made for this patient?
    (A) Chronic moderate generalized periodontitis
    (B) Severe moderate generalized periodontitis
    (C) Mild moderate generalized periodontitis
    (D) Generalized aggressive periodontitis

22. What is the AAP classification for this case?
    (A) Gingivitis
    (B) Type I
    (C) Type 2
    (D) Type 3

23. All of the following are periodontal risk factors **EXCEPT** one. Which one is the **EXCEPTION**?
    (A) Smoking
    (B) Obesity
    (C) High blood pressure and medications
    (D) Biofilm and calculus deposits

24. What would be the **MOST** appropriate way to address this patient's bruxism?
    (A) Adjust her occlusion.
    (B) Refer her to the orthodontist.
    (C) Recommend stress management strategies.
    (D) Fabricate a night guard.

25. What is the **BEST** way to accomplish removal of calculus and biofilm on this patient?
    (A) Gross scaling
    (B) Quadrant debridement with pain management
    (C) Emergency referral to the periodontist
    (D) Complete scaling today; insist upon more frequent maintenance visits.

26. From the results of the second probing during reevaluation, it is clear that the patient did not attain the healing result the hygienist had hoped for. All of the following **EXCEPT** one are contributing factors. Which one is the **EXCEPTION**?
    (A) She is still smoking cigarettes.
    (B) Her home-care efforts are inadequate.
    (C) There are areas of residual calculus.
    (D) The patient has not been wearing her mouth guard.

27. Based on the results of tissue healing and the patient's inability to quit smoking, what is the appropriate next step?
    (A) Put the patient on systemic antibiotics.
    (B) Place the patient on a 2-month recall.
    (C) Give the patient a stern lecture on the need to take better care of herself.
    (D) Refer the patient to the periodontist.

28. During the reevaluation visit, the doctor refers the patient to the periodontist. The patient refuses to go. All of the following are appropriate responses **EXCEPT** one. Which one is the **EXCEPTION**?
    (A) Document the referral carefully, as well as the patient's response.
    (B) Place the patient on a more frequent recall as a compromise.
    (C) Gently remind the patient that she will lose all her teeth if she does not see the specialist.
    (D) Continue smoking-cessation strategies.

29. The patient states at the reevaluation appointment that she refuses to floss her teeth. What is the appropriate hygienist response?
    (A) "Let's try to find an alternative solution to clean in between your teeth."
    (B) "I cannot control your actions, I can only control mine, and I floss every day."
    (C) "I will accept your not flossing daily, but you must do it at least twice a week."
    (D) "There are flat and round toothpicks available. Would you consider using a toothpick?"

30. The patient states that a friend has a Waterpik and loves it. She also says that she would be interested in using it as an alternative to flossing. What is the appropriate hygienist response?
    (A) "Using a Waterpik is not enough and you must floss."
    (B) "I am delighted you want to use a Waterpik. I hope you'll consider flossing too."
    (C) "Get ready for a big mess in your bathroom! Waterpiks spray water all over the place."
    (D) "Why would you want to use a Waterpik? Sonicare is a much better brand."

Directions: Study the case components and answer questions 31–40.

SYNOPSIS OF PATIENT HISTORY

CASE *PT1-4*

Age _60_

Sex _Male_

Height _5'7"_

Weight _165_ lbs

_74.84_ kgs

Vital Signs

Blood pressure _127/83_

Pulse rate _100_

Respiration rate _20_

1. Under Care of Physician
   Yes ☐ No ☑

   Condition: _____

2. Hospitalized within the last 5 years
   Yes ☐ No ☑

   Reason: _____
   _____

3. Has or had the following conditions:
   _____
   _____

4. Current medications:

   Vitamins _____
   _____
   _____

5. Smokes or uses tobacco products
   Yes ☐ No ☑

6. Is pregnant
   Yes ☐ No ☐ N/A ☑

MEDICAL HISTORY:
The patient enjoys excellent health. He exercises regularly and eats right. He is a fitness nut, meditates, and drinks red wine daily.

DENTAL HISTORY:
He comes in regularly for dental cleanings, and has several crowns and restorations.

SOCIAL HISTORY:
He is gay, and lives with a long-term life partner.

CHIEF COMPLAINT:
More tartar build up today.

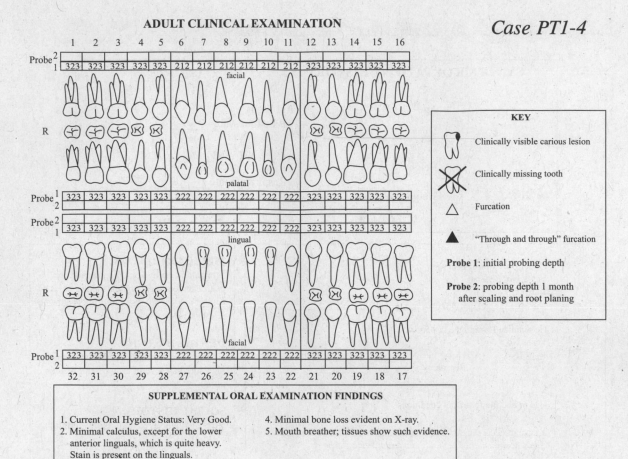

ADULT CLINICAL EXAMINATION

Case PT1-4

KEY

Clinically visible carious lesion

Clinically missing tooth

Furcation

"Through and through" furcation

Probe 1: initial probing depth

Probe 2: probing depth 1 month after scaling and root planing

SUPPLEMENTAL ORAL EXAMINATION FINDINGS

1. Current Oral Hygiene Status: Very Good.
2. Minimal calculus, except for the lower anterior linguals, which is quite heavy. Stain is present on the linguals.
3. 1 mm recession generally, with TB abrasion.
4. Minimal bone loss evident on X-ray.
5. Mouth breather; tissues show such evidence.

31. The patient presents with heavier-than-usual calculus deposits. There is no inflammation present, and his last cleaning was 6 months ago. The hygienist should
(A) recommend a more frequent recall frequency.
(B) work harder at each cleaning and use alternative debridement methods.
(C) recommend a harder toothbrush and give the patient a sample.
(D) recommend an over-the-counter metal pick-type scaler for at home use.

32. All of the following might be recommended to control the patient's calculus and stain build-up **EXCEPT** one. Which one is the **EXCEPTION**?
(A) Tartar control toothpaste
(B) More frequent brushing
(C) Longer brushing time
(D) Increasing pressure to the toothbrush

33. All of the following are reasons why the patient is a good candidate for an automatic toothbrush **EXCEPT** one. Which one is the **EXCEPTION**?
(A) He brushes overzealously as evidenced by his abrasion.
(B) He built up excessive calculus this recall.
(C) He has stain; a brush with a timer encourages longer brushing.
(D) Automatic toothbrushes are superior to manual toothbrushes.

34. Automatic toothbrushes are safe and effective for biofilm removal and stain reduction.

Automatic toothbrushes are considered more abrasive than manual toothbrushes.
(A) Both statements are true.
(B) Both statements are false.
(C) The first statement is true, and the second is false.
(D) The first statement is false, and the second is true.

35. The patient is always 10 minutes late for his appointment. All of the following are effective strategies for handling the patient's consistent tardiness **EXCEPT** one. Which one is the **EXCEPTION**?
(A) Tell him his appointment time is 15 minutes earlier.
(B) Do not run over into the next patient's time frame.
(C) Ask him graciously to be on time next visit so that you can deliver the best treatment.
(D) Fume silently, and work harder.

36. During the patient's cleaning, he experiences dentinal hypersensitivity. What is the **BEST** solution to keep him comfortable during the cleaning?
(A) Use a topical agent.
(B) Polish with a desensitizing paste prior to scaling.
(C) Use oraqix throughout the mouth.
(D) Anesthetize with local anesthesia

37. During the oral cancer screening, the hygienist notices a white lesion on the side of the patient's tongue. All of the following are acceptable responses **EXCEPT** one. Which one is the **EXCEPTION**?
(A) Show the lesion to the patient and ask if he remembers biting his tongue.
(B) Say nothing, and walk out of the room to schedule a biopsy with the oral surgeon.
(C) Bring the lesion to the doctor's attention during the exam, including the information on the patient's recollection of not having bitten his tongue.
(D) Describe the lesion and its location on the patient record.

38. At the next recall, the hygienist notes that the patient still has the lesion, despite the doctor having referred him to a specialist. Which is the **BEST** course of action for the dental hygienist?
(A) Bluntly ask the patient why he did not go to the specialist.
(B) Advise the patient that the lesion is likely cancerous and needs to be addressed immediately.
(C) Say, "I'm concerned that the lesion we referred you to have looked at is still present. Did you get it checked out?" Speak to the doctor about this before he comes in for the exam.
(D) Say nothing to the patient, but tell the doctor in the hallway that the lesion is still present.

39. The patient admits he will not floss his teeth because he cannot maneuver the string. He uses toothpicks, with very good results. All of the following are good substitutes **EXCEPT** one. Which one is the **EXCEPTION**?
(A) A floss-on-a-stick type flosser
(B) Small interdental brush such as go-betweens
(C) Power flosser
(D) A Waterpik

40. All of the following may be contributing to the patient's halitosis **EXCEPT** one. Which one is the **EXCEPTION**?
(A) Periodontal disease
(B) Excess stomach acids
(C) Failure to clean the tongue
(D) Food choices

Directions: Study the case components and answer questions 41–50.

SYNOPSIS OF PATIENT HISTORY

CASE *PT1-5*

Age __3__

Sex __Female__

Height __3'2"__

Weight __40__ lbs

__18.14__ kgs

Vital Signs

Blood pressure __N/A__

Pulse rate __95__

Respiration rate __20__

---

1. Under Care of Physician
   Yes ☑ No ☐

   Condition: __Routine checkups__

2. Hospitalized within the last 5 years
   Yes ☐ No ☑

   Reason: _____

3. Has or had the following conditions:

   _____
   _____

4. Current medications:

   _____
   _____
   _____

5. Smokes or uses tobacco products
   Yes ☐ No ☑

6. Is pregnant
   Yes ☐ No ☐ N/A ☑

MEDICAL HISTORY:
The patient is a 3-year-old child in good physical health.

DENTAL HISTORY:
The patient is here for her first dental visit.

SOCIAL HISTORY:
Unremarkable; she is a pleasant, friendly child who is unafraid.

CHIEF COMPLAINT:
She is here for a cleaning and checkup, as per her mother.

CLINICAL EXAMINATION

Case PT1-5

	1	2	3	4	5	6	7	8	9	10	11	12	13	14	15	16
Probe 2																
Probe 1			868	857		647	646	646	646	646	746		758	868		

facial

R

palatal

	1	2	3	4	5	6	7	8	9	10	11	12	13	14	15	16
Probe 1			868	857		647	646	646	646	646	746		758	868		
Probe 2																

Probe 2		858	757	757		646	646	646	646	646	646		768	868	868	
Probe 1																

lingual

R

facial

Probe 1		858	868	647		746	646	646	546	646	747		868	868	858	
Probe 2																

32	31	30	29	28	27	26	25	24	23	22	21	20	19	18	17

KEY

- Clinically visible carious lesion
- Clinically missing tooth
- △ Furcation
- ▲ "Through and through" furcation

Probe 1: initial probing depth

Probe 2: probing depth 1 month after scaling and root planing

SUPPLEMENTAL ORAL EXAMINATION FINDINGS

1. Current Oral Hygiene Status: Very Good; minimal plaque biofilm; no calculus.
2. Teeth well spaced.
3. Maxillary frenum attached low; diastema between maxillary centrals present, but spacing between all teeth at present.
4. Slight overjet.

41. What is the ideal age in which a child should visit the dentist for the first time?
    - (A) Between 6 months and 1 year
    - (B) Between 1 year and 18 months
    - (C) Between 1 and 2 years
    - (D) Between 2 and 3 years

42. All of the following are familial factors that place a child at risk for oral disease **EXCEPT** one. Which one is the **EXCEPTION**?
    - (A) Low socioeconomic status
    - (B) I.Q. of the child
    - (C) Use of non-fluoridated toothpaste
    - (D) No belief in prevention

43. All of the following dietary considerations place a child at risk for oral disease **EXCEPT** one. Which one is the **EXCEPTION**?
    - (A) Insufficient fluoride in the water supply
    - (B) Bottle or spill-proof cup filled with sweetened liquid in bed
    - (C) Frequent snacking
    - (D) Higher protein diet

44. Which of the following is **NOT** a teething behavior?
    - (A) Sporadic stridor
    - (B) Excessive chewing and drooling
    - (C) Irritability and crying
    - (D) Change in appetite

45. Primary dentition is usually complete when a child is between
    - (A) 6–12 months.
    - (B) 12–24 months.
    - (C) 18–24 months.
    - (D) 2–3 years.

46. Fluorosis is caused by excessive fluoride intake. What is considered the **MOST** critical time of exposure for fluorosis to develop in primary teeth?
    (A) In utero during the final trimester
    (B) During the middle of the first year of life
    (C) During the middle of the second year of life
    (D) During the middle of the third year of life

47. The patient is demonstrating how she brushes her teeth. All of the following comments from the hygienist are appropriate **EXCEPT** one. Which one is the **EXCEPTION**?
    (A) "I knew you could do it!"
    (B) "You are doing great!"
    (C) "You still have a lot to learn!"
    (D) "Well done!"

48. Which of the following is contraindicated when evaluating for caries in posterior teeth?
    (A) Pressing the explorer into pits and fissures to determine if it is soft
    (B) Observing the pits and fissures to determine if they are shallow or deep
    (C) Looking for dark discolorations in the pits and fissures and on proximal surfaces
    (D) Looking for open carious lesions on occlusal and smooth surfaces

49. A parent should assist a child with tooth brushing until the child has reached age
    (A) 4.
    (B) 5.
    (C) 6.
    (D) 7.

50. What is the correct recall frequency for a 3-year-old child with no oral disease?
    (A) 3 months
    (B) 6 months
    (C) Once a year
    (D) 18 months

Directions: Study the case components and answer questions 51–60.

SYNOPSIS OF PATIENT HISTORY

CASE *PT1-6*

Age ___45___

Sex ___Female___

Height _5'3"_

Weight _135_ lbs

_61.23_ kgs

Vital Signs

Blood pressure ___115/78___

Pulse rate ___80___

Respiration rate ___18___

1. Under Care of Physician
   Yes ☑ No ☐

   Condition: _____

2. Hospitalized within the last 5 years
   Yes ☑ No ☐

   Reason: _Various episodes and treatment for a_
   brain tumor, including radiation therapy

3. Has or had the following conditions:

   Brain tumor _____
   _____

4. Current medications:

   Contact MD (she is in a research trial)
   _____
   _____

5. Smokes or uses tobacco products
   Yes ☐ No ☑

6. Is pregnant
   Yes ☐ No ☑ N/A ☐

MEDICAL HISTORY:
The patient was diagnosed with a brain tumor two years ago. She has been in and out of the hospital numerous times for various episodes and treatment of her disease. She is currently stable after having undergone radiation therapy to shrink a tumor. Surgery may or may not be scheduled in the next two months.

DENTAL HISTORY:
The patient has a history of good, regular care. Her decay rate was low historically.

SOCIAL HISTORY:
The patient is married and has one child. She has stopped working because of her illness.

CHIEF COMPLAINT:
Checkup and cleaning. "My mouth feels dry."

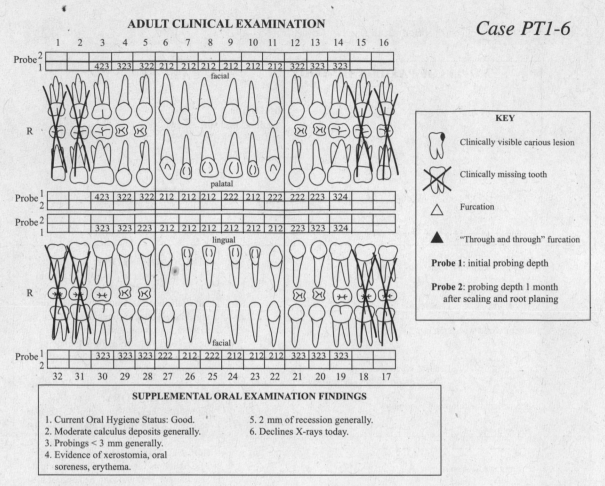

ADULT CLINICAL EXAMINATION

Case PT1-6

SUPPLEMENTAL ORAL EXAMINATION FINDINGS

1. Current Oral Hygiene Status: Good.
2. Moderate calculus deposits generally.
3. Probings < 3 mm generally.
4. Evidence of xerostomia, oral soreness, erythema.
5. 2 mm of recession generally.
6. Declines X-rays today.

51. According to the World Health Organization Oral (WHO) Mucositis Scale, your patient's mucositis is which of the following?
(A) Grade 1
(B) Grade 2
(C) Grade 3
(D) Grade 4

52. During treatment of the patient, the hygienist should do which of the following?
(A) Advise the patient to bring a friend along to take notes during teaching visits.
(B) Provide written instructions for the patient.
(C) Provide positive reinforcement and creativity in helping the patient maintain optimal oral health.
(D) All of the above.

53. Ideally, any dental hygiene treatment should be provided
(A) before the start of cancer therapy.
(B) during cancer therapy.
(C) after cancer therapy is completed.
(D) It does not matter when.

54. This patient is receiving radiation to the head. What is the risk that she will develop oral complications?
(A) Slight risk
(B) Moderate risk
(C) High risk
(D) No significant risk

55. Along with daily biofilm removal, what mouth rinse is important to help her mouth be neutral, and comfortable, given the erythema?
    (A) Baking soda and water, followed by plain water, each 2–3 hours
    (B) Warm water only
    (C) Essential oils
    (D) Chlorhexadine

56. All of the following will help her xerostomia **EXCEPT** one. Which one is the **EXCEPTION**?
    (A) Frequent water sipping or ice chips
    (B) Sugar-free gum or candy, preferably with xylitol
    (C) Saliva substitute spray or gel
    (D) Lemon glycerin swabs

57. All of the following are important to prevent this patient from developing dental caries **EXCEPT** one. Which one is the **EXCEPTION**?
    (A) Fluoride toothpaste used at every brushing, after meals and before bed.
    (B) 1.1 percent neutral NAF gel brushed on teeth after brushing with Fl toothpaste before bedtime. Do not rinse off.
    (C) Rubber tipping to ease, yet stimulate the irritated tissues.
    (D) Custom-made polyvinyl trays and fluoride gel-at-home treatments.

58. All of the following are ingredients of the "magic mouth rinse" used to manage oral pain 30 minutes prior to eating **EXCEPT** one. Which one is the **EXCEPTION**?
    (A) Lidocaine
    (B) Benadryl cough syrup
    (C) A coating agent such as Maalox
    (D) Baking soda

59. For the first 6 months after her radiation therapy, how often should this patient be recalled for debridement and review of oral health instruction?
    (A) Once a week
    (B) Every other week
    (C) Every 4–8 weeks
    (D) Once each quarter

60. You should watch for which of the following potential complications in this patient?
    (A) Trismus
    (B) Bruxing
    (C) Numbness
    (D) Swelling

Directions: Study the case components and answer questions 61–70.

SYNOPSIS OF PATIENT HISTORY

CASE *PT1-7*

Age __85__

Sex __Female__

Height __5'4"__

Weight __135__ lbs

__61.23__ kgs

Vital Signs

Blood pressure __130/82__

Pulse rate __80__

Respiration rate __15__

---

1. Under Care of Physician
   Yes ☑ No ☐

   Condition: *Osteoporosis*

2. Hospitalized within the last 5 years
   Yes ☑ No ☐

   Reason: *Cataract surgery, both eyes,*
   one year apart

3. Has or had the following conditions:

   Osteoporosis

4. Current medications:

   Fosamax

5. Smokes or uses tobacco products
   Yes ☐ No ☑

6. Is pregnant
   Yes ☐ No ☑ N/A ☐

MEDICAL HISTORY:
The patient is basically in good health but is slightly frail. She has had cataract surgery and suffers from osteoporosis. She is somewhat stooped over.

DENTAL HISTORY:
She comes in regularly for cleanings and checkups. She wears a full upper denture and a lower partial. Patient is adamant about having her teeth cleaned no more than 3 times a year.

SOCIAL HISTORY:
She lives alone with her cat. She maintains a cheery "I take one day at a time" attitude toward life. She is on a rigid fixed income.

CHIEF COMPLAINT:
"I am here for a cleaning."

ADULT CLINICAL EXAMINATION

Case PT1-7

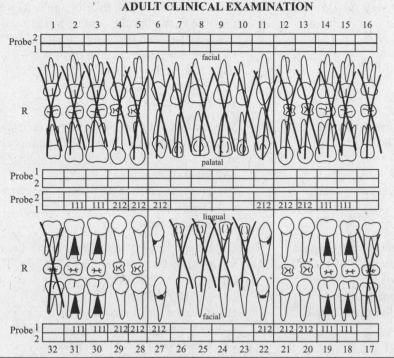

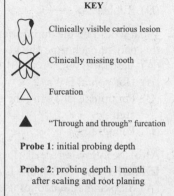

KEY

🦷	Clinically visible carious lesion
⊗	Clinically missing tooth
△	Furcation
▲	"Through and through" furcation

Probe 1: initial probing depth

Probe 2: probing depth 1 month after scaling and root planing

SUPPLEMENTAL ORAL EXAMINATION FINDINGS

1. Full upper denture and lower partial. Remaining lower teeth have a loss of attachment, exhibited by 3-7 mm of recession generally.
2. Probing depths 1-2 mm.
3. Furcation involvement clinically evident on lower molars but teeth appear very stable with no mobility.
4. X-rays show horizontal bone loss generally.
5. Current Oral Hygiene Status: Fair, with light calculus and moderate interproximal debris.
6. Minimal inflammation and bleeding.

61. Given this patient's clinical presentation, what would be the **BEST** maintenance frequency?
(A) 2 months
(B) 3 months
(C) 4 months
(D) 5 months

62. The patient has a clasp-type partial on the lower arch. Which of the following is a concern?
(A) There are no concerns.
(B) Potential for root decay around the teeth where the clasps make contact with the roots.
(C) Her inability to chew properly.
(D) The extrusion of the existing lower dentition.

63. This patient has 4 molars with Class IV furcation involvement. What would be the **BEST** way to scale the furcation of these molars effectively?
(A) Use a gracey 17–18.
(B) Use a right and left microthin ultrasonic tip.
(C) Use any curet.
(D) Use a scaler.

64. What is the **MOST** effective way for the patient to clean the furcations of the molars with Cl IV furcation involvement?
(A) Proxy brush
(B) Toothpick
(C) Superfloss
(D) Pipe cleaner

65. What is the **MOST** effective way for a patient to clean a furcation that shows very early involvement?
   (A) Pipe cleaner
   (B) End tuft brush
   (C) Regular toothbrush
   (D) Rubber tip

66. What would be the appropriate X-rays to take on this patient each time she needs them?
   (A) Vertical BWs
   (B) Horizontal BWs
   (C) Periapicals showing the teeth on the lower arch
   (D) Panograph

67. All of the following are risk factors for osteoporosis **EXCEPT** one. Which one is the **EXCEPTION**?
   (A) Smoking and alcohol use
   (B) Lack of exercise and sedentary lifestyle
   (C) Low lifetime calcium and vitamin C intake
   (D) Early menopause

68. What would be the best fluoride application at the office to strengthen the demineralized areas that make contact with the lower partial clasps?
   (A) Fluoride treatment with trays
   (B) Fluoride rinse
   (C) Fluoride foam
   (D) Fluoride varnish

69. What would be the **BEST** at-home application of fluoride to strengthen these same demineralized areas?
   (A) Fluoride dentifrice
   (B) Prescription-strength fluoride dentifrice
   (C) Desensitizing paste
   (D) Fluoride rinse

70. All of the following would be important in managing this elderly patient **EXCEPT** one. Which one is the **EXCEPTION**?
   (A) Do not rush her.
   (B) Take the time to listen to her.
   (C) Provide extra cushioning as needed.
   (D) Raise your voice to talk with her.

Directions: Study the case components and answer questions 71–80.

SYNOPSIS OF PATIENT HISTORY

CASE *PT1-8*

Age ___78___

Sex ___*Female*___

Height *5'2"*

Weight *138* lbs

___*62.6*___ kgs

Vital Signs

Blood pressure ___*128/80*___

Pulse rate ___70___

Respiration rate ___16___

---

1. Under Care of Physician

    Yes ☑   No ☐

    Condition: *Depression*

2. Hospitalized within the last 5 years

    Yes ☑   No ☐

    Reason: *Treatment for alcohol abuse one year apart*

3. Has or had the following conditions:

    Depression

    _____

4. Current medications:

    Antidepressant, does not know name

    _____

    _____

5. Smokes or uses tobacco products

    Yes ☐   No ☑

6. Is pregnant

    Yes ☐   No ☑   N/A ☐

MEDICAL HISTORY:
This patient is in fair health and is suffering from depression. She is medicated. She entered in house treatment for alcohol abuse three years ago, successfully, and was supposedly attending AA meetings. She states she has lost 15 pounds since her last dental visit.

DENTAL HISTORY:
Patient comes to dental practice once a year for cleaning and checkups.

SOCIAL HISTORY:
Patient lives alone and is widowed.

CHIEF COMPLAINT:
"My gums are bleeding. I know I am overdue for my cleaning."

ADULT CLINICAL EXAMINATION

Case PT1-8

		KEY
	Clinically visible carious lesion
	Clinically missing tooth
	Furcation
	"Through and through" furcation

Probe 1: initial probing depth

Probe 2: probing depth 1 month after scaling and root planing

SUPPLEMENTAL ORAL EXAMINATION FINDINGS

1. Tissues generally inflamed with bleeding.
2. Current Oral Hygiene Status: Fair, with cervical plaque, and food deposits generally.
3. Pocket depths are generally 3–4 mm.
4. Calculus is light but generalized.
5. Stain present.
6. Alcohol is detected on the breath of the patient.
7. X-rays reveal minimal amount of bone loss.
8. She has a large bruise on her face that she states happened when she tripped on the coffee table.

71. Patient had an FMX taken 2 years prior. What films should be taken today to assess for caries and alveolar bone levels per the dentist?
    (A) Panograph
    (B) 2 horizontal BWs
    (C) 4 vertical BWs
    (D) 4 horizontal BWs

72 All of the following may be signs that this patient is drinking excessively **EXCEPT** one. Which one is the **EXCEPTION**?
    (A) Angular cheilitis related to poor nutrition
    (B) Redness of forehead, cheeks, spider petechiae on nose, worsening of rosacea
    (C) Red, baggy eyes; bloated appearance
    (D) Greenish tinge to face from jaundice from liver disease

73. When gently questioned about the bruise on her face, the patient brushes it aside casually. What does the hygienist suspect?
    (A) Someone assaulted this patient.
    (B) The patient may have a form of leukemia.
    (C) She may have fallen while intoxicated.
    (D) She suspects nothing out of the ordinary.

74. Since the patient is a recovering alcoholic, what precaution should the hygienist consider in chairside preparation?
    (A) A plan to carefully avoid any discussion about drinking during the visit
    (B) The use of a nonalcoholic antimicrobial for pre-rinse and rinsing
    (C) A neutral fluoride treatment, if indicated
    (D) Avoidance of moderately abrasive polishing agents

75. What is the appropriate treatment protocol for debridement of this patient?
    (A) Hand scaling followed by polishing
    (B) Hand scaling with no polishing
    (C) Ultrasonic debridement, fine scaling as needed and selective polishing
    (D) Ultrasonic debridement, no polishing

76. If the patient is recommended the use of a mouth rinse, what is important to remember?
    (A) Commercial antibacterial and fluoride mouth rinses may contain up to 30 percent alcohol.
    (B) Since patient is not going to drink the mouth rinse, the ingredients are not significant.
    (C) There would be no need to recommend a mouth rinse for this patient.
    (D) Ask the pharmacist to create a specialized mouth rinse.

77. Is it appropriate for the hygienist to mention to the patient her concern that she may be drinking again?
    (A) No, it is not appropriate.
    (B) It may be appropriate; it is up to the dentist.
    (C) Not at this time; wait and see what happens at the next recare visit.
    (D) Yes, it is appropriate.

78. What would be the **BEST** way to raise your concerns to the patient?
    (A) "Mrs. X., have you been drinking again?"
    (B) "Mrs. X., is anything else you want to make me aware of today…anything going on that you want to talk to me about?"
    (C) "Mrs. X, I can tell you are drinking again."
    (D) Do not raise any concerns to the patient. Have the dentist do it.

79. If the patient still refuses to open up, how should you respond?
    (A) "You need to talk to me, or I'm going to get the doctor in here."
    (B) "I noticed the bruising, I see you have lost weight, and I detect an alcohol odor on your breath. I'm worried about you."
    (C) "You are exhibiting signs of a person who has resumed drinking. What are we going to do about it?"
    (D) Drop the subject, and let her deal with it as she sees fit.

80. What might be the **BEST** way to encourage the patient back into treatment or attending her meetings once the dialogue has opened?
    (A) Suggest she contact her AA "buddy" so that he can get involved and help her get back on track in the way that is best for her.
    (B) Contact the rehabilitation center and set up an appointment without the patient knowing about it.
    (C) Ask the dentist to handle this aspect of the situation.
    (D) Do not get involved at this point. You have already expressed your concerns.

Directions: Study the case components and answer questions 81–90.

SYNOPSIS OF PATIENT HISTORY

CASE *PT1-9*

Age ___20___

Sex ___Female___

Height ___5'7"___

Weight ___130___ lbs

___58___ kgs

Vital Signs

Blood pressure ___120/75___

Pulse rate ___65___

Respiration rate ___17___

---

1. Under Care of Physician
   Yes ☐ No ☑
   Condition: _____

2. Hospitalized within the last 5 years
   Yes ☐ No ☑
   Reason: _____
   _____

3. Has or had the following conditions:
   Asthma _____
   _____

4. Current medications:
   Inhaler, as needed; Birth-control pills ____
   _____
   _____

5. Smokes or uses tobacco products
   Yes ☐ No ☑

6. Is pregnant
   Yes ☐ No ☑ N/A ☐

MEDICAL HISTORY:
The patient is in good health. Her asthma happens infrequently. She has seen a physician only to attain birth control.

DENTAL HISTORY:
Good care, no decay or restorations previously, history of orthodontia, wears retainer at night. Began using a new toothpaste recently.

SOCIAL HISTORY:
Full-time college student lives with parents and commutes from home. Employed part-time at retail store on weekends.

CHIEF COMPLAINT:
"Need teeth cleaned. Gums hurt."

ADULT CLINICAL EXAMINATION

Case PT1-9

	1	2	3	4	5	6	7	8	9	10	11	12	13	14	15	16
Probe 2 / 1		323	323	322	222	212	212	212	212	212	212	222	222	323	323	

facial

R

palatal

	1	2	3	4	5	6	7	8	9	10	11	12	13	14	15	16
Probe 1 / 2		323	323	222	222	222	222	222	222	222	222	222	222	323	323	
Probe 2 / 1		323	323	323	322	222	222	222	222	222	222	222	222	323	323	

lingual

R

facial

	32	31	30	29	28	27	26	25	24	23	22	21	20	19	18	17
Probe 1 / 2		323	323	323	323	323	323	222	222	222	222	222	323	323	323	

KEY

Clinically visible carious lesion

Clinically missing tooth

△ Furcation

▲ "Through and through" furcation

Probe 1: initial probing depth

Probe 2: probing depth 1 month after scaling and root planing

SUPPLEMENTAL ORAL EXAMINATION FINDINGS

1. Current Oral Hygiene Status: Fair.
2. Diffuse, fiery red gingivitis generally.
3. Probes (with difficulty) 1–3 mm.
4. No evidence of bone loss on X-ray.

81. Which of the following is the **MOST** likely diagnosis for this patient's gingival condition?
    (A) Linear gingival erythema
    (B) Lichen planus
    (C) Allergic reaction
    (D) Not enough information to diagnose

82. The American Dental Association (ADA) periodontitis classification for the patient's disease would be
    (A) Type I.
    (B) Type II.
    (C) Type III.
    (D) Type IV.

83. Allergic reactions tend to occur orally to ingredients in all of the following **EXCEPT** one. Which one is the **EXCEPTION**?
    (A) Toothpastes
    (B) Mouthwashes
    (C) Chewing gum
    (D) Floss

84. Allergic reactions are usually the result of
    (A) flavor additives.
    (B) preservatives.
    (C) flavor additives and preservatives.
    (D) neutralizers.

85. Allergic reactions occur most commonly in patients who have a history of all of the following allergic conditions **EXCEPT** one. Which one is the **EXCEPTION**?
    (A) Bee sting reactions
    (B) Hay fever
    (C) Allergic skin rashes
    (D) Asthma

86. What is the **MOST** secret part of the formulation of pastes and mouthwashes, and the most allergenic component?
    (A) Preservative
    (B) Flavor additive
    (C) Neutralizers
    (D) Scent

87. In addition to fiery-red gingivitis on this patient, what clinical manifestation are we also likely to see in allergic reactions?
    (A) Petechaie
    (B) Blisters
    (C) Ulcers
    (D) Pseudomembrane

88. What is the treatment for an allergic reaction to a paste or mouth rinse?
    (A) Discontinue use.
    (B) Discontinue use and switch to a different brand.
    (C) Continue using, but begin using a neutral sodium bicarbonate mouthwash at bedtime.
    (D) Decrease the amount being used.

89. In what other way can the diagnosis of allergic response be confirmed?
    (A) It cannot be confirmed any other way.
    (B) Brush biopsy.
    (C) Tissue biopsy with a diagnosis of plasma cell gingivitis.
    (D) Find out when use is discontinued and gingivitis goes away.

90. Will the patient ever be able to return to this product?
    (A) No
    (B) Yes
    (C) Possibly, in the future
    (D) There is no need for her to use this product again.

Directions: Study the case components and answer questions 91–100.

SYNOPSIS OF PATIENT HISTORY

CASE _PT1-10_

Age ___68___

Sex ___Female___

Height ___5'10"___

Weight ___180___ lbs
___81.65___kgs

Vital Signs

Blood pressure ___140/90___

Pulse rate ___105___

Respiration rate ___17___

1. Under Care of Physician
   Yes ☑   No ☐

   Condition: _Hypertension, angina pectoris_

2. Hospitalized within the last 5 years
   Yes ☑   No ☐

   Reason: _Had heart attack three years ago, followed_
   by catheterization and placement of stent

3. Has or had the following conditions:

   Hypertension, angina, pacemaker

4. Current medications:

   Propanolol, Nitroglycerin (PRN), Loniten

5. Smokes or uses tobacco products
   Yes ☐   No ☑

6. Is pregnant
   Yes ☐   No ☐   N/A ☑

MEDICAL HISTORY:
This patient has a history of cardiovascular disease. He suffered a heart attack three years ago and has made an effort to change his lifestyle.

DENTAL HISTORY:
He has a history of regular dental care. He has had routine cleanings and some crown and bridge work. He has had 2 root canals in recent years. His last cleaning was one year ago.

SOCIAL HISTORY:
The patient retired after the heart attack. He is married with two grown children who do not live at home.

CHIEF COMPLAINT:
"I need my teeth cleaned. My gums are bleeding more lately."

ADULT CLINICAL EXAMINATION

Case PT1-10

	1	2	3	4	5	6	7	8	9	10	11	12	13	14	15	16
Probe 2																
Probe 1			434	535	535	524	524	534	524	524	524	434	434	534		

facial

R

palatal

	1	2	3	4	5	6	7	8	9	10	11	12	13	14	15	16
Probe 1			434	535	535	524	524	534	524	524	524	434	434	534		
Probe 2																

| Probe 2 | | | 546 | 535 | 535 | 535 | 425 | 424 | 424 | 424 | 435 | 434 | 434 | 534 | | |
| Probe 1 | | | | | | | | | | | | | | | | |

lingual

R

facial

Probe 1			546	545	535	535	424	424	423	424	424	545	644	644		
Probe 2																
	32	31	30	29	28	27	26	25	24	23	22	21	20	19	18	17

KEY

- Clinically visible carious lesion
- Clinically missing tooth
- Furcation
- "Through and through" furcation

Probe 1: initial probing depth

Probe 2: probing depth 1 month after scaling and root planing

SUPPLEMENTAL ORAL EXAMINATION FINDINGS

1. Tissues are inflamed in the posteriors; note pocketing on charting.
2. Bleeding upon probing interproximally.
3. Moderate interproximal calculus deposits.
4. Current Oral Hygiene Status: Fair.
5. Bitewings reveal a small amount of bone loss.

91. Your patient **MOST** likely has which of the following conditions?
(A) Chronic localized gingivitis
(B) Chronic generalized mild periodontitis
(C) Necrotizing ulcerative periodontitis (NUP)
(D) Chronic generalized moderate periodontitis

92. The American Association of Periodontology (AAP) classification for this patient's periodontal condition is
(A) Type 1.
(B) Type 2.
(C) Type 3.
(D) Type 4.

93. Which of the following is the **BEST** debridement protocol for this patient?
(A) Half-mouth debridement in two appointments
(B) Quadrant debridement with local anesthesia in one appointment

(C) Gross scaling
(D) Prophylaxis

94. After tissue resolution is achieved, what recall frequency should this patient be placed on?
(A) 2 months
(B) 3 months
(C) 4 months
(D) 6 months

95. You would like to use an ultrasonic scaler followed by hand scaling on this patient. Which of the following is **MOST** appropriate?
(A) Cavitron
(B) Piezo
(C) Cavitron or piezo are both acceptable.
(D) None of the above

96. Which of the following is **BEST** for your patient to use to clean his interproximal surfaces?
    (A) Floss
    (B) Toothpick
    (C) Proxy brush
    (D) End tuft brush

97. All of the following suggest that it is important for this particular patient to minimize the inflammation in his mouth **EXCEPT** one. Which one is the **EXCEPTION**?
    (A) Several research studies indicate consistent associations between periodontal disease and cardiovascular disease.
    (B) Treating periodontal inflammation may help in managing cardiovascular disease.
    (C) Treating periodontal inflammation will decrease the patient's risk of kidney stone, which are linked to cardiovascular disease.
    (D) Periodontal infections result in bacteremias that could possibly have systemic effects on the vascular system.

98. Which of the following bitewings should you take on this patient?
    (A) 2 horizontal
    (B) 4 horizontal
    (C) 2 vertical
    (D) 4 vertical

99. It is important to do which of the following prior to this patient's debridement visit?
    (A) Automatically pre-medicate him.
    (B) Consult with his physician.
    (C) Refer him to a periodontist.
    (D) None of the above

100. If your patient's pacemaker becomes turned off, you should do all of the following **EXCEPT** one. Which one is the **EXCEPTION**?
    (A) Turn off all suspected sources of interference.
    (B) Call for medical assistance because a defibrillator may be needed.
    (C) Position the patient for CPR.
    (D) Offer the patient a large glass of water.

Directions: Study the case components and answer questions 101–110.

SYNOPSIS OF PATIENT HISTORY

CASE *PT1-11*

Age ___8___

Sex ___Male___

Height _4'6"_

Weight _75_ lbs

_34.02_ kgs

Vital Signs

Blood pressure _N/A_

Pulse rate _85_

Respiration rate _20_

1. Under Care of Physician
   Yes ☑ No ☐
   Condition: *Routine checkups*

2. Hospitalized within the last 5 years
   Yes ☑ No ☐
   Reason: *Several surgeries to correct cleft palate and cleft lip*

3. Has or had the following conditions:
   Allergic to metal

4. Current medications:

5. Smokes or uses tobacco products
   Yes ☐ No ☑

6. Is pregnant
   Yes ☐ No ☐ N/A ☑

MEDICAL HISTORY:
The patient was born with a bilateral cleft lip with partial palatal involvement. He has just had a recent surgery on his upper lip.

DENTAL HISTORY:
He has had routine dental checkups since the age of 3. He has several teeth that show signs of demineralization as well as a history of caries.

SOCIAL HISTORY:
He is difficult to understand, as he has speech problems. He also has hearing loss. He is "clinic tired" and nervous in the dental environment.

CHIEF COMPLAINT:
He is here for a 6-month checkup and cleaning. His teeth feel unclean and his parents notice malador.

CLINICAL EXAMINATION   *Case PT1-11*

SUPPLEMENTAL ORAL EXAMINATION FINDINGS

1. Current Oral Hygiene Status: Fair.
2. Biofilm present on many teeth; stain; calculus lower anterior linguals and maxillary first molar buccal surfaces.
3. Tissues inflamed.
4. Shows evidence of dry mouth.
5. Demineralized surfaces exhibited; increased decay this visit.

101. Which of the following is the **BEST** recall frequency for this patient?
(A) 3 months
(B) 4 months
(C) 6 months
(D) 12 months

102. Your patient lives with his parents in a non-fluoridated community. Which of the following is important to prevent caries given his special needs?
(A) Fluoride dentifrice
(B) Fluoride diet supplements
(C) Professional fluoride applications
(D) Fluoride rinses

103. One of the **MOST** important fundamentals for children with cleft lip and/or palate is to preserve teeth because the removal of teeth around the cleft area
(A) creates further complications.
(B) predisposes the child to asthma.
(C) makes it more difficult for the child to breathe.
(D) has been linked to an increased risk of allergies.

104. A prosthesis used for a cleft lip/or cleft palate patient would address all of the following **EXCEPT** one. Which one is the **EXCEPTION**?
(A) Closure of the palate
(B) Scaffolding to fill out the upper lip
(C) Restoration of vertical dimension
(D) Restoration of horizontal dimension

105. Which of the following is the classification for a cleft of the soft and hard palates that continues through the alveolar ridge on both sides, leaving a free premaxilla and usually associated with a bilateral cleft lip?
    (A) Class 4
    (B) Class 5
    (C) Class 6
    (D) Class 7

106. A pregnant mother is at risk for giving birth to a child with a cleft lip/palate formation if she does any of the following **EXCEPT** one. Which one is the **EXCEPTION**?
    (A) Use tobacco.
    (B) Consume alcohol.
    (C) Use teratogenic agents.
    (D) Ingest excess fluoride.

107. A patient with a cleft palate/cleft lip is predisposed to which of the following?
    (A) Strep throat
    (B) GI issues
    (C) Upper-respiratory infections
    (D) Kidney infections

108. The removable prosthesis designed to provide closure of the palatal opening is called a(an)
    (A) palate expander.
    (B) obturative prosthesis.
    (C) opturator.
    (D) palatopharyngeal plate.

109. All of the following are special concerns for the cleft lip/cleft palate patients **EXCEPT** one. Which one is the **EXCEPTION**?
    (A) Increase in caries
    (B) Potential for malador
    (C) Weight loss due to difficulty in swallowing
    (D) Potential for periodontal issues due to greater challenges in biofilm removal

110. Which of the following is **NOT** a facial deformity associated with these patients?
    (A) Sunken eyes due to the depression in the middle of the skull
    (B) Depression of the nostril on the side with the cleft lip
    (C) Deficiency of upper lip, which may be short or retroposed
    (D) Overprominent lower lip

Directions: Study the case components and answer questions 111–120.

SYNOPSIS OF PATIENT HISTORY

CASE *PT1-12*

Age _____48_____

Sex _____Male_____

Height _5'7"_

Weight _150_ lbs

_64.08_kgs

Vital Signs

Blood pressure _____118/78_____

Pulse rate _____95_____

Respiration rate _____23_____

1. Under Care of Physician
   Yes ☐   No ☑

   Condition: _____

2. Hospitalized within the last 5 years
   Yes ☑   No ☐

   Reason: _____
   _____

3. Has or had the following conditions:

   Stomach ulcer _____
   _____

4. Current medications:

   Takes ibuprofen daily _____
   _____
   _____

5. Smokes or uses tobacco products
   Yes ☑   No ☐

6. Is pregnant
   Yes ☐   No ☐   N/A ☑

MEDICAL HISTORY:
This patient had a stomach ulcer three years ago, which he believes was caused by heavy drinking.

DENTAL HISTORY:
He has not seen a dentist in five years. He says he has many cavities. He has made several appointments at this office, but either canceled or did not show. He has noticeable hand tremors. He says he has not had a drink today, but I can smell alcohol on his breath.

SOCIAL HISTORY:
The patient describes himself as a heavy drinker and a partier. He says that he smokes, but just socially. He is divorced twice and lives with a girlfriend. He has no children. He works as a hair stylist at a local salon.

CHIEF COMPLAINT:
"I have a toothache, and my gums bleed sometimes when I brush. My tongue looks yellow."

ADULT CLINICAL EXAMINATION

Case PT1-12

KEY

	Clinically visible carious lesion
	Clinically missing tooth
	Furcation
	"Through and through" furcation

Probe 1: initial probing depth

Probe 2: probing depth 1 month after scaling and root planing

SUPPLEMENTAL ORAL EXAMINATION FINDINGS

1. Current Oral Hygiene Status: Fair/Poor.
2. Some bleeding upon probing.
3. Clinically visible dental caries.
4. Moderate xerostomia.

111. Your patient's dental caries are **MOST LIKELY** caused by which of the following?
(A) Lack of dental care
(B) Excessive drinking
(C) Poor dental self-care
(D) All of the above

112. All of the following may indicate that your patient has a drinking problem **EXCEPT** one. Which one is the **EXCEPTION**?
(A) Hypotension
(B) Xerostomia
(C) Quickened pulse
(D) Trembling hands

113. If this patient tells you that he wants to cut back on or stop drinking, you should refer him to which of the following **FIRST**?
(A) The dentist
(B) Alcoholics Anonymous
(C) A physician
(D) A nutritionist

114. This patient's trembling hands are **MOST LIKELY** due to which of the following?
(A) Anxiety
(B) Pain from a toothache
(C) Alcohol withdrawal
(D) All of the above

115. Suppose your sister frequently visits the salon at which this patient works, and you tell her that he may have a drinking problem. You have just violated which of the following core values?
    (A) Veracity
    (B) Confidentiality
    (C) Societal trust
    (D) Beneficence

116. Which of the following is **MOST LIKELY** the cause of this patient's xerostomia?
    (A) Alcohol
    (B) Tobacco
    (C) Poor oral hygiene
    (D) All of the above

117. Which of the following is the **BEST** course of treatment for this patient's yellow tongue?
    (A) Self-care
    (B) Antibiotic therapy
    (C) Removal of an abscess
    (D) Professional fluoride treatments

118. If your patient continues to drink heavily long term, he is **MOST LIKELY** to develop which of the following in the future?
    (A) Diabetes
    (B) Oral cancer
    (C) Alzheimer's disease
    (D) None of the above

119. Which of the following self-care agents should be recommended for this patient to reduce his risk of additional dental caries?
    (A) Topical paste
    (B) Antiseptic rinse
    (C) Fluoride gel
    (D) Mouth wash

120. This patient's many dental caries are **MOST LIKELY** caused by which of the following?
    (A) Xerostomia
    (B) Smoking
    (C) Drinking
    (D) Ibuprofen

Directions: Study the case components and answer questions 121–130.

SYNOPSIS OF PATIENT HISTORY
CASE *PT1-13*

Age ___23___

Sex ___Female___

Height ___5'4"___

Weight ___125___ lbs

___56.70___kgs

Vital Signs

Blood pressure ___120/80___

Pulse rate ___76___

Respiration rate ___14___

1. Under Care of Physician
   Yes ☐ No ☑
   Condition: _____

2. Hospitalized within the last 5 years
   Yes ☐ No ☑
   Reason: _____
   _____

3. Has or had the following conditions:
   Allergies (hay fever) _____
   _____

4. Current medications:
   Allegra _____
   _____

5. Smokes or uses tobacco products
   Yes ☑ No ☐

6. Is pregnant
   Yes ☐ No ☑ N/A ☐

MEDICAL HISTORY:
Patient takes Allegra daily for allergies. She increases the dosage in the spring and fall.

DENTAL HISTORY:
She is a busy graduate student who has not been at this or other dental office in two years.

SOCIAL HISTORY:
The patient works part-time at a local restaurant and is pursuing a graduate degree in mass communications. She lives with her parents and two brothers. She says she smokes about six cigarettes a day to calm her nerves and enjoys a glass of wine at night.

CHIEF COMPLAINT:
"I have swelling and pain by one of my bottom teeth. I know that I have a cavity there that I never got filled. It hurts to drink anything cold or to eat anything hot. I also have an earache and a bad taste in my mouth. I don't feel like I have any energy."

ADULT CLINICAL EXAMINATION

Case PT1-13

	1	2	3	4	5	6	7	8	9	10	11	12	13	14	15	16
Probe 2																
Probe 1			535	333	333	333	323	323	323	323	323	323	523	424		

facial

R

palatal

Probe 1			535	333	333	323	323	323	323	323	323	323	523	424		
Probe 2																

Probe 2			525	535	333	434	534	535	535	535	434	434	434	525	535	
Probe 1																

lingual

R

facial

Probe 1			525	535	333	434	534	535	535	535	434	434	434	525	535	
Probe 2																

| | 32 | 31 | 30 | 29 | 28 | 27 | 26 | 25 | 24 | 23 | 22 | 21 | 20 | 19 | 18 | 17 |

KEY

Clinically visible carious lesion

Clinically missing tooth

Furcation

"Through and through" furcation

Probe 1: initial probing depth

Probe 2: probing depth 1 month after scaling and root planing

SUPPLEMENTAL ORAL EXAMINATION FINDINGS

1. Current Oral Hygiene Status: Fair; moderate calculus deposits.
2. Clinically visible dental caries.
3. Localized area of swelling distal to #30, which has visible tooth decay.
4. Mild xerostomia.

---

121. Which of the following **BEST** describes your patient's condition?
(A) Chronic gingivitis
(B) Periapical abscess
(C) Periodontal abscess
(D) Acute necrotizing ulcerative gingivitis (ANUG)

122. Your patient's condition is **MOST LIKELY** caused by which of the following?
(A) Tooth decay
(B) Smoking
(C) Allergy medication
(D) None of the above

123. Your patient asks you what she can do to prevent this condition from occurring in the future. Which of the following is the **BEST** recommendation?
(A) Quit smoking.
(B) Avoid alcohol.
(C) Improve brushing.
(D) Visit the dentist regularly.

124. All of the following are symptoms of this patient's condition **EXCEPT** one. Which one is the **EXCEPTION**?
(A) The tooth is slightly extruded from its socket.
(B) The apex of the tooth is acutely inflamed.
(C) Infection occurs where pre-existing periodontitis is present.
(D) The patient may suffer pain, swelling, and fever.

125. Treatment of your patient's condition will likely include which of the following?
(A) Draining of pus through an incision in the gum tissue
(B) Prescription of antibiotics
(C) Injection of an anesthetic into the infected tooth
(D) All of the above

126. Which of the following is **NOT** a common treatment for this patient's condition?
    (A) Root canal therapy
    (B) Bone grafting
    (C) Elimination of infection
    (D) Extraction of the infected tooth

127. While you may take several radiographs of this patient, which of the following is the **BEST** to diagnose this patient's condition?
    (A) Periapical
    (B) Bitewings
    (C) Panoramic
    (D) Full-mouth series

128. On a radiograph, this patient's condition would appear
    (A) light gray.
    (B) white.
    (C) dark.
    (D) fuzzy.

129. Which of the following methods of self-care is **BEST** for this patient while undergoing treatment?
    (A) Apply topical fluoride.
    (B) Rinse with warm salt water.
    (C) Use an antiseptic mouthwash.
    (D) None of the above

130. As a dental hygienist, your role in treating this patient includes all of the following **EXCEPT** one. Which one is the **EXCEPTION**?
    (A) Taking radiographs
    (B) Completing scaling and root planing
    (C) Recommending an antibiotic
    (D) Recommending self-care

Directions: Study the case components and answer questions 131–140.

SYNOPSIS OF PATIENT HISTORY　　　　CASE *PT1-14*

Age ___20___

Sex ___Male___

Height _5'6"_

Weight _140_ lbs

_63.50_kgs

Vital Signs

Blood pressure ___100/60___

Pulse rate ___76___

Respiration rate ___15___

1. Under Care of Physician
   Yes ☑　No ☐

   Condition: _____

2. Hospitalized within the last 5 years
   Yes ☐　No ☑

   Reason: _____
   _____

3. Has or had the following conditions:

   Patient is a diabetic; he undergoes a glycated
   hemoglobin test every three months

4. Current medications:

   Insulin _____
   _____

5. Smokes or uses tobacco products
   Yes ☑　No ☐

6. Is pregnant
   Yes ☐　No ☐　N/A ☑

MEDICAL HISTORY:
The patient was diagnosed with diabetes at age 12. He recently began using an insulin pump.

DENTAL HISTORY:
The patient comes in for regular dental checkups.

SOCIAL HISTORY:
The patient is a full-time college student. He lives with his grandmother. He is active in athletics.

CHIEF COMPLAINT:
He is interested in tooth whitening. He has recently noticed that his gums look different and that they sometimes bleed and feel sore when he brushes.

ADULT CLINICAL EXAMINATION

Case PT1-14

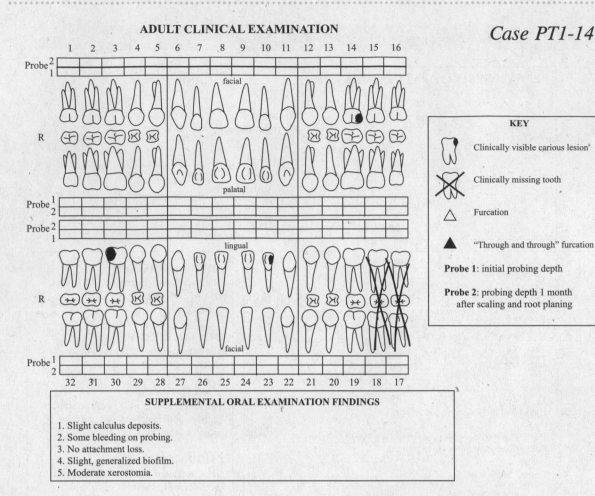

KEY

⌢ Clinically visible carious lesion

⌀ Clinically missing tooth

△ Furcation

▲ "Through and through" furcation

Probe 1: initial probing depth

Probe 2: probing depth 1 month after scaling and root planing

SUPPLEMENTAL ORAL EXAMINATION FINDINGS

1. Slight calculus deposits.
2. Some bleeding on probing.
3. No attachment loss.
4. Slight, generalized biofilm.
5. Moderate xerostomia.

---

131. Based on the American Diabetes Classification system, your patient has which of the following types of diabetes?
(A) Drug-induced
(B) Type 1
(C) Gestational
(D) Type 2

132. According to this patient's dental chart, he has tooth decay on which of the following teeth?
(A) #11
(B) #14
(C) #17
(D) #22

133. Patients with diabetes are at an especially high risk of developing which of the following?
(A) Dental caries
(B) Gingivitis
(C) Periodontal disease
(D) All of the above

134. To prevent periodontal disease, your patient should do all of the following **EXCEPT** one. Which one is the **EXCEPTION**?
(A) Quit smoking.
(B) Maintain good control of diabetes.
(C) Test blood glucose levels every other day.
(D) Maintain good oral hygiene.

135. This patient's xerostomia is **MOST LIKELY** caused by which of the following?
(A) Renal function
(B) Gingivitis
(C) Insulin
(D) Poor oral hygiene

136. Which of the following medical emergencies is **MOST LIKELY** to occur during this patient's treatment?
(A) Diabetic coma
(B) Insulin shock
(C) Hypoglycemia
(D) Hyperglycemia

137. Which of the following recare intervals is **BEST** for this patient?
(A) 1 month
(B) 3 months
(C) 6 months
(D) 12 months

138. When examining a diabetic patient, you should look for changes in which of the following?
(A) The oral cavity
(B) The individual's appearance
(C) Exposed body parts
(D) All of the above

139. All of the following are diabetic-related conditions **EXCEPT** one. Which one is the **EXCEPTION**?
(A) Burning mouth syndrome
(B) Abnormal wound healing
(C) Fungal infections
(D) Tooth abscesses

140. According to the American Dental Association (ADA) classifications, this patient's condition is classified as which of the following?
(A) Type I
(B) Type II
(C) Type III
(D) Type IV

Directions: Study the case components and answer questions 141–150.

SYNOPSIS OF PATIENT HISTORY

CASE *PT1-15*

Age ___69___

Sex *Male*

Height *5'8"*

Weight *157* lbs

71.21 kgs

Vital Signs

Blood pressure ___*152/96*___

Pulse rate ___72___

Respiration rate ___17___

1. Under Care of Physician
    Yes ☑   No ☐

    Condition: _____

2. Hospitalized within the last 5 years
    Yes ☐   No ☑

    Reason: _____
    _____

3. Has or had the following conditions:

    Chronic smoker; high cholesterol
    _____

4. Current medications:

    Zicor for cholesterol
    _____
    _____

5. Smokes or uses tobacco products
    Yes ☑   No ☐

6. Is pregnant
    Yes ☐   No ☐   N/A ☑

MEDICAL HISTORY:
The patient's physician has told him that he must stop smoking, but the patient admits to still smoking more than a pack of cigarettes a day and routinely chews tobacco. He is a recovering alcoholic.

DENTAL HISTORY:
The patient wears a full maxillary denture. He comes in for regular dental checkups and cleanings.

SOCIAL HISTORY:
The patient lives in a retirement community. He is widowed and enjoys fishing. He has seven children and ten grandchildren.

CHIEF COMPLAINT:
He complains of a white area in the muccobuccal fold of the upper lip. He says that the gums underneath his denture are red and sore.

ADULT CLINICAL EXAMINATION

Case PT1-15

KEY

Clinically visible carious lesion

Clinically missing tooth

Furcation

"Through and through" furcation

Probe 1: initial probing depth

Probe 2: probing depth 1 month after scaling and root planing

SUPPLEMENTAL ORAL EXAMINATION FINDINGS

1. Current Oral Hygiene Status: Good.
2. Full upper denture, which is mostly clean.
3. Light calculus on lower arch.
4. Mild recession on lower teeth.
5. Moderate xerostomia.

141. This patient's blood pressure is categorized as which of the following?
(A) Normal
(B) Prehypertension
(C) Stage 1 hypertension
(D) Stage 2 hypertension

142. This patient has all of the following risk factors for developing periodontal disease **EXCEPT** one. Which one is the **EXCEPTION**?
(A) Age
(B) Gender
(C) Smoking
(D) Poor oral hygiene

143. The white lesion in the patient's mouth is **MOST LIKELY** caused by
(A) tobacco.
(B) alcohol.
(C) poor oral hygiene.
(D) All of the above

144. This patient is at an increased risk of developing all of the following **EXCEPT** one. Which one is the **EXCEPTION**?
(A) Oral cancer
(B) Halitosis
(C) Denture stomatitis
(D) Periodontal disease

145. The **BEST** referral for this patient is to a(an)
(A) periodontist.
(B) alcohol-cessation program.
(C) tobacco-cessation program.
(D) nutritionist.

146. This patient's xerostomia is **MOST LIKELY** caused by
(A) sun exposure.
(B) gingivitis.
(C) smoking.
(D) poor oral hygiene.

147. Which of the following is the **BEST** self-care to treat this patient's gums?
(A) Antiseptic rinse
(B) Mouthwash
(C) Warm salt water
(D) None of the above

148. It is important for your patient to remove his dentures at night for which of the following reasons?
(A) To rest the gums
(B) To give the gums air
(C) To give gums contact with saliva
(D) All of the above

149. You should recommend which of the following for your patient to clean his gums and teeth?
(A) A hard-bristled toothbrush
(B) A medium-bristled toothbrush
(C) A soft-bristled toothbrush
(D) A power brush

150. To relieve his xerostomia, this patient should do all of the following **EXCEPT** one. Which one is the **EXCEPTION**?
(A) Drink more water.
(B) Reduce smoking.
(C) Use dry-mouth products.
(D) Suck on hard candy.

ANSWER KEY AND EXPLANATIONS
Component A

1. C	41. D	81. A	121. B	161. C
2. D	42. B	82. B	122. D	162. E
3. D	43. D	83. A	123. B	163. E
4. D	44. B	84. E	124. E	164. A
5. E	45. E	85. C	125. D	165. B
6. A	46. A	86. D	126. B	166. D
7. C	47. B	87. B	127. A	167. B
8. E	48. D	88. D	128. C	168. C
9. D	49. A	89. B	129. A	169. B
10. E	50. C	90. D	130. A	170. E
11. B	51. C	91. E	131. D	171. B
12. A	52. A	92. C	132. A	172. E
13. D	53. A	93. C	133. D	173. E
14. B	54. E	94. B	134. A	174. C
15. E	55. A	95. C	135. B	175. C
16. D	56. A	96. D	136. C	176. B
17. D	57. C	97. A	137. C	177. B
18. D	58. B	98. E	138. B	178. C
19. B	59. D	99. D	139. C	179. C
20. D	60. C	100. B	140. B	180. B
21. D	61. A	101. C	141. B	181. C
22. C	62. A	102. A	142. A	182. C
23. A	63. C	103. A	143. A	183. A
24. B	64. B	104. D	144. D	184. A
25. C	65. A	105. D	145. C	185. A
26. A	66. G	106. C	146. B	186. A
27. A	67. B	107. D	147. D	187. D
28. E	68. A	108. D	148. C	188. C
29. C	69. E	109. C	149. D	189. E
30. C	70. C	110. C	150. A	190. B
31. E	71. E	111. B	151. B	191. A
32. E	72. A	112. B	152. D	192. D
33. D	73. D	113. D	153. E	193. B
34. D	74. E	114. A	154. D	194. D
35. C	75. C	115. C	155. B	195. C
36. B	76. A	116. C	156. B	196. E
37. A	77. C	117. D	157. C	197. A
38. C	78. D	118. B	158. A	198. C
39. C	79. A	119. D	159. A	199. D
40. B	80. E	120. C	160. A	200. A

1. **The correct answer is (C).** Pain intensity is primarily determined by the number of fibers stimulated.

2. **The correct answer is (D).** Penumbra refers to a partial shadow. The penumbra must be reduced to make clear images, which leads to more accurate diagnoses. This can be done by reducing the distance between the object or focal point and the film.

3. **The correct answer is (D).** Chicken pox is caused by the varicella zoster virus and is a member of the herpes family. The incubation period for the virus is generally 2 to 3 weeks, but the virus can also stay dormant in the dorsal root ganglia for many years and cause shingles later in life.

4. **The correct answer is (D).** Dental hygiene professionals can evaluate the overall quality of an individual article or a publication by considering factors such as whether the journal is connected to a professional group, if there is an editorial review board for the publication, and if the data used to write the article is current. The cost of an article or journal is not necessarily indicative of its quality.

5. **The correct answer is (E).** Acetaminophen is an over-the-counter drug that can reduce pain and lower body temperature. Alcohol increases the risk that acetaminophen will have toxic effects on the body (particularly the liver), so patients taking acetaminophen should avoid consuming alcohol.

6. **The correct answer is (A).** One of the main characteristics of enamel hypoplasia is pitted enamel. Other characteristics include a yellow–dark brown color and a thinner matrix layer.

7. **The correct answer is (C).** During metaphase, the chromosomes line up along the midplane. Metaphase is the second of mitosis's four phases. The first phase of mitosis is prophase, the third phase is anaphase, and the fourth phase is telophase. Interphase is the phase a cell stays in while it is not undergoing mitosis.

8. **The correct answer is (E).** The tonsils are part of the lymph system. Tonsils protect against invading antigens. The tonsils drain through the superior deep cervical nodes.

9. **The correct answer is (D).** To be an effective infection-control strategy, gloves should be changed after every patient—regardless of how long the dental hygienist was with that patient—and during lengthy appointments. Glove defects generally begin to appear after about 1 hour.

10. **The correct answer is (E).** A gingivoplasty is a type of excisional surgery that reshapes gingival tissues during periodontitis. It is different from a gingivectomy, which simply removes gingival tissue without altering the shape.

11. **The correct answer is (B).** Because panoramic films often lack definition of detail since they are taken outside of the mouth, it is best to use periapical X-rays to get a better view of the anterior and posterior teeth in addition to the area surrounding a particular problem tooth.

12. **The correct answer is (A).** Teleological or utilitarian ethics establishes ethical rules based on the usefulness of actions and whether they will result in the greatest good. Deontologic ethics focuses more on whether the act itself (as opposed to the outcome) was right or wrong.

13. **The correct answer is (D).** There are 46 chromosomes in the human nucleus. Half of these chromosomes come from the mother and the other half come from the father.

14. **The correct answer is (B).** Tetracyclines bind to the 30S ribosome and impede protein synthesis, which is the mechanism of action of this class of drugs. Tetracyclines often lead to suprainfections, because they are broad spectrum antibiotics that kill many different types of bacteria, something that can alter the healthy balance of bacteria in the body.

15. **The correct answer is (E).** Flossing is important to prevent carious lesions, and floss holders are aids that can help those who have problems with dexterity. Threaders are useful for those who have bridges, while knitting yarn can be used on diastemas and dental implants.

16. **The correct answer is (D).** Protozoa are singled-celled eukaryotes that form protective cysts to survive harsh environments. These cysts allow the protozoa to survive outside of the host. Protozoa are the smallest of all living, single-celled animals.

17. **The correct answer is (D).** Methotraxate is a commonly prescribed chemotherapeutic agent and an antimetabolite. Antimetabolites work by inhibiting cell division and slowing, or stopping, the growth of tumors.

18. **The correct answer is (D).** Several groups are consistently found to be at high risk for oral problems. These groups include the elderly, those with mental or physical challenges, preschool or school-aged children, pregnant women, those with low incomes, and individuals who live in rural areas or inner-city communities.

19. **The correct answer is (B).** Dental hygiene professionals should avoid entering a patient's first zone of personal space (0 to 18 inches) but may usually enter a patient's second zone of personal space (18 inches to 4 feet). The third zone of personal space extends from about 4 feet away from an individual to approximately 12 feet.

20. **The correct answer is (D).** Auscultation is the act of listening to sounds made by the body, such as a clicking jaw, to determine diagnosis and treatment. It does not rely on the sense of touch to assess the patient.

21. **The correct answer is (D).** The mandibular second deciduous molar erupts, or emerges, around age 20 months.

22. **The correct answer is (C).** Periodontal flap surgery is a type of incisional surgery that exposes the underlying bone for modification, as well as the root surface of the tooth for removal of residual calculus. It is used to remove deeper diseased tissues such as epithelial and connective tissue.

23. **The correct answer is (A).** When people suffer from metabolic syndrome, their bodies often fail to use insulin efficiently, which puts them at a greater risk for developing a number of conditions including coronary heart disease, type 2 diabetes, peripheral vascular disease, and stroke. Chronic obstructive pulmonary disease, or COPD, makes it difficult for people to breathe, but it is not a risk factor associated with metabolic syndrome.

24. **The correct answer is (B).** Both statements are false. Dental diagnosis identifies specific oral diseases, while dental hygiene diagnosis identifies human-needs deficits.

25. **The correct answer is (C).** After cleaning the pits and fissures, other steps include etching occlusal surfaces, pits, and fissures with 37 percent phosphoric acid; washing occlusal surfaces for 5 to 10 seconds; and drying the etched area with clean air spray. These steps must be completed before applying the sealant to ensure the sealant adheres to the teeth.

26. **The correct answer is (A).** A patient with braces on his teeth will benefit from a professionally applied fluoride varnish. Since fluoride varnish is applied with a brush, the placement of the varnish can be controlled and applied where it will be most advantageous.

27. **The correct answer is (A).** The main advantage of the Bass technique is that it is very efficient at removing plaque, which is an issue for the patient in the scenario. This brushing technique involves orienting the bristles at a 45-degree angle apically into the sulcus and using a back-and-forth movement.

28. **The correct answer is (E).** Based on the location of the staining and the dark color, the stains Beth observed are most likely caused by tobacco. Pulp necrosis, bacteria, food pigments, and coffee can also alter the appearance of or stain teeth, but they often result in a yellow biofilm, not brown staining.

29. **The correct answer is (C).** Choice (C) is the best answer because the patient can use it to make positive changes and lower his risk of developing future carious lesions. Choices (A), (B), and (D) may be too technical for some patients and they will not likely relate personally to the information, and choice (E) is incorrect.

30. **The correct answer is (C).** A blurred image is the result of patient movement during radiographic exposure. Asking the patient to remain still will ensure a clear image.

31. **The correct answer is (E).** Patients with a history of bulimia do not commonly present with hyperplasia of the adenoids or tonsils. They may present with parotid gland swelling, severe caries, burning tongue, and perimylolysis, or decalcification of teeth.

32. **The correct answer is (E).** When communicating with individuals who have hearing impairments,

some techniques that can improve the quality of communications include eliminating background noise, speaking slowly, and using visual aids and gestures when appropriate. Those who are hearing impaired often respond better to cognitive techniques, will likely find it easier to focus on a single individual, and will probably not want the hygienist to invade their personal space.

33. **The correct answer is (D).** A lipoma is a soft tissue lesion composed of a circumscribed mass of mature fat cells covered by a thin epithelium. Typical lipomas range in size from one to six centimeters. They are soft, easily moveable, and most common in people between the ages of 40 and 60.

34. **The correct answer is (D).** Although patients with recurrent aphthous stomatitis do often present with oval or round ulcerations with a yellow-white fibrous surface encircled by a red halo, exposure to *Bacillus fusiformis* or *Borreliavincentii* commonly causes necrotizing ulcerative gingivitis.

35. **The correct answer is (C).** A patient suffering from hyperparathyroidism would be particularly likely to develop a brown tumor, which is a lesion similar in nature to a central giant cell reparative granuloma.

36. **The correct answer is (B).** Digitalis glycosides, which can be used to treat congestive heart failure and arrhythmias, make the heart work more efficiently by increasing the strength of heartbeats and (usually) decreasing the number of heartbeats. Antianginal agents reduce the amount of blood that is returned to the heart, and antihypertensives such as angiotensin II blockers and vasodilators reduce blood pressure.

37. **The correct answer is (A).** When providing oral health education, dental hygiene professionals can communicate more effectively by sitting beside or at a diagonal angle to patients. Facing patients while sitting or standing may be interpreted as confrontational, providing information while working inside a patient's mouth tends to make patients uncomfortable, and filling out a chart while speaking will likely make the patient feel that the dental hygiene professional is not giving his or her full attention to the conversation.

38. **The correct answer is (C).** Patients can be exposed to another patient's infections when they come into contact with contaminated instruments and surfaces. Aside from sterilizing dental instruments, dental hygiene professionals should disinfect surfaces, use disposable items when appropriate, change face masks after every patient visit, and decontaminate protective eyewear for patients to minimize the risk of cross contamination.

39. **The correct answer is (C).** Because molars have many pits and grooves, a beneficial way to prevent tooth decay is by using a dental sealant. Although saliva washes the teeth to prevent decay, it is difficult for saliva to get deep into the grooves of molars. Pit-and-fissure sealants, therefore, prevent particles from settling in the grooves and initiating tooth decay.

40. **The correct answer is (B).** Severe bacterial infections can cause septic shock when large quantities of cytokines can cause cardiovascular failure and hypoglycemia; therefore, although severe bacterial infections can trigger high levels of leukocytes, the leukocytes are not responsible for septic shock.

41. **The correct answer is (D).** Disclosing agents make plaque visible, which helps with patient education because the dental hygiene professional can see what aspects of oral hygiene the client needs to work on most and tailor instruction accordingly. While iodine solutions were commonly used as disclosing agents at one time, they are not used much today because they have the potential to cause serious allergic reactions.

42. **The correct answer is (B).** The primary purpose of polishing a restoration is to remove surface irregularities. This practice is of vital importance because surface irregularities can retain plaque, which may result in gingivitis or the corrosion of material.

43. **The correct answer is (D).** Water fluoridation is effective in reducing tooth decay by 20–40 percent. This process prevents cavities in both children and adults and is especially important and beneficial to those who cannot see a dentist regularly.

44. **The correct answer is (B).** Proteins are nutrients that are made up of thousands of amino acids. When proteins are broken down in the body, the

body uses the amino acids from the food. Complete proteins such as meat and eggs include more amino acids than incomplete proteins such as legumes and leafy greens.

45. **The correct answer is (E).** *Campylobacter* is a Gram-negative genus of bacteria. A Gram-negative bacteria is one that does not turn a violet color during a Gram staining test. *Listeria, Actinomyces, Strepococcus,* and *Staphlococcus* are all Gram-positive genera of bacteria.

46. **The correct answer is (A).** Lectures or informative talks tend to stifle the creativity of learners because they do not require students to actively participate, and most communication is one-way. The other choices are disadvantages of lectures that include demonstrations to illustrate essential information visually.

47. **The correct answer is (B).** The body's clotting system is part of the body's natural healing process. The clotting system is activated by chemicals such as collagen and protease. It helps from thrombin (an enzyme that helps clot blood) and it clots the blood. When it clots the blood, the system localizes microorganisms and helps prevent the spread of infection. The plasma proteins kininogens and kallikreins are produced during the kinin system (or the kinin-kallikrein system), not the clotting system.

48. **The correct answer is (D).** Small doses of barbiturates administered orally or intramuscularly can be used in dentistry to sedate patients and relieve anxiety. In larger doses, barbiturates administered intravenously can be used to induce general anesthesia.

49. **The correct answer is (A).** Educating students about the long-term physical effects of smoking, the social consequences, and strategies students can use when confronted with peer pressure to smoke are educational strategies that may prevent students from picking up the habit. Choices (B), (C), and (D) are more disciplinary in nature, and choice (E) may help students stop smoking, but will not prevent them from starting.

50. **The correct answer is (C).** Mean (or average) is calculated by adding up all of the values in a data set and then dividing the total by the number of values. In this case the average is calculated as follows: $9 + 9 + 5 + 8 + 4 = 35$; $35 \div 5 = 7$.

51. **The correct answer is (C).** While it is true that a patient who is allergic to one ester will have an allergic reaction to all other anesthetics derived from ester, the reason for this is that all *esters* are cross-reactive. Anesthetics made with amides are not cross-reactive.

52. **The correct answer is (A).** The normal resting heart rate of a healthy adult is 60–100 beats per minute. Athletes' heart rates are typically as low as 40 beats per minute. Many factors affect heart rate, such as activity level, fitness level, air temperature, body position, and emotions.

53. **The correct answer is (A).** Root debridement procedures should be performed as a series of appointments focusing on each quadrant of the mouth at 2-week intervals. The final reevaluation of pockets is made 6 weeks after the final root debridement procedure.

54. **The correct answer is (E).** About 95 percent of enamel is inorganic. The rest of tooth enamel is made up of organic material and water.

55. **The correct answer is (A).** Patients who are actively taking MAO inhibitors may have a limited ability to metabolize vasoconstrictors. These medications inhibit the production of monoamine oxidase (MAO), the enzyme responsible for biotransformation.

56. **The correct answer is (A).** Both the statement and the reason are correct and related. Fluoride in the body obtained through systemic sources such as fluoridated drinking water is present in saliva, which continuously remineralizes the surface of teeth to prevent decay.

57. **The correct answer is (C).** The statement is correct, but the reason is NOT. While it is true that acidulated phosphate fluoride should not be used on patients with crowns, bridges, veneers, or composite restorations, the reason for this is because its acidity causes a layer of enamel to demineralize.

58. **The correct answer is (B).** Dental sealants are a way of preventing dental caries in children and teenagers, and are recommended for individuals

in this age group whether they live in areas with fluoridated or nonfluoridated water. Sealants are typically covered by third-party payers.

59. **The correct answer is (D).** Cirrhosis, or scarring of the liver, is the most likely ailment to cause fibrosis. Fibrosis is a condition in which excess fibrosis connective tissue forms in tissues or organs.

60. **The correct answer is (C).** While the Internet can be a valuable educational aid, its public nature means online information may be incomplete or inaccurate. Because of this, those involved in community programs may want to consider using other educational aids such as CD-ROMs, books, models, and pamphlets instead.

61. **The correct answer is (A).** Carious enamel lesions occur when the mouth's pH level is 4.5–5.5. Root caries can occur when the mouth pH is 6.0–6.7. The normal pH of the mouth is 6.75–7.25.

62. **The correct answer is (A).** The internal carotid artery supplies the brain, eyes, and orbital cavities with blood.

63. **The correct answer is (C).** Folate (or folic acid), vitamin C, thiamin (or vitamin B1), and biotin (or vitamin H) are all water-soluble vitamins. Vitamin E, however, is a fat-soluble vitamin. Fat-soluble vitamins can build up in fat stores in the body, and people who ingest too much of these vitamins can experience vitamin toxicity.

64. **The correct answer is (B).** Nursing-bottle decay does not typically affect the mandibular anterior teeth, because the tongue protects these teeth and prevents milk from pooling on them. Because milk tends to pool on the maxillary anterior teeth, these teeth are the first to see the effects of nursing-bottle decay.

65. **The correct answer is (A).** Dental hygienists should be aware if patients have heart damage. This is because people with heart conditions are susceptible to endocarditis. These patients should be treated with an antibiotic before undergoing dental procedures.

66. **The correct answer is (C).** Incidental curettage involves removing a thin layer of diseased pocket epithelium tissue. This process usually occurs at the same time as root debridement as the first line of therapy against periodontitis.

67. **The correct answer is (B).** Formal activities include events, curricula, programs, etc., that are specifically designed to encourage certain behaviors that will enhance oral health. Informal activities result in accidental learning that can also encourage behaviors that may prevent disease, and include conversations and interactions with family, friends, and of course oral health professionals.

68. **The correct answer is (A).** The three types of SANS receptors are β-1, β-2, and β-3. The β-1 receptors are involved in constricting smooth muscles and blood vessels. β-2 and β-3 receptors carry out functions such as relaxing smooth muscles, and breaking down lipids.

69. **The correct answer is (E).** Prostaglandins are chemical mediators released from mast cells. These chemical mediators work by causing vaso-dilatation, pain, and fever.

70. **The correct answer is (C).** Xylitol is a sweetener with many dental health benefits, including a reduction in childhood caries related to maternal consumption of the sweetener, a reduction in the adhesiveness of plaque, and enamel reminer-alization. Choices (A), (B), (D), and (E) are all names of common artificial sweeteners, but none are associated with the dental health benefits of xylitol.

71. **The correct answer is (E).** When administering an injected anesthetic, it is necessary to record all of the above information, except for the type of syringe used. This information will not be necessary if the patient's record is reevaluated at a later date.

72. **The correct answer is (A).** Viruses are not eukaryotic cells. Scientists are still trying to classify viruses, as they are neither eukaryotic nor exactly prokaryotic. Although the virus's classification is still unclear, scientists have agreed that it is not a eukaryotic cell because it does not have nuclei.

73. **The correct answer is (D).** Bile is the bodily secretion that breaks down fat during digestion. Pepsin and trypsin are enzymes that help break down protein. Saliva helps break down starches in the mouth. Mucus that is secreted during

digestion helps protect the body from acid that is also produced.

74. **The correct answer is (E).** A patient's medical history should include information about allergies, tobacco use, alcohol or drug use, daily medications, and medical conditions, including cardiovascular disease or diabetes. Information about oral habits, such as grinding or clenching teeth, is part of the dental history of a patient, which should be updated at each visit. The dental history also should include the patient's chief complaint; past orthodontic, endodontic, or periodontal treatments; areas of pain or discomfort; and other factors.

75. **The correct answer is (C).** Bell's palsy is a form of facial paralysis, but it does not affect the trigeminal nerve. Bell's palsy affects the facial nerve (VII).

76. **The correct answer is (A).** HIV-associated periodontitis is not an example of a genetic disorder that brings about periodontitis. Instead, it is a condition in which viral infection of the Human Immunodeficiency Virus leads to the exacerbation of inflammation in the periodontium.

77. **The correct answer is (C).** The normal respiration rate for healthy adults is 14 to 20 breaths per minute. For children, the rate is 18 to 30 breaths per minute. Respiration rate is determined by counting the number of breaths for 30 seconds and then multiplying by 2. If the rate after 30 seconds is deemed irregular, then respiration rate should be taken again for 1 minute. A breath is considered one exhalation and one inhalation.

78. **The correct answer is (D).** The scientific method consists of a set of ordered steps that can be used to conduct almost any type of research. The steps, in order, are identifying the problem; creating a hypothesis; collecting, organizing, and analyzing data; forming conclusions; and rejecting, accepting, or modifying the original hypothesis.

79. **The correct answer is (A).** The first branchial arch gives rise to the sphenoid bone, which is part of the skull. The sphenoid articulates with six other bones to form the orbit.

80. **The correct answer is (E).** The hypothalamus regulates the body's homeostasis. This gland controls body temperature, emotions, hunger, thirst, and sleep.

81. **The correct answer is (A).** A procedure conducted under indirect or close supervision must be authorized by a licensed dentist before it is performed. The dentist must also remain on the premises while the hygienist is performing the procedure.

82. **The correct answer is (B).** A drug's degree of ionization and lipid solubility and other factors such as a client's age and gender all have an influence on drug absorption. Drugs that are more ionized are absorbed less readily by the body, while drugs that are more lipid soluble are absorbed more readily by the body.

83. **The correct answer is (A).** A case presentation is a formal communication between the health-care provider and his or her patients. The main purpose of a case presentation is to meet legal and ethical requirements, reach a treatment agreement, and obtain informed consent.

84. **The correct answer is (E).** Three types of strokes differ by the amount of lateral pressure applied to the tooth and by the length and direction of stroke movement. The walking stroke is used with probes since EA varies in depth and contour. Walking strokes use an up-and-down motion while moving around the tooth in small steps. The exploratory stroke is used with all instruments for assessment purposes. The working stroke uses the most pressure.

85. **The correct answer is (C).** Desensitizing toothpastes contain a variety of active ingredients, including the ones mentioned in choices (A), (B), (D), and (E) as well as potassium oxalate and ferric oxalate. Other strategies for managing tooth hypersensitivity at home include fluoride gels that can be brushed onto the teeth and fluoride rinses.

86. **The correct answer is (D).** The main goal of oral health promotion and education is prevention. By showing patients how to floss properly, for instance, dental hygiene professionals may be able to avoid the need to diagnose, treat, and cure a variety of oral health problems.

87. **The correct answer is (B).** The U. S. Public Health Service recommends 0.7–1.2 parts per million in drinking water as a safe way to aid in the prevention of tooth decay.

88. **The correct answer is (D).** The Vickers test is designed to determine the hardness of a dental material through the use of a square-based diamond point. The Knoops and Brinell tests are also hardness tests, but they utilize a diamond indenter and a steel ball, respectively. The Rockwell test measures the difference in depth caused by two different forces. Mohs refers to the Mohs scale, which provides a means of measuring rigidity and resistance to pressure and scratching.

89. **The correct answer is (B).** Air polishers and ultrasonic scalers should not be used on patients with cerebral palsy, because these tools use large quantities of water. Patients with cerebral palsy may experience dysphagia, or difficulty swallowing. The danger of using these tools lies in the fact that the patient could easily aspirate the fluids, which could lead to pneumonia.

90. **The correct answer is (D).** The Leonard method of tooth brushing is not recommended because of its up and down motion from maxillary to mandibular teeth. The toothbrush is held at a 90-degree angle along the long axis of the tooth.

91. **The correct answer is (E).** Corticosteroids are usually prescribed for the treatment of lichen planus to decrease ulcerations and inflammation.

92. **The correct answer is (C).** The resources section of a program plan should outline the location, facilities, equipment, materials, and personnel needed for a community program. Resources should be evaluated based on their appropriateness, adequacy, effectiveness, and whether they are likely to be efficient in terms of helping with the cost effective and timely completion of program tasks.

93. **The correct answer is (C).** The word part *strepto* indicates bacteria are arranged in chains. The bacteria *Streptococcus pyogenes*, for example, can form chains. The word part *diplo* indicates bacteria forms in pairs. The word part *spirillum* indicates a bacterium is a coil or spiral shape. The word part *coccus* indicates a bacterium is a round shape. The word part *staphylo* indicates the bacteria form into clusters.

94. **The correct answer is (B).** A patient who receives a dental prosthesis should eat only liquid foods for the first 24 hours. Keeping a patient on this liquid diet for 24 hours will help her oral muscles become accustomed to the prosthesis before she tries to eat soft, solid foods.

95. **The correct answer is (C).** A PSR score of 2 indicates that a patient has calculus deposits. The PSR scale, which is used to determine whether periodontal disease is present, ranges from 0 (no deposits) to 4 (subgingival calculus).

96. **The correct answer is (D).** The trigeminal nerve is the largest nerve in the body. It has three branches that divide into even smaller branches.

97. **The correct answer is (A).** A Grade IV furcation involvement is the most severe, which includes severe involvement and complete loss of inter-radicular bone. The difference between Grade IV and Grade III involvement is a visible through-and-through furcation in Grade IV. In Grade III the probe has entered the root and is just visible on the opposite side.

98. **The correct answer is (E).** To analyze the significance of results, an experiment will usually include an experimental group and a control group. The experimental group receives the variable being investigated (in this case the mouthwash), while the control group will receive no treatment, a traditional, or a placebo (in this case water).

99. **The correct answer is (D).** The safest area in which to stand is 90–135 degrees at the side of the patient and away from the primary beam. It is also important for the mother to wear a lead apron that is 0.25 mm in thickness or stand behind a lead barrier.

100. **The correct answer is (B).** A bitewing will show any decay or problems with the patient's teeth. Since the patient has his 6-year-old molars, a bitewing will allow the dentist to see if any decay is located between the back teeth and will also show if the teeth are aligned correctly.

101. **The correct answer is (C).** By adjusting the tube to an average angulation of +8 degrees and directing the central ray to pass straight through to the center of the film at the level of the occlusal plane, an accurate image of the molars will be taken.

102. **The correct answer is (A).** The FDA guidelines recommend radiographs on young children at the first dental visit if the proximal surfaces (sides of the teeth) cannot be seen well or explored with a dental instrument. Since decay is likely to occur on the sides of the teeth where it is difficult to see, radiographs can be postponed until later if the child's teeth are spaced far apart and there is no clinical evidence of decay.

103. **The correct answer is (A).** Cortical plate surgery is not a type of surgery used after initial therapy to correct refractory areas. Excisional surgery, periodontal flap surgery, mucogingival surgery, and osseous surgery are all types of surgery used after initial treatment for periodontitis.

104. **The correct answer is (D).** *Staphylococcal* food poisoning often incurs when people eat unrefrigerated dairy products; however, a fever is not a symptom of *staphylococcal* food poisoning. Symptoms of this type of food poisoning include nausea, vomiting, and diarrhea.

105. **The correct answer is (D).** Patients have certain rights with respect to their records, including the right to review records, the right to copy them, and the right to know about information that was disclosed without authorization. Patients also have the right to request that health-care information be changed (but not removed) when appropriate.

106. **The correct answer is (C).** The maximum permissible dose per year for any hygienist regardless of his or her age is 5 rem.

107. **The correct answer is (D).** The main dental health benefit of water fluoridation is a reduction in dental caries, but other benefits include fewer missing teeth and fewer cases of malocclusion. Even with water fluoridation, however, individuals still need to have check-ups and cleanings on a regular basis to maintain good oral health.

108. **The correct answer is (D).** Responsibilities that dental hygienists have to their communities and to society include reporting illegal activities by health-care providers or incidences of substandard care to authorities, complying with all laws related to public health and safety, and complying with laws and regulations related to the dental hygiene profession. Choices (A), (B), (C), and (E) all describe professional responsibilities dental hygienists have to the dental hygiene profession.

109. **The correct answer is (C).** When applied topically, a varnish will impregnate a tooth with fluoride for 3–4 hours. Fluoride varnishes are used to prevent tooth decay, mineralize the surface of teeth, and treat tooth sensitivity.

110. **The correct answer is (C).** Chief cells produce pepsinogen. This enzyme eventually becomes pepsin, which aids in the digestion of proteins by breaking them down into peptides.

111. **The correct answer is (B).** Prescriptions for schedule II drugs can be phoned in during an emergency, but the pharmacy will need to receive the signed prescription within 3 days. No refills are permitted for schedule II drugs; prescriptions for schedule III drugs can be refilled up to five times over a 6-month period.

112. **The correct answer is (B).** Root debridement therapy sessions should be given to a patient with periodontitis. After each root debridement procedure, the pocket should be reevaluated for antibiotic therapy.

113. **The correct answer is (D).** Inflammation occurs when the immune system reacts to an injury, and the classic symptoms of inflammation (heat, pain, redness, and swelling) occur because of the immune system's response. Bleeding is not a sign of inflammation because it is not one of the immune system's responses to injury.

114. **The correct answer is (A).** Although a timetable and deadlines are important parts of any program plan, there should be some amount of flexibility to allow for unforeseen circumstances that could delay project implementation. Program plans should also identify relevant strengths, weaknesses, opportunities, and threats (SWOT analysis).

115. **The correct answer is (C).** Fungi are microorganisms that are classified as eukaryotes. Fungi,

however, are not classified as photosynthetic organisms. Because fungi do not use photosynthesis to create their own food, they are non-photosynthetic organisms.

116. **The correct answer is (C).** Glucose, fructose, dextrose, and galactose are all monosaccharides; however, lactose is a disaccharide. Disaccharides form when two monosaccharides are linked together. Lactose is made up of glucose and galactose.

117. **The correct answer is (D).** The cost of treatment should not be listed on a dental hygiene treatment plan. This detail would be listed on the patient's bill.

118. **The correct answer is (B).** Systematic sampling is a random sampling technique. A list of an entire population arranged in random order is used, and then every *n*th subject is selected to compile study data.

119. **The correct answer is (D).** The vomer bone has no muscle attachments. Most of the anterior nasal septum is made of cartilage.

120. **The correct answer is (C).** The normal respiratory rate for a toddler is 20–35 breaths per minute. Adults have a lower respiratory rate.

121. **The correct answer is (B).** According to the ASA's physical status classification, a healthy patient with extreme anxiety falls into Category II. To reduce the patient's anxiety on subsequent visits, consider scheduling a morning appointment and be sure to record the patient's vital signs at each visit.

122. **The correct answer is (D).** The plaque index (PI) is used to assess how much plaque a patient has on his or her teeth and is a good indicator of how well the patient cares for his or her teeth at home. A PI score between 0.1 and 0.9 is rated as "good." This suggests that the patient has good home care.

123. **The correct answer is (B).** Fremitus is movement or vibration in the teeth that happens during occlusion, when the upper and lower teeth contact each other. If fremitus cannot be seen or felt in the teeth, the patient's fremitus classification should be N. This means that everything was normal and no movement was seen or felt.

124. **The correct answer is (E).** HIV-associated periodontitis progresses rapidly and can cause significant loss of attachment (9 to 12 mm) in just half a year. Treatment and management measures can include antibiotics, specifically tetracyclines, scalings, and possible surgery.

125. **The correct answer is (D).** Trauma does not cause periodontal disease but rather exacerbates inflammation associated with periodontal disease. The reason is correct because trauma can cause teeth to become more mobile from widening of the periodontal ligament.

126. **The correct answer is (B).** Both statements are false. Viruses are generally smaller than bacteria. In fact, the smallest bacteria are about the same size as the largest viruses. Furthermore, viruses are less complex than bacteria.

127. **The correct answer is (A).** A negative correlation means that an increase in an independent variable—in this case the number of minutes spent brushing—is associated with a decrease in a dependent variable—in this case the number of fillings required before adulthood. Choice (B) describes a positive correlation, which is when an increase in the independent variable is associated with an increase in the dependent variable.

128. **The correct answer is (C).** The placement of implants would fall into phase II of dental care planning, which focuses on surgical treatments.

129. **The correct answer is (A).** Scaling and root debridement involves the removal of all hard and soft deposits of plaque as well as the biofilm from the root and coronal surfaces of teeth. Scaling and root debridement are usually the initial therapy for all periodontal disease.

130. **The correct answer is (A).** Ultrasonic tools are becoming more common than handheld tools for periodontal debridement. These tools are versatile because they come in a number of different sizes and shapes. They also have either internal or external water conduits.

131. **The correct answer is (D).** The tooth buds begin to develop around week 8. This is when rapid proliferation of the dental lamia forms the primary dentition.

132. **The correct answer is (A).** Fat from foods can coat the teeth and prevent food particles from sticking to the teeth. Periodontal disease is unrelated to consuming a high-fat diet because fat does not negatively affect teeth. Diets high in carbohydrates are more likely to cause periodontal disease and other dental problems.

133. **The correct answer is (D).** The reevaluation procedures to determine the clinical health of tissues do not take into account the amount of neutrophils, or cells that migrate to attack foreign bacteria. If the amount of neutrophils is decreased, that is actually a sign of reduced infection.

134. **The correct answer is (A).** The median palatine suture is a radiolucent line between the maxillary incisors. It is the juncture of the horizontal plates of the palatine bone.

135. **The correct answer is (B).** Excluding the pharynx, the tongue is the location of the majority of oral carcinomas. Thirty-seven to 50 percent of all diagnosed oral carcinomas occur on the tongue.

136. **The correct answer is (C).** Anticholinergic agents such as atropine and dicyclomine are favorable in the practice of dentistry because they reduce salivary flow. They should not be used, however, with patients who have prostatic hypertrophy (enlarged prostate) since urinary retention is one of the adverse effects.

137. **The correct answer is (C).** Chlorhexidine gluconate is the most effective antimicrobial agent for reducing plaque and gingivitis in the long term. It is the gold standard for topical antimicrobial mouth rinses and contains a relatively high amount of alcohol.

138. **The correct answer is (B).** The hormone norepinephrine produces the fight-or-flight response. Norepinephrine increases heart rate, raises blood pressure, and redirects blood away from the digestive tract.

139. **The correct answer is (C).** Although in most situations interactions between the hygienist and patient must be kept confidential, certain exceptions exist. These include suspected cases of elder or child abuse and gunshot wounds.

140. **The correct answer is (B).** Ethically, a dental hygienist must maintain client confidentiality and respect a client's right to privacy at all times; however, situations exist in which dental hygiene professionals are legally obligated to break client confidentiality, such as when they suspect elderly individuals or children are being abused.

141. **The correct answer is (B).** Autonomy means that individuals are permitted to make their own health-care–related decisions. The dental hygienist in this situation must respect the client's decision even though she does not agree with it.

142. **The correct answer is (A).** Obtaining informed consent is an important ethical matter in the dental hygiene profession. The patient must be made aware of the risks and benefits associated with a treatment, alternative treatments, and other information they may find relevant when making a decision about whether to have a treatment or procedure.

143. **The correct answer is (A).** Fidelity, also known as role fidelity, is a universal moral principle stating that health-care providers must refrain from providing services outside of their scope of practice. Dental hygienists are not permitted to do fillings—this activity would therefore violate the principle of fidelity.

144. **The correct answer is (D).** Patients with some form of thyroid disease commonly present with deterioration of the alveolar bone, as well as accelerated or delayed dental development.

145. **The correct answer is (C).** External resorption first starts on the root surface with loss and a flat rather than conical appearance when viewed on radiographs. However, the bone and the lamina dura appear normal.

146. **The correct answer is (B).** Beats per minute are taken from the radial artery if a patient is conscious and from the common carotid artery if the patient is unconscious and an adult. Only EMS personnel should determine the BPM on an infant from the brachial artery. If the BPM are regular, then they should be taken for 30 seconds. If irregular, BPMs should be taken for one additional minute. Regular is considered 60 to 90 BPM for adults and 80 to 110 BPM for children.

147. **The correct answer is (D).** The Oath of Hippocrates was developed during the fifth century BC to guide the actions of physicians. Aside from being associated with the statement "Above all, do no harm," it stated that physicians should protect the rights of patients and maintain confidentiality.

148. **The correct answer is (C).** Affective learning is tied to emotions and attitudes, so encouraging a feeling of pride that is related to practicing good oral health habits is likely to be effective with this learner. Choice (B) would be a good technique to use with psychomotor learners, while choices (A), (D), and (E) would be good techniques to use when interacting with cognitive learners.

149. **The correct answer is (D).** When making an impression using an alginate hydrocolloid, distortion can best be avoided by removing the mold using a quick pulling motion.

150. **The correct answer is (A).** On a periodontal exam chart, a zigzag red arrow in the interproximal space between two teeth indicates food impaction. Deficient contacts are indicated by a single blue line in the interproximal space between two teeth. A missing tooth is indicated by a blue X over the tooth. An impacted tooth is circled in red. Decalcification is indicated by a zigzag red line over the affected area.

151. **The correct answer is (B).** Orthostatic hypotension may occur when a patient sits up too quickly after being in the supine position for a while. Orthostatic hypotension is the second most common cause of unconsciousness in a dental setting. If a patient loses consciousness because he sat up too quickly, check his vital signs and administer oxygen at 5 liters per minute. Once the patient feels better, reposition him slowly from the supine position, and discontinue any dental procedure. Orthostatic hypotension can be prevented by bringing all patients up slowly at the conclusion of their dental examination.

152. **The correct answer is (D).** A community profile gives professionals planning a program a comprehensive overview of the area where a target group resides. Compiling the profile includes gathering data regarding population size, the political atmosphere in the community, funding and availability of health services, and factors that may limit access to health care.

153. **The correct answer is (E).** The drawbacks of written questionnaires include the fact that respondents may not interpret questions as intended, may be dishonest, or may simply not return the questionnaire. Advantages of this method include the fact that questionnaires are relatively quick and inexpensive to administer and can help researchers obtain general statistics about a population.

154. **The correct answer is (D).** Written questionnaires are useful for everything mentioned in the answer choices except studying behavior. Psychomotor activity and behaviors (including ones individuals might not self-report) are assessed using direct observation techniques such as checklists and videotape recordings.

155. **The correct answer is (B).** When assessing a population, one of the most important tasks is to identify the target group. This is the group that will be the focus of a particular health program. In this instance, it is the group at the highest risk of developing a specific condition.

156. **The correct answer is (B).** The earliest manifestations of Behcet syndrome usually appear in the oral cavity. Common symptoms of Behcet syndrome include mouth and skin sores, swelling in parts of the eye, and swelling and stiffness in the joints.

157. **The correct answer is (C).** Fluoride mouthwashes containing sodium fluoride, acidulated phosphate fluoride, and stannous fluoride are effective at preventing dental caries. They should be swished around the mouth for a period of 1 minute before being spit out.

158. **The correct answer is (A).** Both the statement and the reason are correct and related. All dental personnel in the dental office must know the emergency procedures to be followed, as well as the location and use of the emergency kit and oxygen. In addition, some personnel should know how to use a portable defibrillator and pulse oximeter. All personnel should be able to provide basic life support, however, as it is the main way to manage emergency situations. Any drugs that are given to the patient are of secondary concern behind basic life-support provisions.

159. **The correct answer is (A).** Both the statement and the reason are correct and related. When bacteria

multiply in the body, the hypothalamus reacts by increasing the body's temperature. Since bacteria thrive at about the same temperature as humans, the increased body temperature kills the bacteria.

160. **The correct answer is (A).** Glass ionomer dental cement is widely considered to be ideal for use on patients with a high rate of caries because of its ability to leach fluoride.

161. **The correct answer is (C).** The first bone lost in periodontal disease is the alveolar crest bone. The alveolar crest bone is at the coronal rim of alveolar bone.

162. **The correct answer is (E).** The dependent variable is the factor that changes in response to changes in the independent variable. In this case the study is investigating whether the number of dental surgeries will change in response to the presence of free dental clinics.

163. **The correct answer is (E).** If the temperature is not warm enough, the radiograph will be underdeveloped or too light. It is important to monitor the temperature to produce a clear image. In manual processing, the temperature should be 68 degrees for 5 minutes or 72 degrees for 4 minutes.

164. **The correct answer is (A).** Bent film will create a black streak on a radiograph. It is important to make sure the film is flat and smooth.

165. **The correct answer is (B).** When communicating with patients, the dental hygiene professional should remember that they can only absorb so much information in a given period of time. In the situation, speaking faster will cause information overload for the patient, so the hygienist should be selective about what information she presents.

166. **The correct answer is (D).** Fluoridated toothpaste is a source of topical fluoride. Topical fluoride provides protection on the tooth surface, whereas systemic fluoride sources are those ingested into the body.

167. **The correct answer is (B).** Iontophoresis is used most often in the treatment of hypersensitivity. In this procedure, an electrical current is used to aid impregnation of the fluoride ion into the tooth surface.

168. **The correct answer is (C).** Salivation, nausea, and vomiting can occur when a person ingests too much fluoride in non-lethal doses. Such symptoms can result from ingestion of 250 milligrams to 450 milligrams, equaling the amount in one gel capsule.

169. **The correct answer is (B).** To avoid tissue injury, a toothbrush with soft bristles should be used. The diameter of the bristles should be between 0.007 and 0.009 inches and the tips should be rounded.

170. **The correct answer is (E).** On a periodontal exam chart, furcation involvement is indicated by Roman numerals I–IV, depending on the class of involvement, written in red ink on the affected area. Class IV indicates through-and-through furcation involvement with complete bone loss between roots.

171. **The correct answer is (B).** The new theory of debridement emphasizes debriding deep pockets first, followed by a series of root debridement sessions. No antibiotics are administered during the initial debridement session.

172. **The correct answer is (E).** Hypercementosis is characterized by an excessive formation of cementum on the root surface. This may give the tooth a larger appearance. The cause of this condition is unknown.

173. **The correct answer is (E).** Bisphenol A glycidyl methacrylate is used in many dental sealants as a monomer to help the sealant flow into fissures and grooves in the teeth.

174. **The correct answer is (C).** During the periodontal evaluation, probing is used to evaluate the health of subgingival areas. However, periodontal probing depths should be measured on six tooth sites, not four. The six sites are distofacial, facial, mesiofacial, distolingual, lingual, and mesiolingual.

175. **The correct answer is (C).** Xerostomia, often commonly known as dry mouth, is caused by a lack of saliva. Measures that can effectively address xerostomia include sucking on ice chips or candy, avoiding alcohol and caffeine, using saliva substitutes, and increasing water intake.

176. **The correct answer is (B).** HPV, a virus that may cause cervical cancer in women, is not a concern in the dental environment as it is spread through

sexual contact. Aside from the types of vaccinations identified in choices (A), (C), (D), and (E), oral health–care workers should also be protected against measles, mumps, and tetanus.

177. **The correct answer is (B).** Cracked lips, which should be checked during the oral evaluation, are often a symptom of a vitamin B deficiency.

178. **The correct answer is (C).** Healthy gingival tissue should follow the contour of the teeth. Gingival margins that appear knife-edged are healthy. If the gingival margins appear blunted, cratered, rolled, or bulbous, periodontal disease could be present in the patient.

179. **The correct answer is (C).** Chlorhexidine (Periochip) is not an antibiotic designed to disrupt the multiplication of bacterial growth. It gains entry into bacteria by disrupting the bacterial cell wall and causes the bacterial cells that are present to lyse and die.

180. **The correct answer is (B).** All of the choices represent characteristics of trigeminal neuralgia except for permanent paralysis of the face. This is more often a characteristic of Bell's palsy.

181. **The correct answer is (C).** A systolic blood pressure reading of 140–159 or a diastolic reading of 90–99 is classified as Stage I hypertension. In a blood pressure reading of 151/97, both the systolic and diastolic readings fall within the specified ranges for Stage I hypertension.

182. **The correct answer is (C).** While unethical actions are also often illegal, this is not always the case. If a hygienist's actions were unethical but not illegal, an administrative body, such as the state dental board, may impose sanctions. Although the hygienist could be fired by his or her employer for unethical actions, the employer would not impose sanctions.

183. **The correct answer is (A).** Syncope, which is also known as fainting, is the most common emergency that occurs in a dental setting. Syncope is most often associated with stress and is caused by a decreased flow of oxygen to the brain. Before fainting, patients may feel dizzy or nauseous and may have a peculiar pallor. Hyperventilation and airway obstruction are other common dental setting emergencies.

184. **The correct answer is (A).** Type 1 examinations are very thorough, and may involve percussion and laboratory tests. They are time consuming, expensive, and require numerous personnel, which makes them unrealistic for most public health applications.

185. **The correct answer is (A).** The rubella virus is in the Tagoviride family of viruses. Rubella, which is also called German measles, is a contagious infection that causes a rash on the skin. Most children in America are immunized against this virus at a young age.

186. **The correct answer is (A).** Periodontal flap surgery is not part of the routine reassessment procedures for chronic periodontal disease or aggressive periodontitis. During the reevaluation procedure after six weeks, reassessment procedures include culturing of bacteria, occlusal equilibration, and treatment with antibiotics.

187. **The correct answer is (D).** Erythromycin is a macrolide that works by inhibiting protein synthesis. It is used to treat infections cause by Gram-positive bacteria, including strains of *Rickettsia*, *Mycoplasma pneumoniae*, and *Legionella pneumophila*.

188. **The correct answer is (C).** Dilaceration is a sharp bend of a root thought to be caused by trauma. This trauma changes the position of the root, which causes the rest of the tooth to form at an angle.

189. **The correct answer is (E).** Situational ethics involves making decisions based upon the unique set of circumstances related to a dilemma. When making a decision, a dental hygiene professional might consider the characteristics of the patient, the quality of his or her relationship with the patient, and whether an action is humanistic.

190. **The correct answer is (B).** A darkened area on a tooth indicates decay. Because decay dissolves part of the tooth, more of the radiation will penetrate that area, making that part of the tooth darker on the radiograph.

191. **The correct answer is (A).** Ultrasonic tools are becoming more popular than handheld tools for periodontal debridement for a number of reasons. One reason is because ultrasonic tools do not require a specific angle to be maintained between the tooth and the tool.

192. **The correct answer is (D).** Pericoronitis is an infection of the tissue surrounding the mandibular third molar. This is a common problem in young adults with impacted or partially impacted teeth.

193. **The correct answer is (B).** Hand hygiene is a vital aspect of infection control, and during hand washing the hands should be lathered with soap for at least 15 seconds, not 45. While hand sanitizers are an effective way to remove bacteria from the hands and are sometimes more effective than soap and water, they should only be used if no visible soil on the hands exists.

194. **The correct answer is (D).** A type I error occurs when a researcher incorrectly rejects a null hypothesis, meaning the researcher concludes there is a statistically significant difference when there is not. The mode is the number that occurs most frequently in a data set. The number 1 is found 3 times in the data set given.

195. **The correct answer is (C).** The human body can survive without water for approximately 3 days. Water is a vital nutrient for the body and without it the body begins to shut down. Therefore, dehydration should be treated immediately.

196. **The correct answer is (E).** Cells in the lymphocytes, or white blood cells, are most sensitive to exposure to radiation. Though cells in the kidneys, muscles, connective tissue, and salivary glands can be affected by radiation exposure, it is most damaging to lymphocytes.

197. **The correct answer is (A).** Many patients diagnosed with internal resorption often present with pink tooth, which is pink coloration of the crown because of the vascularity of the lesion inside the tooth.

198. **The correct answer is (C).** Certain individuals should not have their teeth polished, including those with communicable diseases, hypersensitive teeth, gingiva that are inflamed and bleeding, or areas of demineralization. The main purpose of polishing is to improve the appearance of teeth—the stains removed during polishing do not increase a patient's risk for oral health problems.

199. **The correct answer is (D).** Diseased gingiva may be red or a mixture of blue and red or purple and red (the latter two are due to an increase in the number of capillaries). The other choices describe characteristics of healthy gingiva, which is pink or pink-brown in color.

200. **The correct answer is (A).** The "fight or flight" response causes the bronchi and the pupils to dilate, respiration and breathing to increase, and perspiration and blood pressure to increase. This is controlled specifically by the sympathetic nervous system, which is part of the autonomic (or visceral) nervous system.

Component B

1. D	31. A	61. C	91. B	121. B
2. C	32. D	62. B	92. B	122. A
3. B	33. D	63. B	93. A	123. D
4. B	34. C	64. D	94. B	124. C
5. B	35. D	65. B	95. B	125. D
6. C	36. B	66. C	96. A	126. B
7. C	37. B	67. C	97. C	127. A
8. B	38. C	68. D	98. B	128. C
9. A	39. D	69. B	99. B	129. B
10. B	40. A	70. D	100. D	130. C
11. B	41. A	71. D	101. A	131. B
12. C	42. B	72. D	102. D	132. B
13. C	43. D	73. C	103. A	133. D
14. D	44. A	74. B	104. D	134. C
15. A	45. D	75. C	105. C	135. A
16. A	46. B	76. A	106. D	136. C
17. B	47. C	77. D	107. C	137. B
18. B	48. A	78. B	108. C	138. D
19. C	49. D	79. B	109. C	139. D
20. B	50. B	80. A	110. A	140. A
21. A	51. A	81. D	111. D	141. C
22. C	52. D	82. A	112. A	142. D
23. B	53. A	83. D	113. C	143. A
24. D	54. C	84. C	114. C	144. C
25. B	55. A	85. A	115. B	145. C
26. D	56. D	86. B	116. D	146. C
27. D	57. C	87. C	117. A	147. C
28. C	58. D	88. B	118. B	148. D
29. A	59. C	89. C	119. C	149. C
30. B	60. C	90. C	120. A	150. D

1. **The correct answer is (D).** For those patients with implants, X-rays should be taken at least once per year. Take X-rays more often in patients where periodontal breakdown was previously noted around the implant. For patients with implants, X-rays are taken in order to evaluate levels of bone loss and the fit and integrity of the implant or prosthesis components.

2. **The correct answer is (C).** The best indicator for implant failure is the presence of mobility. Other indicators include pocketing, BoP, exudate, progression of bone loss, dull sound on percussion, and radiographic evidence of periimplant radiolucency. The failure of dental implants is most often related to failure to osseointegrate correctly.

3. **The correct answer is (B).** Purulence has to do with the amount of pus contained within the surrounding tissue. When evaluating implant health, purulence is not an indicator. Dental personnel should assess the tissue around an implant for the presence of periimplantitis, because periimplant tissues are at risk for invasion by microorganisms just as natural periodontium are.

4. **The correct answer is (B).** The periapical view examines from the cementoenamel junction to the root. It is used to diagnose pathological changes in a specific tooth by examining its root and the surrounding bone. The paralleling technique is an intraoral technique that requires that film be placed parallel to the long axis of the tooth and the primary beam perpendicular to the film and the long axis. These techniques allow for optimum analysis when compared with previous film.

5. **The correct answer is (B).** Part of a dental hygienist's responsibility is to work well with patients and develop a good rapport with them. In a case such as this, it is wise to hear the patient's concerns, and alert the general practitioner or dentist before he or she comes in to do the exam.

6. **The correct answer is (C).** Professional maintenance for implants is crucial. Maintenance procedures include tissue assessment, probing implant sulcus depths, checking for BoP and mobility, assessing dental biofilm and calculus deposits and removing them, and taking annual radiographs. In this case, the implant has been well maintained for 6 years. Normal maintenance includes a 3-month recare interval for at least the first year after placement of an implant. This patient is well beyond the suggested recare time period.

7. **The correct answer is (C).** Curets are known as being the most versatile instrument. It is the best tool to promote tissue safety because of its design. It also has excellent cutting and smoothing abilities for traditional root planning. There are, however, special considerations when caring for implants. One of the major concerns is that an implant cannot be scratched or else the periodontal health of a patient might be compromised.

8. **The correct answer is (B).** As with natural teeth, rubber-cup polishing with a fine powder or a fine-grit commercial polishing paste may be used selectively to polish implants. Only instruments made specifically for the removal of hard and soft deposits on implants should be used. Sonic and ultra-sonic instrumentation, as well as air-powered polishing instruments, should not be used. The only exception for the use of these instruments is if implant plastic tips are used.

9. **The correct answer is (A).** There is some controversy surrounding pocket depth probing of implants. Any probing should be done with a plastic probe and light pressure. If bleeding occurs during probing, it should be noted. Tissue color and consistency should also be noted during probing. To say that probing should never be done on implants is a false statement.

10. **The correct answer is (B).** Dental floss is always the best tool for cleaning the interproximal areas between the teeth. In this case, it adapts well along the margin of the crown. It also adapts well into the sulcus and around the abutment.

11. **The correct answer is (B).** Patients in good dental health should visit the dentist every 6 months for a routine cleaning and check-up. In fact, most insurance companies will not cover dental visits prior to the 6-month mark unless there is an issue that needs to be addressed before that.

12. **The correct answer is (C).** The dentist is responsible for setting and prescribing the frequency with which X-rays are taken. Based on this patient's clinical presentation and history, bitewing X-rays should be taken once per 18-month period.

13. **The correct answer is (C).** Power toothbrushes are as effective in dental care as manual toothbrushes if they are used correctly. When using a powered toothbrush, patients should hold the head at a 45-degree angle. Smaller heads are used to target specific teeth and require more time to clean all teeth. Powered toothbrushes are recommended for those with orthodontic appliances, malposed teeth, periodontal disease, arthritis, and other grasping challenges. They are also recommended for caregivers who must brush someone else's teeth.

14. **The correct answer is (D).** This patient visits the dentist regularly and has good oral hygiene habits. Any scaling instrument will be effective on this patient's teeth.

15. **The correct answer is (A).** A dental hygienist should always use positive reinforcement while emphasizing the best preventive practices. In this case, the hygienist compliments the patient for her good oral hygiene while reminding her that the best way to prevent future dental problems is to floss daily.

16. **The correct answer is (A).** The purposes of polishing are to improve the appearance of teeth and increase a patient's overall satisfaction. Sometimes polishing is used to prepare teeth for sealants. Polishing should not be considered part of the routine oral examination according to the "Position Paper on Polishing" by the American Dental Hygienists' Association (ADHA).

17. **The correct answer is (B).** There are several advantages for both patient and hygienist when correct patient positioning is consistently practiced. It improves visibility and access to the treatment area, increases treatment efficiency, and increases overall patient and hygienist comfort reducing the risk of injury to the hygienist. When examining the maxillary arch, the light should be positioned over the patient's chest so the light shines into the patient's mouth at an angle.

18. **The correct answer is (B).** There are many mouth rinses available to consumers today. The best mouth rinses, however, are ADA-recommended antimicrobial rinses with fluoride. They help prevent caries as well as periodontal diseases and other concerns.

19. **The correct answer is (C).** This patient does not smoke. Therefore, cigarettes cannot cause the staining. The patient also mentioned that she is currently not taking any medications. Therefore, the antibiotic tetracycline can be ruled out. The patient is 32 years old. Staining due to age does not begin to occur until much later. Tea is a natural staining agent and is most likely the cause of the staining.

20. **The correct answer is (B).** Dentifrices or toothpastes are meant to assist in the removal of dental plaque and other deposits that collect on the teeth and gingiva. It is the mechanical action of brushing, not the dentifrice, which is the major contributor to the removal of soft deposits on the teeth. Any toothpaste is acceptable as long as it is ADA approved. This ensures that it meets all safe levels of abrasiveness.

21. **The correct answer is (A).** Based on the findings of the clinical examination, it can be determined that the patient be diagnosed with chronic moderate generalized periodontitis. Chronic periodontitis is classified as slight if 1–2 mm of attachment loss is present, moderate if 3–4 mm attachment loss, and severe if more than 5 mm of attachment loss is present. It is also characterized by the presence of periodontal pockets, bone loss, and tooth mobility. In addition, it is most commonly exhibited by horizontal interdental bone loss, which this patient exhibits according to the supplemental oral examination findings.

22. **The correct answer is (C).** The American Dental Association (ADA) developed a system primarily based on the severity of attachment loss. Type II classification is also referred to as early periodontitis. During Stage II, the progression of gingival inflammation into the marginal bone results in mild bone loss and mild to moderate pocket formation. In Type II classification, there is usually no increased tooth mobility.

23. **The correct answer is (B).** There are many factors that contribute to gingivitis and periodontitis. Some factors are able to be modified, while others are not. Smoking is one of those factors that affect periodontal health that can also be modified and controlled. Medications, especially adverse reactions to them, can affect periodontal health. Biofilm

and calculus deposits lead to gingivitis, which normally precedes periodontitis. Obesity does not affect periodontitis. However, poor eating habits can lead to gingivitis, which again, often precedes periodontitis.

24. **The correct answer is (D).** Bruxism is tooth grinding. Bruxism can be mild to severe and may not require treatment. This patient has evidence of severe bruxism and requires treatment. A night mouth guard may help the patient's night grinding.

25. **The correct answer is (B).** Since this patient has Type II periodontitis, the best way to accomplish removal of calculus and biofilm is quadrant debridement with pain management. This allows for thorough debridement with reinforcement of home-care strategies and smoking-cessation efforts.

26. **The correct answer is (D).** The patient should be wearing a mouth guard at night to control her severe bruxism. The mouth guard, however, is not a factor in assisting in the healing process after the debridement procedure. Smoking, home hygiene care, and calculus all contribute to the severity of periodontitis.

27. **The correct answer is (D).** In this instance, co-management with the periodontist will benefit the patient. The periodontist is an expert in this area and will be able to offer valuable information and advice to the patient, as well as offer some other care alternatives.

28. **The correct answer is (C).** It is never all right to even slightly threaten a patient. Telling the patient that she will lose all her teeth if she does not see the specialist is not only a lie but also a threat. Scaring patients into doing something that you know will benefit them in the long run is never an acceptable practice.

29. **The correct answer is (A).** It is always best to use a positive, solution-oriented approach when dealing with patients. This patient refuses to use floss. It is the hygienist's responsibility to remain positive with this patient, yet be creative in thinking of an alternative solution such as using antibacterial mouthwashes twice a day.

30. **The correct answer is (B).** Dental hygienist must always strive to be positive and solution-oriented in their responses to patients. By first stating how delighted you are the patient wants to use a Waterpik, you are offering positive feedback about a choice the patient is making. Then, by mentioning the recommended daily practice of flossing, you are taking a solution-oriented approach.

31. **The correct answer is (A).** The patient has good overall dental hygiene. Therefore, recommending more frequent visits is the best way to handle the patient's increased calculus deposits. The patient's visitation frequency can be reevaluated at each subsequent visit.

32. **The correct answer is (D).** Increased pressure in brushing is not a good recommendation, because it serves no purpose and will only abrade the tooth surfaces. The patient should use a tartar control toothpaste that has been ADA approved, and should brush more frequently for a longer period with regular pressure.

33. **The correct answer is (D).** There is no documented proof that a power or automatic toothbrush is better than a manual toothbrush. There are instances when a power toothbrush might be better for a patient to use, however, and abrasion from overzealous brushing, excessive calculus build up, and a built-in timer may be reasons to explore the power toothbrush as an option.

34. **The correct answer is (C).** Power toothbrushes are safe and effective tools for removing biofilm and stain at home. Power toothbrushes are not more abrasive than manual toothbrushes and are often recommended to patients who are too aggressive in their brushing because power toothbrushes can be gentler on teeth.

35. **The correct answer is (D).** It is never a good idea to keep anger inside. Better ways to handle a patient's consistent tardiness are to either tell him his appointment is 15 minutes earlier, keep his appointments within their allotted time frame so as not to run into the next patient's appointment, or ask him nicely to be on time for his next visit so he can receive the best treatment. Effective treatment requires the full allotted appointment time.

36. **The correct answer is (B).** Polishing with a desensitizing agent should be the first option. It is the

most conservative option and should be tried first before more aggressive options like anesthesia are utilized.

37. **The correct answer is (B).** The patient should always be involved and questioned about anything that may be out of the ordinary. In addition, the dentist should first be made aware of any possible concerns. Then the dentist will determine what the next course of action should be. All irregularities should be noted on the patient's chart. However, to schedule a biopsy with the oral surgeon before mentioning anything to the patient or dentist is rash and inappropriate.

38. **The correct answer is (C).** By mentioning concerns to the patient, the hygienist is able to hear the patient's response regarding his follow up with a specialist. By doing this, the hygienist is able to offer more information to the dentist before he or she comes in to examine the patient. Perhaps by hearing concerns from both the hygienist and the dentist, the patient will realize the importance of scheduling a follow-up visit with a specialist.

39. **The correct answer is (D).** A Waterpik is useful in reducing inflammation but does not replace flossing. Unfortunately for this patient, there aren't any alternatives to flossing. A floss-on-a-stick type flosser, small interdental brush, or power flosser are options that the patient can try that will be effective and might be easier for the patient to maneuver.

40. **The correct answer is (A).** Generally, periodontal disease may contribute to halitosis, but this patient does not have periodontal disease. According to the patient's history and clinical presentation, periodontal disease is not present and is, therefore, not an option. Other general factors that may contribute to halitosis are excess stomach acids, failure to clean the tongue while brushing, and food choices.

41. **The correct answer is (A).** According to the American Association of Pediatric Dentistry, the ideal age for a child's first dental visit is between 6 months and 1 year of age. Parents should schedule a child's first visit when the first tooth comes in. Generally, this milestone occurs between 6 and 12 months of age. Dental problems can begin early. The biggest concern is early childhood caries. This was formerly known as baby-bottle tooth decay or nursing caries. Once a child's diet includes anything other than breast milk, erupted teeth are at risk for decay.

42. **The correct answer is (B).** The I.Q. of a child is not a factor for oral disease at age 3. Later, when the child becomes more self-sufficient and is responsible for her dental care, I.Q. may be a factor. At age 3, however, low socioeconomic status, the use of non-fluoridated toothpastes, and familial beliefs in cavity prevention will all play into whether or not oral disease is a risk factor.

43. **The correct answer is (D).** Higher protein will not negatively affect a child's oral health. Protein is essential in muscle development. Insufficient fluoride in a community water supply, a bottle or spill-proof cup with sweetened liquid in bed, and frequent snacking will all place a child at risk for oral disease.

44. **The correct answer is (A).** Stridor is a high-pitched sound that results from turbulent air flow in the upper airway. Sporadic stridor does not occur all the time. Stridor is irrelevant to teething. Children who are teething will often chew or drool excessively, be more irritable than usual, and sometimes eat less because of the discomfort caused to their gums and mouths during eating.

45. **The correct answer is (D).** Although children develop at different stages and ages, primary dentition is usually complete between 2 and 3 years of age. After that, children generally lose their first tooth between the ages of 4 and 6.

46. **The correct answer is (B).** The most critical period of exposure for fluorosis is during the middle of the first year of life, or about 6 months. The dental effects of fluorosis develop much earlier than the skeletal effects. Fluorosis is later characterized by staining and pitting of the teeth. More severe cases may show damaged enamel.

47. **The correct answer is (C).** Even with adult patients, negative reinforcement is never appropriate. However, with young patients, positive reinforcement is all that should be used. "I knew you could do it!," "You are doing great!," and "Well done!" are all great examples of comments that offer positive reinforcement to let the young patient know she is doing a good job at her first attempts at brushing her own teeth.

48. **The correct answer is (A).** Pressing the explorer into pits and fissures to determine if it is soft may cause cavitation. Caries mainly involve primary maxillary anterior teeth because of nipple contact. The tongue and saliva help cleanse other teeth. Young patients are often evaluated through observation rather than through the use of instrumentation.

49. **The correct answer is (D).** A parent should assist a child with tooth brushing until approximately age 7. Generally, when children have reached 7 years of age, their fine motor skills have developed enough for them to effectively clean their teeth by themselves.

50. **The correct answer is (B).** A child should follow the same recall frequency as an adult with no oral disease, which is every 6 months. Adults and children should only be seen more frequently if there are dental issues that must be addressed or monitored more frequently.

51. **The correct answer is (A).** The patient presents with oral soreness and erythema. According to the World Health Association (WHO) Mucositis Scale, her condition would be classified as Grade 1.

52. **The correct answer is (D).** During treatment, the hygienist should offer helpful suggestions that will enhance the patient's experience and help her to improve her oral health. Advising the patient to bring a friend to take notes, providing written instructions, and providing positive reinforcement and creativity in helping the patient maintain optimal oral health are all examples of such suggestions.

53. **The correct answer is (A).** Ideally, dental hygiene treatment of a cancer patient should begin before the patient undergoes cancer therapy, so that the patient begins therapy in good oral health and with appropriate instruction for care during therapy.

54. **The correct answer is (C).** Receiving radiation treatments to the head places the patient at high risk of developing oral complications.

55. **The correct answer is (A).** In order to maintain oral neutrality and comfort, patients with erythema should rinse with baking soda and water, followed by plain water, every 2 to 3 hours.

56. **The correct answer is (D).** Lemon glycerin swabs will not help the patient's xerostomia, because the lemon will be highly irritating.

57. **The correct answer is (C).** The use of rubber tipping to ease and stimulate the irritated tissues is not indicated for the prevention of dental caries.

58. **The correct answer is (D).** Baking soda is not one of the ingredients contained in "magic mouthrinse".

59. **The correct answer is (C).** During the first 6 months following her radiation therapy, this patient should be recalled for debridement and review of oral health instruction every 4–8 weeks, at the discretion of the hygienist.

60. **The correct answer is (C).** This patient should be closely monitored for the development of trismus, which may arise as a result of radiation therapy.

61. **The correct answer is (C).** Every 3 or 4 months would be an appropriate frequency for oral maintenance, but since the patient presents with light calculus and minimal pocketing and requests fewer recare visits, every 3 months would be best.

62. **The correct answer is (B).** The potential for root decay around the teeth where the clasps make contact with the roots is a concern because the clasps may contribute to food retention and decalcification in the area where she has recession.

63. **The correct answer is (B).** The best way to scale the furcation of these molars would be to use a right and left microthin ultrasonic tip, as this will effectively debride contours and provide lavage.

64. **The correct answer is (D).** A pipe cleaner would be the most effective way for the patient to clean the affected molars because of its length and ease of manipulation.

65. **The correct answer is (B).** Using an end tuft brush would be the most effective way for a patient to clean a furcation that shows very early involvement because it is gentle and can reach into the concavity.

66. **The correct answer is (C).** Periapicals showing the teeth on the lower arch would be the most appropriate type of X-rays to take on this patient each time she needs them because these would allow for assessment of bone heights and apices, as well as caries.

67. **The correct answer is (C).** A patient's risk of developing osteoporosis is increased by a low lifetime intake of vitamin D, not calcium and vitamin C.

68. **The correct answer is (D).** A fluoride varnish would be the best in-office fluoride application to use to strengthen the demineralized areas that make contact with the lower partial clasps because it is targeted, effective, and retentive.

69. **The correct answer is (B).** The best at-home application of fluoride to strengthen these same demineralized areas would be a prescription-strength fluoride dentifrice because the patient can place it on the afflicted areas, without rinsing, before going to bed.

70. **The correct answer is (D).** Since the patient is not hard of hearing, it would not be necessary to raise your voice while talking with her.

71. **The correct answer is (D).** Four horizontal BWs should be taken, as these should be sufficient to assess for caries and bone levels, given the presence of the 3rd molars, as well as minimal bone loss.

72. **The correct answer is (D).** Although a patient who drinks excessively may present with discoloration caused by jaundice from liver disease, she would show a light yellowish brown tinge, rather than a greenish one.

73. **The correct answer is (C).** Based on other signs that the patient may be drinking excessively, the hygienist would likely suspect that she may have fallen while intoxicated.

74. **The correct answer is (B).** Since the patient is a recovering alcoholic, the hygienist should be sure to use a nonalcoholic antimicrobial for pre-rinse and rinsing, rather than one that contains alcohol.

75. **The correct answer is (C).** Because of the amount of calculus deposits and the tissue conditions, ultrasonic debridement, fine scaling as needed, and selective polishing would be indicated for this patient.

76. **The correct answer is (A).** When recommending the use of a mouth rinse, it is important to remember that commercial antibacterial and fluoride mouth rinses may contain up to 30 percent alcohol, so the patient's apparent history of alcohol abuse would contraindicate the use of such a product.

77. **The correct answer is (D).** It would be appropriate for the hygienist to mention to the patient her concern that she may be drinking again because the patient has exhibited signs that are detrimental to her health and the hygienist has the right to be concerned.

78. **The correct answer is (B).** The best way to raise your concerns to the patient would be to gently and nonjudgmentally ask if there "is anything else you want to make me aware of today...anything going on that you want to talk to me about?"

79. **The correct answer is (B).** If the patient still refuses to open up, you should make a gentle, nonjudgmental, concerned statement, such as "I noticed the bruising, I see you have lost weight, and I detect an alcohol odor on your breath. I'm worried about you."

80. **The correct answer is (A).** Once the dialogue has opened, the best way to encourage the patient back into treatment or attending her meetings would be to suggest that she contact her AA "buddy" so that he can get involved and help her get back on track in the way that is best for her. This approach addresses the patient in a caring, gentle, non-judgmental, helpful, and concerned manner.

81. **The correct answer is (D).** There is not enough information to properly diagnose the patient, though preliminary evidence would suggest an allergic reaction.

82. **The correct answer is (A).** The American Dental Association (ADA) periodontitis classification for the patient's disease would be Type I, which is the gingival disease category.

83. **The correct answer is (D).** There is no documented evidence to suggest that floss contains any additives that may cause an allergic reaction.

84. **The correct answer is (C).** Both flavor additives and preservative have been documented as the causes of allergic reactions.

85. **The correct answer is (A).** Allergic reactions occur most commonly in patients who have a history of all of the given, except for bee sting reactions.

There is no correlation between bee sting reactions and other allergic reactions.

86. **The correct answer is (B).** The flavor additive is the most secret part of the formulation of pastes and mouthwashes and the most likely part to cause an allergic reaction.

87. **The correct answer is (C).** In addition to fiery-red gingivitis, allergic reactions are also likely to cause ulcers on the gingiva.

88. **The correct answer is (B).** The best treatment for an allergic reaction to a paste or mouth rinse is to recommend that the patient discontinue use and switch to a different brand.

89. **The correct answer is (C).** The only true way to diagnose an allergic reaction is through a tissue biopsy with a diagnosis of plasma cell gingivitis.

90. **The correct answer is (C).** The patient may be able to return to this product again in the future because manufacturers often change the flavoring agents or additives in their products when they learn that they are causing allergic reactions.

91. **The correct answer is (B).** Chronic generalized mild periodontitis is consistent with this patient's pocket and bone loss.

92. **The correct answer is (B).** This patient's signs and symptoms indicate a Type 2 classification.

93. **The correct answer is (A).** Half-mouth debridement in two appointments is most appropriate for this patient based on the amount of calculus and pocketing. Topical or oraqix should be used to manage pain.

94. **The correct answer is (B).** A 3-month recall is best for this patient. However, it is anticipated that this patient can be upgraded to a 4-month recall after the next visit.

95. **The correct answer is (B).** Piezo is most appropriate because of the patient's pacemaker.

96. **The correct answer is (A).** This patient's pockets are not deep and he has minimal interdental space, so dental floss is best for him to use to clean his interproximal surfaces.

97. **The correct answer is (C).** There is no known correlation between kidney stones and cardiovascular disease.

98. **The correct answer is (B).** Four horizontal bite-wings are sufficient to view the bone height around all teeth and to open all contacts to view decay.

99. **The correct answer is (B).** Consulting with his physician is ideal given this patient's history of cardiovascular disease.

100. **The correct answer is (D).** Offering the patient a large glass of water is not recognized as protocol. In addition to the actions in choices (A), (B), and (C), you should observe the patient carefully.

101. **The correct answer is (A).** Because of his special needs and the increase in decay, 3 months is preferable to 4 months for this patient's recall frequency.

102. **The correct answer is (D).** Fluoride rinses are the best option as long as the patient is able to rinse without swallowing.

103. **The correct answer is (A).** Removing teeth in a child with a cleft palate creates further complications. The optimum arch is enabled when teeth are preserved.

104. **The correct answer is (D).** A prosthesis would not address restoration of horizontal dimension. In addition to closure of the palate, scaffolding to fill out the upper lip, and restoration of vertical dimension, a prosthesis would address masticatory function.

105. **The correct answer is (C).** The classification is Class 6, which is known as a complete cleft.

106. **The correct answer is (D).** Ingesting fluoride does not put an expectant mother at risk of giving birth to a child with a cleft lip/palate. Another risk factor other than those stated in the answer options is a folic-acid deficiency.

107. **The correct answer is (C).** A patient with a cleft palate/lip is predisposed to upper-respiratory and middle-ear infections.

108. **The correct answer is (C).** An opturator is an appliance that is frequently necessary for palatal cleft closure.

109. **The correct answer is (C).** Swallowing difficulties are not an issue for patients with a cleft lip/palate.

110. **The correct answer is (A).** Sunken eyes are not a deformity associated with a cleft lip/palate.

111. **The correct answer is (D).** This patient has not seen a dentist in 5 years, is a heavy drinker, and has oral hygiene that is only fair/poor. All of these most likely contributed to his many dental caries.

112. **The correct answer is (A).** This patient's blood pressure is only slightly below normal, so he does not have hypotension. Hypotension is also not a sign of a drinking problem.

113. **The correct answer is (C).** This patient may have underlying medical problems that might determine a particular course of treatment. He should see a physician before changing his lifestyle.

114. **The correct answer is (C).** It is likely that this patient has not had a drink in a few hours, so he is going into alcohol withdrawal. His trembling hands and rapid pulse support this theory.

115. **The correct answer is (B).** If you tell your sister about this patient's condition, you have violated his right to confidentiality.

116. **The correct answer is (D).** Alcohol, tobacco, and poor oral hygiene are likely all factors in this patient's xerostomia.

117. **The correct answer is (A).** Self-care is usually all that is needed to treat yellow tongue. The patient should brush his tongue with one part hydrogen peroxide and five parts water and then rinse thoroughly. If this does not take care of the problem, he should see a physician, as this may be a sign of a liver or gall bladder problem.

118. **The correct answer is (B).** If your patient continues to drink heavily long term, he has a higher-than-average chance of developing oral cancer.

119. **The correct answer is (C).** This patient should not use self-care agents containing alcohol; the best choice for him is a fluoride gel as this will help reduce the development of additional dental caries.

120. **The correct answer is (A).** Xerostomia, or dry mouth, is most likely the cause of this patient's dental caries. A lack of saliva in the mouth allows for an overgrowth of bacteria, which causes dental caries.

121. **The correct answer is (B).** Your patient most likely has a periapical abscess, which refers to a tooth in which the pulp is infected. This type of abscess is usually caused by tooth decay.

122. **The correct answer is (A).** This patient's symptoms indicate a periapical abscess, which is caused by tooth decay.

123. **The correct answer is (D).** Since a periapical abscess is caused by tooth decay, and your patient has untreated dental caries, you should recommend that she visit the dental regularly.

124. **The correct answer is (C).** This patient's condition appears to be a periapical abscess. A periodontal abscess is characterized by infection that occurs where pre-existing periodontitis is present.

125. **The correct answer is (D).** Treatment of a periapical abscess usually involves making an incision in the gum to drain the pus. Draining may also be achieved by enlarging the hole in the tooth. The patient will be prescribed antibiotics to combat infection. To relieve pain, which is often intense, an anesthetic is often injected into the tooth.

126. **The correct answer is (B).** Patients with a periapical abscess will take antibiotics to combat infection. They typically require root canal therapy or extraction of the infected tooth. Bone grafting, a treatment of periodontitis, is not required to treat their condition.

127. **The correct answer is (A).** Periapical radiographs are the best for this patient because they show the entire tooth, including the tip of the root and the bone surrounding the tooth.

128. **The correct answer is (C).** An abscess would appear as a dark area on a radiograph.

129. **The correct answer is (B).** Rinsing with warm salt water will soothe the patient's gum tissue and help her heal.

130. **The correct answer is (C).** The dentist would recommend and prescribe an antibiotic. Penicillin VK, Amoxicillin, or Erythromycin is often prescribed.

131. **The correct answer is (B).** Patients who must take insulin daily have Type 1 diabetes. These patients

must test their blood glucose levels several times a day.

132. **The correct answer is (B).** The patient has tooth decay on #14, #23, and #30.

133. **The correct answer is (D).** Diabetic patients are far more likely to develop dental caries, gingivitis, and periodontal disease than other patients.

134. **The correct answer is (C).** Patients with Type I diabetes should test their blood glucose levels several times a day.

135. **The correct answer is (A).** Diabetic patients typically have an increased urine volume, resulting in a loss of saliva.

136. **The correct answer is (C).** If a patient has taken insulin, but not eaten a meal, hypoglycemia, or low blood sugar, may occur. Dental hygienists should keep sugar on hand when treating diabetic patients.

137. **The correct answer is (B).** Since this patient is diabetic and has developed gingivitis, he should be seen more often than every 6 months. The best recare interval for him is 3 months.

138. **The correct answer is (D).** When examining a diabetic patient, you should look for changes in all areas, not just the oral cavity. Any type of change might indicate a problem in a diabetic patient.

139. **The correct answer is (D).** Diabetic patients are not at a higher-than-average risk of developing tooth abscesses, but they are at an increased risk of developing burning mouth syndrome, abnormal wound healing, fungal infections, along with other conditions such as dental caries and gingivitis.

140. **The correct answer is (A).** This patient's gums bleed and he has no attachment loss. Based on these findings, he has Type 1 gingivitis.

141. **The correct answer is (C).** This patient's blood pressure is 152/96. This falls into the range for Stage 1 hypertension, which is systolic 140–159 and diastolic 90–99.

142. **The correct answer is (D).** This patient's oral hygiene is indicated as good, so this is not a risk factor of periodontal disease.

143. **The correct answer is (A).** The patient's lesion is most likely leukoplakia, which is caused by chewing tobacco. He should have it screened to ensure that it is not precancerous.

144. **The correct answer is (C).** Denture stomatitis is caused by ill-fitting dentures. There is no indication that this patient is having problems with the fit of his dentures.

145. **The correct answer is (C).** The patient's smoking and tobacco chewing are most likely to cause him serious problems in the future. His first referral should be to a tobacco-cessation program.

146. **The correct answer is (C).** Smoking is a major cause of xerostomia, or dry mouth.

147. **The correct answer is (C).** Since this patient is a recovering alcoholic, he should not use products containing alcohol. Rinsing with warm salt water will soothe his gums.

148. **The correct answer is (D).** All of the following are important reasons to remove dentures at night: to rest the gums and give them air, to give gums contact with saliva, and to prevent the growth of fungus.

149. **The correct answer is (C).** The patient should gently brush his gums and teeth with a soft-bristled toothbrush.

150. **The correct answer is (D).** Hard candy contains sugar, which can make the patient's dry mouth worse.

ANSWER SHEET PRACTICE TEST 3

Component A

1. Ⓐ Ⓑ Ⓒ Ⓓ Ⓔ	41. Ⓐ Ⓑ Ⓒ Ⓓ Ⓔ	81. Ⓐ Ⓑ Ⓒ Ⓓ Ⓔ	121. Ⓐ Ⓑ Ⓒ Ⓓ Ⓔ	161. Ⓐ Ⓑ Ⓒ Ⓓ Ⓔ
2. Ⓐ Ⓑ Ⓒ Ⓓ Ⓔ	42. Ⓐ Ⓑ Ⓒ Ⓓ Ⓔ	82. Ⓐ Ⓑ Ⓒ Ⓓ Ⓔ	122. Ⓐ Ⓑ Ⓒ Ⓓ Ⓔ	162. Ⓐ Ⓑ Ⓒ Ⓓ Ⓔ
3. Ⓐ Ⓑ Ⓒ Ⓓ Ⓔ	43. Ⓐ Ⓑ Ⓒ Ⓓ Ⓔ	83. Ⓐ Ⓑ Ⓒ Ⓓ Ⓔ	123. Ⓐ Ⓑ Ⓒ Ⓓ Ⓔ	163. Ⓐ Ⓑ Ⓒ Ⓓ Ⓔ
4. Ⓐ Ⓑ Ⓒ Ⓓ Ⓔ	44. Ⓐ Ⓑ Ⓒ Ⓓ Ⓔ	84. Ⓐ Ⓑ Ⓒ Ⓓ Ⓔ	124. Ⓐ Ⓑ Ⓒ Ⓓ Ⓔ	164. Ⓐ Ⓑ Ⓒ Ⓓ Ⓔ
5. Ⓐ Ⓑ Ⓒ Ⓓ Ⓔ	45. Ⓐ Ⓑ Ⓒ Ⓓ Ⓔ	85. Ⓐ Ⓑ Ⓒ Ⓓ Ⓔ	125. Ⓐ Ⓑ Ⓒ Ⓓ Ⓔ	165. Ⓐ Ⓑ Ⓒ Ⓓ Ⓔ
6. Ⓐ Ⓑ Ⓒ Ⓓ Ⓔ	46. Ⓐ Ⓑ Ⓒ Ⓓ Ⓔ	86. Ⓐ Ⓑ Ⓒ Ⓓ Ⓔ	126. Ⓐ Ⓑ Ⓒ Ⓓ Ⓔ	166. Ⓐ Ⓑ Ⓒ Ⓓ Ⓔ
7. Ⓐ Ⓑ Ⓒ Ⓓ Ⓔ	47. Ⓐ Ⓑ Ⓒ Ⓓ Ⓔ	87. Ⓐ Ⓑ Ⓒ Ⓓ Ⓔ	127. Ⓐ Ⓑ Ⓒ Ⓓ Ⓔ	167. Ⓐ Ⓑ Ⓒ Ⓓ Ⓔ
8. Ⓐ Ⓑ Ⓒ Ⓓ Ⓔ	48. Ⓐ Ⓑ Ⓒ Ⓓ Ⓔ	88. Ⓐ Ⓑ Ⓒ Ⓓ Ⓔ	128. Ⓐ Ⓑ Ⓒ Ⓓ Ⓔ	168. Ⓐ Ⓑ Ⓒ Ⓓ Ⓔ
9. Ⓐ Ⓑ Ⓒ Ⓓ Ⓔ	49. Ⓐ Ⓑ Ⓒ Ⓓ Ⓔ	89. Ⓐ Ⓑ Ⓒ Ⓓ Ⓔ	129. Ⓐ Ⓑ Ⓒ Ⓓ Ⓔ	169. Ⓐ Ⓑ Ⓒ Ⓓ Ⓔ
10. Ⓐ Ⓑ Ⓒ Ⓓ Ⓔ	50. Ⓐ Ⓑ Ⓒ Ⓓ Ⓔ	90. Ⓐ Ⓑ Ⓒ Ⓓ Ⓔ	130. Ⓐ Ⓑ Ⓒ Ⓓ Ⓔ	170. Ⓐ Ⓑ Ⓒ Ⓓ Ⓔ
11. Ⓐ Ⓑ Ⓒ Ⓓ Ⓔ	51. Ⓐ Ⓑ Ⓒ Ⓓ Ⓔ	91. Ⓐ Ⓑ Ⓒ Ⓓ Ⓔ	131. Ⓐ Ⓑ Ⓒ Ⓓ Ⓔ	171. Ⓐ Ⓑ Ⓒ Ⓓ Ⓔ
12. Ⓐ Ⓑ Ⓒ Ⓓ Ⓔ	52. Ⓐ Ⓑ Ⓒ Ⓓ Ⓔ	92. Ⓐ Ⓑ Ⓒ Ⓓ Ⓔ	132. Ⓐ Ⓑ Ⓒ Ⓓ Ⓔ	172. Ⓐ Ⓑ Ⓒ Ⓓ Ⓔ
13. Ⓐ Ⓑ Ⓒ Ⓓ Ⓔ	53. Ⓐ Ⓑ Ⓒ Ⓓ Ⓔ	93. Ⓐ Ⓑ Ⓒ Ⓓ Ⓔ	133. Ⓐ Ⓑ Ⓒ Ⓓ Ⓔ	173. Ⓐ Ⓑ Ⓒ Ⓓ Ⓔ
14. Ⓐ Ⓑ Ⓒ Ⓓ Ⓔ	54. Ⓐ Ⓑ Ⓒ Ⓓ Ⓔ	94. Ⓐ Ⓑ Ⓒ Ⓓ Ⓔ	134. Ⓐ Ⓑ Ⓒ Ⓓ Ⓔ	174. Ⓐ Ⓑ Ⓒ Ⓓ Ⓔ
15. Ⓐ Ⓑ Ⓒ Ⓓ Ⓔ	55. Ⓐ Ⓑ Ⓒ Ⓓ Ⓔ	95. Ⓐ Ⓑ Ⓒ Ⓓ Ⓔ	135. Ⓐ Ⓑ Ⓒ Ⓓ Ⓔ	175. Ⓐ Ⓑ Ⓒ Ⓓ Ⓔ
16. Ⓐ Ⓑ Ⓒ Ⓓ Ⓔ	56. Ⓐ Ⓑ Ⓒ Ⓓ Ⓔ	96. Ⓐ Ⓑ Ⓒ Ⓓ Ⓔ	136. Ⓐ Ⓑ Ⓒ Ⓓ Ⓔ	176. Ⓐ Ⓑ Ⓒ Ⓓ Ⓔ
17. Ⓐ Ⓑ Ⓒ Ⓓ Ⓔ	57. Ⓐ Ⓑ Ⓒ Ⓓ Ⓔ	97. Ⓐ Ⓑ Ⓒ Ⓓ Ⓔ	137. Ⓐ Ⓑ Ⓒ Ⓓ Ⓔ	177. Ⓐ Ⓑ Ⓒ Ⓓ Ⓔ
18. Ⓐ Ⓑ Ⓒ Ⓓ Ⓔ	58. Ⓐ Ⓑ Ⓒ Ⓓ Ⓔ	98. Ⓐ Ⓑ Ⓒ Ⓓ Ⓔ	138. Ⓐ Ⓑ Ⓒ Ⓓ Ⓔ	178. Ⓐ Ⓑ Ⓒ Ⓓ Ⓔ
19. Ⓐ Ⓑ Ⓒ Ⓓ Ⓔ	59. Ⓐ Ⓑ Ⓒ Ⓓ Ⓔ	99. Ⓐ Ⓑ Ⓒ Ⓓ Ⓔ	139. Ⓐ Ⓑ Ⓒ Ⓓ Ⓔ	179. Ⓐ Ⓑ Ⓒ Ⓓ Ⓔ
20. Ⓐ Ⓑ Ⓒ Ⓓ Ⓔ	60. Ⓐ Ⓑ Ⓒ Ⓓ Ⓔ	100. Ⓐ Ⓑ Ⓒ Ⓓ Ⓔ	140. Ⓐ Ⓑ Ⓒ Ⓓ Ⓔ	180. Ⓐ Ⓑ Ⓒ Ⓓ Ⓔ
21. Ⓐ Ⓑ Ⓒ Ⓓ Ⓔ	61. Ⓐ Ⓑ Ⓒ Ⓓ Ⓔ	101. Ⓐ Ⓑ Ⓒ Ⓓ Ⓔ	141. Ⓐ Ⓑ Ⓒ Ⓓ Ⓔ	181. Ⓐ Ⓑ Ⓒ Ⓓ Ⓔ
22. Ⓐ Ⓑ Ⓒ Ⓓ Ⓔ	62. Ⓐ Ⓑ Ⓒ Ⓓ Ⓔ	102. Ⓐ Ⓑ Ⓒ Ⓓ Ⓔ	142. Ⓐ Ⓑ Ⓒ Ⓓ Ⓔ	182. Ⓐ Ⓑ Ⓒ Ⓓ Ⓔ
23. Ⓐ Ⓑ Ⓒ Ⓓ Ⓔ	63. Ⓐ Ⓑ Ⓒ Ⓓ Ⓔ	103. Ⓐ Ⓑ Ⓒ Ⓓ Ⓔ	143. Ⓐ Ⓑ Ⓒ Ⓓ Ⓔ	183. Ⓐ Ⓑ Ⓒ Ⓓ Ⓔ
24. Ⓐ Ⓑ Ⓒ Ⓓ Ⓔ	64. Ⓐ Ⓑ Ⓒ Ⓓ Ⓔ	104. Ⓐ Ⓑ Ⓒ Ⓓ Ⓔ	144. Ⓐ Ⓑ Ⓒ Ⓓ Ⓔ	184. Ⓐ Ⓑ Ⓒ Ⓓ Ⓔ
25. Ⓐ Ⓑ Ⓒ Ⓓ Ⓔ	65. Ⓐ Ⓑ Ⓒ Ⓓ Ⓔ	105. Ⓐ Ⓑ Ⓒ Ⓓ Ⓔ	145. Ⓐ Ⓑ Ⓒ Ⓓ Ⓔ	185. Ⓐ Ⓑ Ⓒ Ⓓ Ⓔ
26. Ⓐ Ⓑ Ⓒ Ⓓ Ⓔ	66. Ⓐ Ⓑ Ⓒ Ⓓ Ⓔ	106. Ⓐ Ⓑ Ⓒ Ⓓ Ⓔ	146. Ⓐ Ⓑ Ⓒ Ⓓ Ⓔ	186. Ⓐ Ⓑ Ⓒ Ⓓ Ⓔ
27. Ⓐ Ⓑ Ⓒ Ⓓ Ⓔ	67. Ⓐ Ⓑ Ⓒ Ⓓ Ⓔ	107. Ⓐ Ⓑ Ⓒ Ⓓ Ⓔ	147. Ⓐ Ⓑ Ⓒ Ⓓ Ⓔ	187. Ⓐ Ⓑ Ⓒ Ⓓ Ⓔ
28. Ⓐ Ⓑ Ⓒ Ⓓ Ⓔ	68. Ⓐ Ⓑ Ⓒ Ⓓ Ⓔ	108. Ⓐ Ⓑ Ⓒ Ⓓ Ⓔ	148. Ⓐ Ⓑ Ⓒ Ⓓ Ⓔ	188. Ⓐ Ⓑ Ⓒ Ⓓ Ⓔ
29. Ⓐ Ⓑ Ⓒ Ⓓ Ⓔ	69. Ⓐ Ⓑ Ⓒ Ⓓ Ⓔ	109. Ⓐ Ⓑ Ⓒ Ⓓ Ⓔ	149. Ⓐ Ⓑ Ⓒ Ⓓ Ⓔ	189. Ⓐ Ⓑ Ⓒ Ⓓ Ⓔ
30. Ⓐ Ⓑ Ⓒ Ⓓ Ⓔ	70. Ⓐ Ⓑ Ⓒ Ⓓ Ⓔ	110. Ⓐ Ⓑ Ⓒ Ⓓ Ⓔ	150. Ⓐ Ⓑ Ⓒ Ⓓ Ⓔ	190. Ⓐ Ⓑ Ⓒ Ⓓ Ⓔ
31. Ⓐ Ⓑ Ⓒ Ⓓ Ⓔ	71. Ⓐ Ⓑ Ⓒ Ⓓ Ⓔ	111. Ⓐ Ⓑ Ⓒ Ⓓ Ⓔ	151. Ⓐ Ⓑ Ⓒ Ⓓ Ⓔ	191. Ⓐ Ⓑ Ⓒ Ⓓ Ⓔ
32. Ⓐ Ⓑ Ⓒ Ⓓ Ⓔ	72. Ⓐ Ⓑ Ⓒ Ⓓ Ⓔ	112. Ⓐ Ⓑ Ⓒ Ⓓ Ⓔ	152. Ⓐ Ⓑ Ⓒ Ⓓ Ⓔ	192. Ⓐ Ⓑ Ⓒ Ⓓ Ⓔ
33. Ⓐ Ⓑ Ⓒ Ⓓ Ⓔ	73. Ⓐ Ⓑ Ⓒ Ⓓ Ⓔ	113. Ⓐ Ⓑ Ⓒ Ⓓ Ⓔ	153. Ⓐ Ⓑ Ⓒ Ⓓ Ⓔ	193. Ⓐ Ⓑ Ⓒ Ⓓ Ⓔ
34. Ⓐ Ⓑ Ⓒ Ⓓ Ⓔ	74. Ⓐ Ⓑ Ⓒ Ⓓ Ⓔ	114. Ⓐ Ⓑ Ⓒ Ⓓ Ⓔ	154. Ⓐ Ⓑ Ⓒ Ⓓ Ⓔ	194. Ⓐ Ⓑ Ⓒ Ⓓ Ⓔ
35. Ⓐ Ⓑ Ⓒ Ⓓ Ⓔ	75. Ⓐ Ⓑ Ⓒ Ⓓ Ⓔ	115. Ⓐ Ⓑ Ⓒ Ⓓ Ⓔ	155. Ⓐ Ⓑ Ⓒ Ⓓ Ⓔ	195. Ⓐ Ⓑ Ⓒ Ⓓ Ⓔ
36. Ⓐ Ⓑ Ⓒ Ⓓ Ⓔ	76. Ⓐ Ⓑ Ⓒ Ⓓ Ⓔ	116. Ⓐ Ⓑ Ⓒ Ⓓ Ⓔ	156. Ⓐ Ⓑ Ⓒ Ⓓ Ⓔ	196. Ⓐ Ⓑ Ⓒ Ⓓ Ⓔ
37. Ⓐ Ⓑ Ⓒ Ⓓ Ⓔ	77. Ⓐ Ⓑ Ⓒ Ⓓ Ⓔ	117. Ⓐ Ⓑ Ⓒ Ⓓ Ⓔ	157. Ⓐ Ⓑ Ⓒ Ⓓ Ⓔ	197. Ⓐ Ⓑ Ⓒ Ⓓ Ⓔ
38. Ⓐ Ⓑ Ⓒ Ⓓ Ⓔ	78. Ⓐ Ⓑ Ⓒ Ⓓ Ⓔ	118. Ⓐ Ⓑ Ⓒ Ⓓ Ⓔ	158. Ⓐ Ⓑ Ⓒ Ⓓ Ⓔ	198. Ⓐ Ⓑ Ⓒ Ⓓ Ⓔ
39. Ⓐ Ⓑ Ⓒ Ⓓ Ⓔ	79. Ⓐ Ⓑ Ⓒ Ⓓ Ⓔ	119. Ⓐ Ⓑ Ⓒ Ⓓ Ⓔ	159. Ⓐ Ⓑ Ⓒ Ⓓ Ⓔ	199. Ⓐ Ⓑ Ⓒ Ⓓ Ⓔ
40. Ⓐ Ⓑ Ⓒ Ⓓ Ⓔ	80. Ⓐ Ⓑ Ⓒ Ⓓ Ⓔ	120. Ⓐ Ⓑ Ⓒ Ⓓ Ⓔ	160. Ⓐ Ⓑ Ⓒ Ⓓ Ⓔ	200. Ⓐ Ⓑ Ⓒ Ⓓ Ⓔ

Component B

1. Ⓐ Ⓑ Ⓒ Ⓓ	31. Ⓐ Ⓑ Ⓒ Ⓓ	61. Ⓐ Ⓑ Ⓒ Ⓓ	91. Ⓐ Ⓑ Ⓒ Ⓓ	121. Ⓐ Ⓑ Ⓒ Ⓓ
2. Ⓐ Ⓑ Ⓒ Ⓓ	32. Ⓐ Ⓑ Ⓒ Ⓓ	62. Ⓐ Ⓑ Ⓒ Ⓓ	92. Ⓐ Ⓑ Ⓒ Ⓓ	122. Ⓐ Ⓑ Ⓒ Ⓓ
3. Ⓐ Ⓑ Ⓒ Ⓓ	33. Ⓐ Ⓑ Ⓒ Ⓓ	63. Ⓐ Ⓑ Ⓒ Ⓓ	93. Ⓐ Ⓑ Ⓒ Ⓓ	123. Ⓐ Ⓑ Ⓒ Ⓓ
4. Ⓐ Ⓑ Ⓒ Ⓓ	34. Ⓐ Ⓑ Ⓒ Ⓓ	64. Ⓐ Ⓑ Ⓒ Ⓓ	94. Ⓐ Ⓑ Ⓒ Ⓓ	124. Ⓐ Ⓑ Ⓒ Ⓓ
5. Ⓐ Ⓑ Ⓒ Ⓓ	35. Ⓐ Ⓑ Ⓒ Ⓓ	65. Ⓐ Ⓑ Ⓒ Ⓓ	95. Ⓐ Ⓑ Ⓒ Ⓓ	125. Ⓐ Ⓑ Ⓒ Ⓓ
6. Ⓐ Ⓑ Ⓒ Ⓓ	36. Ⓐ Ⓑ Ⓒ Ⓓ	66. Ⓐ Ⓑ Ⓒ Ⓓ	96. Ⓐ Ⓑ Ⓒ Ⓓ	126. Ⓐ Ⓑ Ⓒ Ⓓ
7. Ⓐ Ⓑ Ⓒ Ⓓ	37. Ⓐ Ⓑ Ⓒ Ⓓ	67. Ⓐ Ⓑ Ⓒ Ⓓ	97. Ⓐ Ⓑ Ⓒ Ⓓ	127. Ⓐ Ⓑ Ⓒ Ⓓ
8. Ⓐ Ⓑ Ⓒ Ⓓ	38. Ⓐ Ⓑ Ⓒ Ⓓ	68. Ⓐ Ⓑ Ⓒ Ⓓ	98. Ⓐ Ⓑ Ⓒ Ⓓ	128. Ⓐ Ⓑ Ⓒ Ⓓ
9. Ⓐ Ⓑ Ⓒ Ⓓ	39. Ⓐ Ⓑ Ⓒ Ⓓ	69. Ⓐ Ⓑ Ⓒ Ⓓ	99. Ⓐ Ⓑ Ⓒ Ⓓ	129. Ⓐ Ⓑ Ⓒ Ⓓ
10. Ⓐ Ⓑ Ⓒ Ⓓ	40. Ⓐ Ⓑ Ⓒ Ⓓ	70. Ⓐ Ⓑ Ⓒ Ⓓ	100. Ⓐ Ⓑ Ⓒ Ⓓ	130. Ⓐ Ⓑ Ⓒ Ⓓ
11. Ⓐ Ⓑ Ⓒ Ⓓ	41. Ⓐ Ⓑ Ⓒ Ⓓ	71. Ⓐ Ⓑ Ⓒ Ⓓ	101. Ⓐ Ⓑ Ⓒ Ⓓ	131. Ⓐ Ⓑ Ⓒ Ⓓ
12. Ⓐ Ⓑ Ⓒ Ⓓ	42. Ⓐ Ⓑ Ⓒ Ⓓ	72. Ⓐ Ⓑ Ⓒ Ⓓ	102. Ⓐ Ⓑ Ⓒ Ⓓ	132. Ⓐ Ⓑ Ⓒ Ⓓ
13. Ⓐ Ⓑ Ⓒ Ⓓ	43. Ⓐ Ⓑ Ⓒ Ⓓ	73. Ⓐ Ⓑ Ⓒ Ⓓ	103. Ⓐ Ⓑ Ⓒ Ⓓ	133. Ⓐ Ⓑ Ⓒ Ⓓ
14. Ⓐ Ⓑ Ⓒ Ⓓ	44. Ⓐ Ⓑ Ⓒ Ⓓ	74. Ⓐ Ⓑ Ⓒ Ⓓ	104. Ⓐ Ⓑ Ⓒ Ⓓ	134. Ⓐ Ⓑ Ⓒ Ⓓ
15. Ⓐ Ⓑ Ⓒ Ⓓ	45. Ⓐ Ⓑ Ⓒ Ⓓ	75. Ⓐ Ⓑ Ⓒ Ⓓ	105. Ⓐ Ⓑ Ⓒ Ⓓ	135. Ⓐ Ⓑ Ⓒ Ⓓ
16. Ⓐ Ⓑ Ⓒ Ⓓ	46. Ⓐ Ⓑ Ⓒ Ⓓ	76. Ⓐ Ⓑ Ⓒ Ⓓ	106. Ⓐ Ⓑ Ⓒ Ⓓ	136. Ⓐ Ⓑ Ⓒ Ⓓ
17. Ⓐ Ⓑ Ⓒ Ⓓ	47. Ⓐ Ⓑ Ⓒ Ⓓ	77. Ⓐ Ⓑ Ⓒ Ⓓ	107. Ⓐ Ⓑ Ⓒ Ⓓ	137. Ⓐ Ⓑ Ⓒ Ⓓ
18. Ⓐ Ⓑ Ⓒ Ⓓ	48. Ⓐ Ⓑ Ⓒ Ⓓ	78. Ⓐ Ⓑ Ⓒ Ⓓ	108. Ⓐ Ⓑ Ⓒ Ⓓ	138. Ⓐ Ⓑ Ⓒ Ⓓ
19. Ⓐ Ⓑ Ⓒ Ⓓ	49. Ⓐ Ⓑ Ⓒ Ⓓ	79. Ⓐ Ⓑ Ⓒ Ⓓ	109. Ⓐ Ⓑ Ⓒ Ⓓ	139. Ⓐ Ⓑ Ⓒ Ⓓ
20. Ⓐ Ⓑ Ⓒ Ⓓ	50. Ⓐ Ⓑ Ⓒ Ⓓ	80. Ⓐ Ⓑ Ⓒ Ⓓ	110. Ⓐ Ⓑ Ⓒ Ⓓ	140. Ⓐ Ⓑ Ⓒ Ⓓ
21. Ⓐ Ⓑ Ⓒ Ⓓ	51. Ⓐ Ⓑ Ⓒ Ⓓ	81. Ⓐ Ⓑ Ⓒ Ⓓ	111. Ⓐ Ⓑ Ⓒ Ⓓ	141. Ⓐ Ⓑ Ⓒ Ⓓ
22. Ⓐ Ⓑ Ⓒ Ⓓ	52. Ⓐ Ⓑ Ⓒ Ⓓ	82. Ⓐ Ⓑ Ⓒ Ⓓ	112. Ⓐ Ⓑ Ⓒ Ⓓ	142. Ⓐ Ⓑ Ⓒ Ⓓ
23. Ⓐ Ⓑ Ⓒ Ⓓ	53. Ⓐ Ⓑ Ⓒ Ⓓ	83. Ⓐ Ⓑ Ⓒ Ⓓ	113. Ⓐ Ⓑ Ⓒ Ⓓ	143. Ⓐ Ⓑ Ⓒ Ⓓ
24. Ⓐ Ⓑ Ⓒ Ⓓ	54. Ⓐ Ⓑ Ⓒ Ⓓ	84. Ⓐ Ⓑ Ⓒ Ⓓ	114. Ⓐ Ⓑ Ⓒ Ⓓ	144. Ⓐ Ⓑ Ⓒ Ⓓ
25. Ⓐ Ⓑ Ⓒ Ⓓ	55. Ⓐ Ⓑ Ⓒ Ⓓ	85. Ⓐ Ⓑ Ⓒ Ⓓ	115. Ⓐ Ⓑ Ⓒ Ⓓ	145. Ⓐ Ⓑ Ⓒ Ⓓ
26. Ⓐ Ⓑ Ⓒ Ⓓ	56. Ⓐ Ⓑ Ⓒ Ⓓ	86. Ⓐ Ⓑ Ⓒ Ⓓ	116. Ⓐ Ⓑ Ⓒ Ⓓ	146. Ⓐ Ⓑ Ⓒ Ⓓ
27. Ⓐ Ⓑ Ⓒ Ⓓ	57. Ⓐ Ⓑ Ⓒ Ⓓ	87. Ⓐ Ⓑ Ⓒ Ⓓ	117. Ⓐ Ⓑ Ⓒ Ⓓ	147. Ⓐ Ⓑ Ⓒ Ⓓ
28. Ⓐ Ⓑ Ⓒ Ⓓ	58. Ⓐ Ⓑ Ⓒ Ⓓ	88. Ⓐ Ⓑ Ⓒ Ⓓ	118. Ⓐ Ⓑ Ⓒ Ⓓ	148. Ⓐ Ⓑ Ⓒ Ⓓ
29. Ⓐ Ⓑ Ⓒ Ⓓ	59. Ⓐ Ⓑ Ⓒ Ⓓ	89. Ⓐ Ⓑ Ⓒ Ⓓ	119. Ⓐ Ⓑ Ⓒ Ⓓ	149. Ⓐ Ⓑ Ⓒ Ⓓ
30. Ⓐ Ⓑ Ⓒ Ⓓ	60. Ⓐ Ⓑ Ⓒ Ⓓ	90. Ⓐ Ⓑ Ⓒ Ⓓ	120. Ⓐ Ⓑ Ⓒ Ⓓ	150. Ⓐ Ⓑ Ⓒ Ⓓ

Practice Test 3

COMPONENT A

Directions: Choose the option that best answers the questions.

1. The type of hepatitis that can be contracted only in the presence of hepatitis B is
   (A) hepatitis A.
   (B) hepatitis C.
   (C) hepatitis D.
   (D) hepatitis E.
   (E) hepatitis G.

2. The first measurement of attached gingiva is the CEJ to the mucogingival line.

   The second measurement of attached gingiva is the CEJ to the gingival margin.
   (A) Both statements are true.
   (B) Both statements are false.
   (C) The first statement is true, but the second statement is false.
   (D) The first statement is false, but the second statement is true.

3. Which of the following **BEST** describes the lag phase of bacterial replication?
   (A) Cells do not change.
   (B) Cells grow and divide.
   (C) Cells do not grow but do divide.
   (D) Cells grow but do not divide.
   (E) Cells replicate at the same pace they die.

4. One possible disadvantage of using discovery learning as a dental health education method would be that
   (A) learning is difficult to monitor because students spend so much time outside the classroom.
   (B) learners must be carefully monitored to maintain focus.

   (C) strong personalities may come to dominate the group dynamic.
   (D) students must be guided toward the correct conclusions.
   (E) careful planning and adequate facilities are required.

5. Airway obstructions or foreign body airway obstruction occurs more easily in a dental setting **BECAUSE** patients are typically in the supine position.
   (A) Both the statement and reason are correct and related.
   (B) Both the statement and reason are correct but NOT related.
   (C) The statement is correct, but the reason is NOT.
   (D) The statement is NOT correct, but the reason is correct.
   (E) NEITHER the statement NOR the reason is correct.

6. Which of the following drugs would be the most effective treatment for gastroesophageal reflux disease?
   (A) Famotidine
   (B) Flunisolide
   (C) Aerobid
   (D) Triamcinolone
   (E) Fluticasone

7. Tooth mobility is measured during the periodontal assessment because it is a risk factor for the progression of periodontal disease.

Mobility is measured by bidigital palpitation only when the teeth are not occluded.
(A) Both statements are true.
(B) Both statements are false.
(C) The first statement is true, the second is false.
(D) The first statement is false, the second is true.

8. Which of the following are mobile cells in the periodontal pocket that "sense" an invading microbe by the smell of their chemicals?
(A) Peripheral cells
(B) Cementocytes
(C) Neutrophils
(D) Keratocytes
(E) Fibroblasts

9. Each of the following is considered an environmental factor of a disease state **EXCEPT** one. Which one is the **EXCEPTION**?
(A) Food sources
(B) Pollution and sanitation
(C) Climate and geography
(D) Parasitic population
(E) Socioeconomic conditions

10. Which of the following contains not only bacteria but also protozoa, mycoplasmas, and yeasts?
(A) Coccus
(B) Pellicle
(C) Plaque biofilm
(D) Calculus
(E) Proline

11. Local anesthesia blocks the perception of pain by
(A) keeping potassium locked inside neurons.
(B) deactivating selected neurons.
(C) neutralizing the charges of neurons.
(D) preventing sodium from entering neurons.
(E) flooding neurons with excess potassium.

12. Which sampling method is used to achieve a proportionate representation of subgroups in a sample when their existence in the population is established?
(A) Purposive sample
(B) Stratified sample
(C) Random sample
(D) Convenience sample
(E) Systematic sample

13. Phase I therapy would focus on which of the following?
(A) Endodontic therapy
(B) Deposit removal
(C) Placement of implants
(D) Self-care education
(E) Periodontal surgery

14. The primary purpose of assessing a population as part of developing a community health program is to
(A) identify a prevalent health issue.
(B) demonstrate the makeup of the community.
(C) isolate a target group.
(D) find the source of a health issue.
(E) reach a conclusion for solving the problem.

15. Which of the following has a pH between 7 and 8 and may irritate connective tissues when used?
(A) Glass ionomer cement
(B) Resin cement
(C) Zinc oxide-eugenol
(D) Calcium hydroxide
(E) Polycarboxylate cement

16. Which of the following **BEST** describes a cell's flagellum?
(A) A body that stores chemicals
(B) A jelly-like substance inside the cell
(C) A part that produces the cell's power
(D) A cylinder that supports the cell's structure
(E) A filament connected to the cell wall that allows mobility

17. Which of the following anticonvulsant agents is used to treat petit mal seizures?
(A) Dilantin
(B) Tegretol
(C) Phenytoin
(D) Carbamazepine
(E) Ethosuximide

18. How many bones are found in the adult human body?
    (A) 195
    (B) 206
    (C) 227
    (D) 278
    (E) 300

19. A blunted papilla would be indicated on a periodontal assessment by drawing which of the following?
    (A) A crater-shaped symbol
    (B) A straight vertical line
    (C) The letters EX
    (D) A zigzag line
    (E) A straight horizontal line

20. Each of the following is a symptom of chronic leukemia **EXCEPT** one. Which one is the **EXCEPTION**?
    (A) Gingival pallor
    (B) Purpuric spots
    (C) Ecchymosis
    (D) Enlarged gingival tissue
    (E) Candidiasis

21. Which number radiograph film should be used on adults who are having both their periapicals and their bitewings filmed?
    (A) 0
    (B) 1
    (C) 2
    (D) 3
    (E) 4

22. A dental condition that may be treated with an adrenocorticosteroid is
    (A) bruxism.
    (B) TMJ disease.
    (C) odontogenic cysts.
    (D) periodontitis.
    (E) canker sores.

23. An injury to the buccinator muscle could cause food to get trapped in the cheek **BECAUSE** the buccinator muscle aids in whistling.
    (A) Both the statement and reason are correct and related.
    (B) Both the statement and the reason are correct but NOT related.
    (C) The statement is correct, but the reason is NOT.

(D) The statement is NOT correct, but the reason is correct.
(E) NEITHER the statement NOR the reason is correct.

24. Patients taking calcium channel blockers such as nifedipine, verapamil, or ditiazem, run an increased risk of gingival hyperplasia.

Current dental research shows that periodontal disease and coronary artery disease are not linked.
    (A) Both statements are true.
    (B) Both statements are false.
    (C) The first statement is true, the second is false.
    (D) The first statement is false, the second is true.

25. The objective of a health education plan plays a vital role in dynamic teaching for students and teachers alike **BECAUSE** it provides a basis on which both teaching and learning can be assessed, designed, implemented, and evaluated.
    (A) Both the statement and the reason are correct and related.
    (B) Both the statement and the reason are correct but NOT related.
    (C) The statement is correct, but the reason is NOT.
    (D) The statement is NOT correct, but the reason is correct.
    (E) NEITHER the statement NOR the reason is correct.

26. Which type of palpitation involves the simultaneous use of the index finger of one hand and the fingers and thumb of the other hand to move or compress the tissue of the floor of the client's mouth?
    (A) Bidigital
    (B) Manual
    (C) Bilateral
    (D) Digital
    (E) Bimanual

27. Body language plays an important role in communication in the dental hygiene profession. Each of the follow is an example of body language **EXCEPT** one. Which one is the **EXCEPTION**?
    (A) Paralanguage
    (B) Posture
    (C) Gestures
    (D) Facial expression
    (E) Eye contact

28. Periapical (PA), bitewing (BW), occlusal, and full-mouth series (FMX) are all
    (A) intraoral radiographic views.
    (B) intraoral examination techniques.
    (C) extraoral examination techniques.
    (D) types of panoramic imaging.
    (E) cephalometric radiographic projections.

29. Which of the following is thought to be most responsible for the noted decrease in dental caries over the last few decades?
    (A) Improved oral hygiene practices
    (B) Greater focus on preventive care
    (C) Enhanced dental hygiene products
    (D) Increased exposure to fluoride
    (E) Better dietary habits

30. When patients are hesitant to make eye contact with dental hygiene professionals, it often means they aren't being entirely honest.

    Two individuals having a general conversation typically maintain eye contact about 50 percent of the time.
    (A) Both statements are true.
    (B) Both statements are false.
    (C) The first statement is true, the second is false.
    (D) The first statement is false, the second is true.

Use the following scenario to answer questions 31–34.

Clara is a dental hygienist for a busy dental practice. On Monday, she goes out for dinner with her friend and shares a made-up story about her male boss harassing her at work. On Tuesday, a client's wife calls Clara and asks for information about the nature of her husband's recent appointments. Since it is the patient's spouse, Clara reveals this information. On Wednesday, she faxes some patient information requested by Workers' Compensation that is related to a recent claim made by the patient. Finally, on Thursday, she performs a dental procedure on a 10-year-old patient, but not before getting him to sign a consent form.

31. If Clara's boss decided to bring her to court because of her actions while she was out at dinner, what charge would he **MOST LIKELY** file against her?
    (A) Appropriation
    (B) Slander
    (C) Libel
    (D) Fraud
    (E) Battery

32. What type of legal violation did Clara commit by revealing the details of a client's visits to that client's spouse?
    (A) Intrusion upon seclusion
    (B) Appropriation
    (C) Defamation
    (D) Publicity of private life
    (E) False light

33. The patient who filed a Workers' Compensation claim threatens to take the hygienist to court for revealing confidential information without consent. If this happens, the **BEST** defense for the hygienist to use is
    (A) statute of limitations.
    (B) privilege.

    (C) disclosure statutes.
    (D) implied consent.
    (E) necessity.

34. The 10-year-old patient met the basic requirements related to competency of consent.

    The 10-year-old patient could have given oral consent as an alternative to signing a consent form.
    (A) Both statements are true.
    (B) Both statements are false.
    (C) The first statement is true, the second is false.
    (D) The first statement is false, the second is true.

35. Which of the following symptoms is an indication of a phosphorus deficiency in a patient?
    (A) Glossitis
    (B) Bleeding gums
    (C) Halitosis
    (D) Tongue ulcers
    (E) Dental caries

36. In the American Dental Hygienists' Association's Code of Ethics, which of the following is an ethical duty hygienists have to clients?
    (A) Avoid actions that are or may be perceived as discriminatory.
    (B) Try to manage and resolve conflicts in a constructive way.
    (C) Help other hygienists promote preventive oral care.
    (D) Try to create a safe work environment for other hygienists.
    (E) Comply with the obligation to provide pro bono services.

37. A multi-therapeutic regimen to administering fluoride is the most effective approach to prevent caries.

    Such an approach includes a fluoridated water supply, a professional application of fluoride, and fluoride toothpaste.
    (A) Both statements are true.
    (B) Both statements are false.
    (C) The first statement is true, the second is false.
    (D) The first statement is false, the second is true.

38. Which of the following **BEST** describes the procedure of osseous surgery?
    (A) An excisional surgery that removes diseases gingival tissue.
    (B) A surgery that corrects diseased pocket beyond the mucogingival junction.
    (C) An incisional surgery that exposes underlying bone and root surface for removal of diseased tissue.
    (D) A surgery that corrects bone defects by resculpting the bone.
    (E) An excisional surgery that reshapes gingival tissues.

39. Each of the following is a type of dental implant **EXCEPT** one. Which one is the **EXCEPTION**?
    (A) Titanium implants
    (B) Endosseous implants
    (C) Subperiosteal implants
    (D) Transosteal implants
    (E) Soft-tissue implants

40. Which angle should be used when polishing the occlusal tooth surfaces?
    (A) 90-degree angle
    (B) 80-degree angle
    (C) 75-degree angle
    (D) 60-degree angle
    (E) 45-degree angle

41. The final state or condition the student can demonstrate following an instructional event is referred to as the
    (A) terminal product.
    (B) expected outcome.
    (C) end-result.
    (D) terminal behavior.
    (E) course objective.

42. Dental hygienists have an ethical duty to themselves as individuals to spend time promoting the profession.

    Dental hygienists have an ethical duty to themselves as professionals to maintain a healthy lifestyle.
    (A) Both statements are true.
    (B) Both statements are false.
    (C) The first statement is true, the second is false.
    (D) The first statement is false, the second is true.

43. Which stage may produce the anomaly hyperdontia?
    (A) Initiation stage
    (B) Bud stage
    (C) Cap stage
    (D) Bell stage
    (E) Maturation

44. It is **NOT** a good idea to use a scaler subgingivally during periodontal debridement because
    (A) it is so small and difficult to work with.
    (B) it will not work the gingival tissue enough.
    (C) its tip won't easily adapt to the tooth.
    (D) its rigid shanks make it difficult to feel.
    (E) its tip is too curved to correctly touch the tooth surface.

45. Each of the following is a dental abnormality that occurs during the cap stage **EXCEPT** one. Which one is the **EXCEPTION**?
    (A) Enamel pearls
    (B) Dens in dente
    (C) Gemination
    (D) Tubercles
    (E) Fusion

46. A patient in a dental office has a thiamin deficiency. Which of the following foods should the patient eat more of to increase thiamin intake?
    (A) Whole grains
    (B) Dairy products
    (C) Red meat
    (D) Citrus fruits
    (E) Leafy vegetables

47. Which of the following lower respiratory infections is caused in humans by bacteria found in infected bird excretions?
    (A) Legionnaire's disease
    (B) Tuberculosis
    (C) Pneumococcal pneumonia
    (D) Psittacosis
    (E) Whooping cough

48. Which type of cysts can be treated with root canal therapy?
    (A) Nonodontogenic
    (B) Demoid
    (C) Lymphoepithelial
    (D) Primordial
    (E) Radicular

49. Which of the following human needs categories relates to the presence of plaque and calculus?
    (A) Biologically sound and functional dentition
    (B) Protection from health risks
    (C) Wholesome facial image
    (D) Responsibility for oral health
    (E) Conceptualization and understanding

50. If the temperature is 68 degrees Fahrenheit, the number of minutes the film should stay in the developer is
    (A) 2.5 minutes.
    (B) 3 minutes.
    (C) 4.5 minutes.
    (D) 5 minutes.
    (E) 6.5 minutes.

51. Discrete data can be measured using which pair of scales?
    (A) Nominal and ordinal
    (B) Ratio and interval
    (C) Interval and ordinal
    (D) Nominal and ratio
    (E) Ordinal and interval

52. Which of the following procedures involves the removal of one root on a multirooted tooth with the crown still intact?
    (A) Guided-tissue regeneration
    (B) Root hemisection
    (C) Root resection
    (D) Pedicle soft tissue graft
    (E) Free soft tissue graft

53. A female patient taking oral contraceptives must have a wisdom tooth extracted. The best day of her oral contraceptive cycle to perform this procedure would be day
    (A) 5.
    (B) 10.
    (C) 15.
    (D) 20.
    (E) 25.

54. Which of the following parts of the oral cavity is **NOT** part of the periodontium?
    (A) Gingiva
    (B) Periodontal ligament
    (C) Cementum
    (D) Pulp cavity
    (E) Alveolar bone

55. Photopolymerizing refers to
    (A) curing by oxidation.
    (B) curing on occlusal surfaces.
    (C) self-curing.
    (D) curing by physical light.
    (E) curing by biocompatible substances.

56. Laws tend to emphasize behaviors that benefit an entire society.

    The concept of ethics is related to the overt conduct and behaviors of individuals.
    (A) Both statements are true.
    (B) Both statements are false.
    (C) The first statement is true, the second is false.
    (D) The first statement is false, the second is true.

57. Dentin makes up the majority of the tooth structure.

Dentin forms throughout life.
(A) Both statements are true.
(B) Both statements are false.
(C) The first statement is true, the second is false.
(D) The first statement is false, the second is true.

58. A dental hygienist is educating a patient on how dentifrices can be used to prevent gingivitis. They also discuss the properties of the various substances found in dentifrices. Which of the following substances uses a foaming action to help loosen plaque from the patient's teeth?
(A) Preservatives
(B) Polishing agents
(C) Humectants
(D) Cleaning agents
(E) Detergents

59. The range of vibrations per second for most ultrasonic debridement tools is usually
(A) 1,000–5,000.
(B) 5,000–10,000.
(C) 15,000–25,000.
(D) 20,000–30,000.
(E) 30,000–50,000.

60. During the extraoral examination, the client's thyroid gland can be assessed for asymmetry and enlargement through a combination of
(A) manual palpitation and direct observation.
(B) bilateral palpitation and auscultation.
(C) bimanual and bilateral palpitation.
(D) bidigital palpitation and circular compression.
(E) digital palpitation and olfaction.

61. Each of the following is true about the modified pen grasp **EXCEPT** one. Which one is the **EXCEPTION**?
(A) Three fingers are used in this grasp.
(B) The middle finger is very important and stops the instrument from slipping.
(C) The ring finger guides the instrument from tooth to tooth.
(D) The index finger is used in this grasp as the fulcrum.
(E) The ring finger should be used to balance the hand.

62. Periapical cemento-osseous dysplasia would be **MOST LIKELY** to occur in a patient of which age?
(A) 25
(B) 35
(C) 45
(D) 55
(E) 65

63. Which penetration site should be used to anesthetize the anterior superior alveolar nerve?
(A) Mucobuccal fold distal to the maxillary second and third molars
(B) Mucocuccal fold mesial to the canine eminence
(C) Base of the incisive papillae
(D) Anterior to the greater palatine foramen and distal to the maxillary second molar
(E) Mucobuccal fold near the apex of the maxillary second premolar

Use the following scenario to answer questions 64–67.

Kim, a dental hygiene professional, and a team of other oral health professionals are in the process of planning a community program. The program targets men between the ages of 25 and 36 who are employed in blue-collar professions. Statistics show that these individuals are up to three times more likely to smoke than males who work in other fields. Therefore, Kim and her team want to create a program that will educate these men about the oral health issues associated with smoking. The team hopes this knowledge will encourage these men to quit.

64. The team relied mainly on primary sources when assessing the oral health status of the target population as they planned the program described above. Which of the following did the team **MOST LIKELY** use during their preliminary research?
(A) Data from Oral Health America
(B) Data from a state census
(C) Data from Gallup polls
(D) Data from the American Dental Association
(E) Data from dental indices

65. During the program planning phase, every member of the team created several possible objectives for the community program using the SMART formula. Which of the following objectives **BEST** meets the requirements outlined in the SMART formula?
(A) By the end of the 6-week program, at least 75 percent of program participants will be able to describe five oral health issues associated with smoking.
(B) By the end of the 6-week program, 100 percent of program participants will have stopped smoking for at least three weeks.
(C) A few months after the program, many of the program participants will have successfully quit smoking or attempted to quit.
(D) A year after the program, the individuals who participated will be practicing a healthier lifestyle overall.
(E) By the time the program is well underway, participants will have a good knowledge of many different oral health issues.

66. While designing the program, the team used many strategies to help them achieve their objectives. Kim presented a cartoon in which Cyl Cigar was the villain and a tube of toothpaste and a healthy white tooth were the superheroes. Which principle of teaching did Kim fail to consider when she chose this activity?
(A) The learners' needs must be identified.
(B) The audience level must be considered.
(C) The objectives of activities must be stated.
(D) The learning tasks must be based on objectives.
(E) The lesson must include an evaluation activity.

67. Which of the following would be an effective evaluation method for the community program described above?
(A) Give participants an assignment that asks them to describe the connection between smoking and cancer.
(B) Conduct a study in the local community to determine the percentage of residents who are smokers.
(C) Distribute a survey after the program that asks participants if they are smoking, exercising, and eating right.
(D) Perform oral inspections on all participants to determine which oral health issues are present.
(E) Issue multiple-choice tests after each unit to assess knowledge of smoking-related oral diseases.

68. Patients with which condition often exhibit an unusually low rate of caries and a plaque accumulation with increased calculus deposits?
(A) Muscular dystrophy
(B) Down syndrome
(C) Multiple sclerosis
(D) Myasthenia gravis
(E) Cystic fibrosis

69. An article that appears in a journal published by a professional society would be preferred over one appearing in a journal published by a commercial firm **BECAUSE** the published data should indicate only the most current data related to the subject.
    (A) Both the statement and the reason are correct and related.
    (B) Both the statement and the reason are correct but NOT related.
    (C) The statement is correct, but the reason is NOT.
    (D) The statement is NOT correct, but the reason is correct.
    (E) NEITHER the statement NOR the reason is correct.

70. Which of the following bacteria arrange themselves into clumps or clusters?
    (A) *Streptococcus mutans*
    (B) *Moraxella catarrhalis*
    (C) *Streptococcus pneumoniae*
    (D) *Neisseria gonorrhoeae*
    (E) *Staphylococcus aureus*

71. A microorganism feeding off decaying plant matter is an example of
    (A) syntrophism.
    (B) competition.
    (C) commensalism.
    (D) symbiosis.
    (E) parasitism.

72. Which of the following **BEST** describes why redness occurs at a sight with inflammation?
    (A) Excretion of fluid
    (B) Release of inflammatory mediators
    (C) Increased blood flow
    (D) Stretching of pain receptors and nerves
    (E) Loss of function

73. An individual would **MOST LIKELY** take a diuretic to treat
    (A) hypokalemia.
    (B) hyperglycemia.
    (C) hypertension.
    (D) hypoglycemia.
    (E) hyperuricemia.

74. Which of the following uses geometry to determine the angulation of the X-ray tube head?
    (A) Bisecting technique
    (B) Parallel technique
    (C) Horizontal angulation
    (D) Vertical angulation
    (E) Perpendicular technique

75. Which of the following is true about the cancellous bone?
    (A) It surrounds the root that is lined by the cribriform plate.
    (B) It fills in bone between the cortical bone and alveolar bone.
    (C) It attaches the periodontal ligament.
    (D) It makes up the cortical plates on the facial and lingual aspects of teeth.
    (E) It acts as the thin line of bone surrounding the root of the teeth.

76. Each of the following is a term used to describe unusual heart rates **EXCEPT** one. Which one is the **EXCEPTION**?
    (A) Tachycardia
    (B) Bradycardia
    (C) Dyspnea
    (D) Pulsus alternans
    (E) Premature ventricular contractions

77. Which of the following should be administered if a large amount of fluoride has been ingested?
    (A) Water
    (B) Milk
    (C) Food
    (D) Acetaminophen
    (E) Antacids

78. Acidulated phosphate fluoride should ideally be applied once
    (A) per month.
    (B) every 3 months.
    (C) every 6 months.
    (D) every 9 months.
    (E) per year.

79. One of the core values of the dental hygiene profession is nonmalfeasance. This means that dental hygienists have a professional responsibility to
    (A) support practices that distribute health-care resources equitably.
    (B) be truthful and honest at all times while interacting with others.
    (C) protect clients during treatment and reduce harm when possible.
    (D) keep confidential any client information obtained on the job.
    (E) give patients the information needed to make informed decisions.

80. Which of the following can be caused by a vitamin K deficiency?
    (A) Gastrointestinal disorders
    (B) Respiratory disorders
    (C) Bleeding disorders
    (D) Neurological disorders
    (E) Muscular disorders

81. What do lines or stripes of Retzius indicate?
    (A) Enamel rods
    (B) Enamel pearls
    (C) Gradual change in enamel
    (D) Weakened areas of enamel
    (E) Reduced enamel epithelium

82. An endemic is a disease of a notable greater prevalence than usual that quickly spreads through a demographic segment of the general public.

    A pandemic is an ongoing problem that involves average disease prevalence with a predictable number of cases remaining indigenous to a given population or area.
    (A) Both statements are true.
    (B) Both statements are false.
    (C) The first statement is true, the second is false.
    (D) The first statement is false, the second is true.

83. Which of the following represents the vessel with the greatest pressure?
    (A) Renal vein
    (B) Jugular
    (C) Iliac vein
    (D) Aorta
    (E) Subclavian vein

84. Which muscle depresses the tongue?
    (A) Transverse
    (B) Intrinsic
    (C) Genioglossus
    (D) Styloglossus
    (E) Hyoglossus

85. Glands of the head aid in digestion.

    These glands also strengthen the immune system.
    (A) Both statements are true.
    (B) Both statements are false.
    (C) The first statement is true, the second statement is false.
    (D) The first statement is false, the second statement is true.

86. The frontal sinuses drain through the
    (A) Stensen's duct.
    (B) nasal conchae.
    (C) middle nasal meatus.
    (D) lacrimal ducts.
    (E) sublingual caruncle.

87. Which of the following is **MOST LIKELY** to have abnormalities?
    (A) Maxillary central incisor
    (B) Maxillary lateral incisor
    (C) Mandibular second premolar
    (D) Mandibular first molar
    (E) Mandibular second molar

88. Which of the following conditions is characterized by the presence of an excess number of roots?
    (A) Fused roots
    (B) Enamel pearls
    (C) Hypercementosis
    (D) Dilaceration
    (E) Supernumerary roots

89. The medulla oblongata is part of the peripheral nervous system.

    The medulla oblongata regulates the respiratory system and the circulatory system.
    (A) Both statements are true.
    (B) Both statements are false.
    (C) The first statement is true, the second is false.
    (D) The first statement is false, the second is true.

90. Patients with gout can be treated with a low-protein diet **BECAUSE** high-protein diets create a buildup of potassium in the body.
    (A) Both the statement and the reason are correct and related.
    (B) Both the statement and the reason are correct but NOT related.
    (C) The statement is correct but the reason is NOT.
    (D) The statement is NOT correct, but the reason is correct.
    (E) NEITHER the statement NOR the reason is correct.

91. Which of the following data-collection methods would be most effective for gathering information about the status quo in the population being assessed?
    (A) Personal interview
    (B) Written questionnaire
    (C) Epidemiologic survey
    (D) Direct observation
    (E) Records search

92. Each of the following is a type of noninjectable drug that should be included in a basic emergency kit **EXCEPT** one. Which one is the **EXCEPTION**?
    (A) Nitroglycerin
    (B) Bronchodilator
    (C) Glucose source
    (D) Aspirin
    (E) Diphenhydramine

93. The presence of which of the following affects the outcome of Gram stains?
    (A) Cell wells
    (B) Circular bacteria
    (C) Viruses
    (D) Prokaryotic cells
    (E) Fungi

94. *Cheilitis* is **BEST** described as the swelling of the
    (A) lips.
    (B) tongue.
    (C) muscles.
    (D) gums.
    (E) vessels.

95. Each of the following is an autosomal dominant disorder **EXCEPT** one. Which one is the **EXCEPTION**?
    (A) Rett syndrome
    (B) Marfan syndrome
    (C) Polycystic kidney disease
    (D) Ehlers-Danlos syndrome
    (E) Huntington disease

96. A female patient was recently diagnosed with mild periodontitis, and a dental hygiene professional is educating the patient on how the condition will be managed. The course of treatment he is presenting is based on the American Academy of General Dentistry's guidelines for treating adult periodontal disease. Which strategy will be used first during the management of this disease?
    (A) Writing a prescription for antibiotics
    (B) Scaling and root planing affected areas
    (C) Performing a full-mouth debridement
    (D) Completing an occlusal equilibration
    (E) Taking bacterial cultures from the gums

97. A type of graph that is used to depict interval- or ratio-scaled variables that are continuous in nature is called a
    (A) frequency polygon.
    (B) histogram.
    (C) bar graph.
    (D) scatter plot.
    (E) pie graph.

98. Couples who are predisposed to genetic disorders should be referred to genetic counseling **BECAUSE** genetic counseling involves determining genetic risks in future offspring.
    (A) Both the statement and reason are correct and related.
    (B) Both the statement and reason are correct but NOT related.
    (C) The statement is correct, but the reason is NOT.
    (D) The statement is NOT correct, but the reason is correct.
    (E) NEITHER the statement NOR the reason is correct.

99. Which of the following dental defects is a type of fusion that takes place after root formation has been completed?
(A) Dens evaginatus
(B) Gemination
(C) Dilaceration
(D) Concrescence
(E) Dens in dente

Use the following scenario to answer questions 100–103.

A 37-year-old male patient complains of swollen gums. His medical history indicates that he was recently diagnosed with hypertension, for which he takes a calcium channel blocker. During the periodontal exam, the dental hygienist notes that the gingiva appear pink and stippled and records a PSR score of 0. The patient's PI and CI-S scores are also 0. The hygienist notes that minor gingival hyperplasia is present.

100. The patient's complaint of swollen gums, or gingival hyperplasia, is **MOST LIKELY** caused by
(A) advanced periodontal disease.
(B) inadequate oral hygiene.
(C) occlusal trauma.
(D) medication.
(E) class IV furcation involvement.

101. The patient's PSR score suggests that during the periodontal screening, the dental hygienist discovered
(A) plaque, but no calculus.
(B) plaque and calculus.
(C) supragingival calculus.
(D) subgingival calculus.
(E) no plaque or calculus.

102. What do the patient's PI and CI-S scores indicate?
(A) The patient has excellent home care.
(B) The patient has slight tooth mobility.
(C) The patient has an overbite.
(D) The patient shows signs of fremitus.
(E) The patient shows evidence of an occlusal trauma.

103. Which of the following would be considered an elevated heart rate for this patient?
(A) 65
(B) 73
(C) 94
(D) 100
(E) 108

104. Each of the following observations is made during the head and neck examination **EXCEPT** one. Which one is the **EXCEPTION**?
(A) Check for skin discoloration.
(B) Assess symmetry of head, face, and nose.
(C) Check pupil size.
(D) Observe the patient swallowing.
(E) Examine hard and soft palate.

105. Each of the following is one of the eight human needs related to oral health and disease **EXCEPT** one. Which one is the **EXCEPTION**?
(A) Wholesome facial image
(B) Freedom from respiratory difficulties
(C) Biologically sound and functional dentition
(D) Protection from health risks
(E) Skin and mucus membrane integrity of head and neck

106. In a darkroom, the safelight bulb in the room should be 20 watts or less.

The safelight should be at least 2 feet from the film.
(A) Both statements are true.
(B) Both statements are false.
(C) The first statement is true, the second is false.
(D) The first statement is false, the second is true.

107. Patients with Parkinson's disease may encounter problems with dental prosthesis retention **BECAUSE** of reduced oral motor functions and personal hygiene skills.
    (A) Both the statement and the reason are correct and related.
    (B) Both the statement and the reason are correct, but NOT related.
    (C) The statement is correct, but the reason is NOT.
    (D) The statement is NOT correct, but the reason is correct.
    (E) NEITHER the statement NOR the reason is correct.

108. The maxillary anterior teeth will be obscured when the
    (A) chin is tilted downward.
    (B) chin is tilted upward.
    (C) chin is positioned farther from the focal trough.
    (D) midline is positioned closer to the film assembly.
    (E) midline is not centered.

109. A dental hygiene professional is educating a patient on using fluoride for the prevention of dental caries and discussing the options offered by the dental practice. When educating the patient about neutral sodium fluoride, the dental hygiene professional will **MOST LIKELY** mention which of the following?
    (A) Neutral fluoride is not recommended for people undergoing chemo.
    (B) Neutral fluoride is unsuitable for people who have xerostomia.
    (C) Neutral fluoride is safe to use on porcelain veneers.
    (D) Neutral fluoride is available in a two-part rinse.
    (E) Neutral fluoride can cause gingival sloughing.

110. The greater the dispersion of the scores around the median of the distribution, the greater the standard deviation and variance will be.

    A small standard deviation is an indication that the distribution of scores is clustered around the mean.
    (A) Both statements are true.
    (B) Both statements are false.

(C) The first statement is true, the second is false.
(D) The first statement is false, the second is true.

111. A dental hygiene professional noticed that a patient had a large amount of debris in between the teeth during his last check-up and cleaning. The dental hygienist is planning to educate the patient about proper flossing technique to address this issue. Which of the following instructions will the hygienist **MOST LIKELY** give to the patient during the educational session?
    (A) Do not push floss into the embrasure.
    (B) Use waxed floss made of braided nylon.
    (C) Wrap floss around the tooth surface so it looks like a "C."
    (D) Use a side-to-side motion to clean inter-proximal surfaces.
    (E) Apply firm pressure when sliding floss below the gingival margin.

112. Accumulated radiation accelerates the
    (A) aging process.
    (B) spread of disease.
    (C) damage to DNA.
    (D) rate of mitosis.
    (E) amount of free radicals.

113. A dental hygiene professional is providing a client with general suggestions about strategies that can help prevent dental caries. Which of the following will **MOST LIKELY** be one of the suggestions presented to the client?
    (A) Chew gum sweetened with xylitol.
    (B) Suck on a hard candy after a meal.
    (C) Apply more pressure when brushing.
    (D) Use a tooth whitening gel at home.
    (E) Try to increase carbohydrate intake.

114. Which of the following are scavenger cells that perform phagocytosis to ingest or engulf microbes?
    (A) Neutrophils
    (B) Cementocytes
    (C) Polymorphonuclear leukocytes hoagie
    (D) Macrophages
    (E) Lymphocytes

115. Each of the following is true about ultrasonic debridement tools **EXCEPT** one. Which one is the **EXCEPTION**?

(A) They are effective in a static position.
(B) Their tip is usually 0.75–1.0 mm wide.
(C) They can clean deep periodontal pockets.
(D) Their tips do not require a cutting edge.
(E) They do not require a specific tooth-to-tool angle.

116. Which of the following is the **BEST** description of the Trendelenburg position?

(A) A patient sits in a chair bent at the waist with his head between his knees.
(B) A patient lies on his left side with his feet elevated above his head.
(C) A patient lies on his right side with his feet elevated above his head.
(D) A patient lies on his back with his feet elevated above his head.
(E) A patient sits in a chair with his arms raised above his head.

117. Acidulated phosphate fluoride (APF) gels work by

(A) forming fluoride salts on tooth surface.
(B) providing tong-term fluoride distribution.
(C) strengthening tooth enamel.
(D) distributing fluoride to molars.
(E) producing fluoride-generating substances.

118. Amalgam dental filling is a mixture of metal powders triturated with mercury.

The amount of mercury vapor produced by amalgam filling does not present a health risk to any patients.

(A) Both statements are true.
(B) Both statements are false.
(C) The first statement is true, the second is false.
(D) The first statement is false, the second is true.

119. Ultrasonic cleaning is the preferred method of removing stains from dental implants **BECAUSE** it prevents any scratching of the implant's surface.

(A) Both the statement and reason are correct and related.
(B) Both the statement and reason are correct but NOT related.

(C) The statement is correct, but the reason is NOT.
(D) The statement is NOT correct, but the reason is correct.
(E) NEITHER the statement NOR the reason is correct.

120. A dental hygienist is counseling a patient about a wisdom tooth extraction that will require the use of a general anesthetic. Because the hygienist doesn't want the patient to be apprehensive, he states that there are no significant risks associated with general anesthesia. The hygienist is

(A) not recognizing the principle of justice.
(B) acting ethically given the circumstances.
(C) violating the moral principle of veracity.
(D) complying with the statutes of most states.
(E) failing to obey the Oath of Hippocrates.

121. If the density of a radiographic film is 1.5 with an mA of 18, and the impulses are 8 at a kVp of 75, how many impulses are required for radiograph with the same density with an mA of 12 and a kVp of 75?

(A) 18
(B) 20
(C) 24
(D) 30
(E) 32

122. A dental hygienist should speak quite loudly when interacting with patients on a one-on-one basis **BECAUSE** it facilitates understanding.

(A) Both the statement and reason are correct and related.
(B) Both the statement and reason are correct but NOT related.
(C) The statement is correct, but the reason is NOT.
(D) The statement is NOT correct, but the reason is correct.
(E) NEITHER the statement NOR the reason is correct.

123. Which type of hepatitis commonly occurs in children and is most often transmitted through contaminated water or food?

(A) Hepatitis A
(B) Hepatitis B
(C) Hepatitis C
(D) Hepatitis D
(E) Hepatitis E

124. When working with patients, dental hygiene professionals may need to employ or educate patients about primary, secondary, and tertiary strategies to prevent or treat oral disease. An example of a primary dental hygiene strategy is
    (A) running oral cancer screenings.
    (B) applying dental sealants.
    (C) performing self-examinations.
    (D) filling a carious lesion.
    (E) completing crown lengthening.

125. When researchers examine a disease based on the number of new cases of the disease that occur within a particular population over a certain period of time, they are studying the disease in terms of its
    (A) count.
    (B) prevalence.
    (C) rate.
    (D) proportion.
    (E) incidence.

126. The epithelial proliferations give rise to the
    (A) lymph nodes.
    (B) dental enamel.
    (C) salivary glands.
    (D) smooth muscles.
    (E) muscles of mastication.

127. A patient at a dental office has cracked lips and an increase in bone density, or bone hypertrophy. Based on these symptoms, the patient **MOST LIKELY** has an excess of
    (A) vitamin A.
    (B) vitamin C.
    (C) vitamin E.
    (D) vitamin H.
    (E) vitamin K.

128. A patient is suffering from a degenerative gum disease that will **MOST LIKELY** cause tooth loss if left untreated. A dental hygienist is discussing a possible treatment with the patient. Each of the following is a piece of information the dental hygienist must provide to obtain informed consent **EXCEPT** one. Which one is the **EXCEPTION**?
    (A) The specific dental diagnosis
    (B) Information on similar conditions
    (C) The chances of treatment success
    (D) Outcome if treatment is refused
    (E) A clearly worded consent form

129. When working with hemihydrates as a replication material, how much water should be added to produce the highest strength stone?
    (A) 37–50 mL/100 g powder
    (B) 31–36 mL/100 g powder
    (C) 28–32 mL/100 g powder
    (D) 25–28 mL/100 g powder
    (E) 19–24 mL/100 g powder

130. A 4-year-old child has white streaks on one of her central incisors. This is **MOST LIKELY** caused by
    (A) too much fluoride.
    (B) not enough fluoride.
    (C) early exposure to fluoride.
    (D) late exposure to fluoride.
    (E) ineffective brushing.

131. The first periodontal ligaments to be lost in periodontal disease are alveolar crest fibers.

    Interradicular fibers are found on only multirooted teeth.
    (A) Both statements are true.
    (B) Both statements are false.
    (C) The first statement is true, but the second statement is false.
    (D) The first statement is false, but the second statement is true.

132. If the source-to-film distance becomes closer, the central ray widens or becomes larger **BECAUSE** an increase in exposure time is needed to create a clearer image.
    (A) Both the statement and the reason are correct and related.
    (B) Both the statement and the reason are correct but NOT related.
    (C) The statement is correct, but the reason is NOT.
    (D) The statement is NOT correct, but the reason is correct.
    (E) Neither the statement NOR the reason is correct.

133. Each of the following conditions might be treated with anticoagulants **EXCEPT** one. Which one is the **EXCEPTION**?
    (A) Von Willebrand disease
    (B) Myocardial infarction
    (C) Thrombophlebitis
    (D) Atrial fibrillation
    (E) Embolism

134. Which of the following **BEST** describes why chronic inflammatory diseases often lead to fibrosis?
(A) The diseases cause persistent tissue damage.
(B) The body suffers only superficial wounds.
(C) The diseases keep tissue framework intact.
(D) The body regenerates its normal structure.
(E) The diseases cause acute injuries.

135. Each of the following is a factor that predisposes a patient to infective endocarditis **EXCEPT** one. Which one is the **EXCEPTION**?
(A) Scarring on heart valves
(B) Clogged arteries
(C) Heart-valve surgery
(D) Drug abuse
(E) Arrhythmia

Use the following scenario to answer questions 136–139.

Brent is a dental hygiene professional who conducts most of the individualized patient education for the busy dental practice where he works. During the upcoming week, he is scheduled to meet with Candy, a young woman who recently got a tongue piercing and wants to find out about any associated dental concerns associated with the piercing. He also has an educational session scheduled with a man who recently received dental implants to replace some missing teeth. Finally, he will educate a mother about the benefits of sealants for her young children.

136. During his session with Candy, Bruce wants to emphasize the risk of infection associated with tongue piercings. Which of the following conditions should he plan to cover during his individualized education session with this patient?
(A) Periodontitis
(B) Ludwig angina
(C) Herpes simplex
(D) Gingivitis
(E) Vincent's angina

137. Bruce is planning to educate the man about at-home care for dental implants. Specifically, he wants to educate the patient about open embrasure areas. Which of the following should Bruce recommend to help the man care for any open embrasure areas?
(A) A rotary toothbrush
(B) Use of the Bass method
(C) Yarn or tufted floss
(D) Use of floss threaders
(E) An interdental brush

138. Bruce conducted an individualized education session with the man before he received his dental implants. The man wanted to know how dental implants would change the nature of his dental visits. Based on this request, which point did Bruce likely include in the list of information he planned to cover when he was preparing for the session?
(A) Steel instruments will be used to remove calculus.
(B) Radiographs will be done every two years.

(C) Oral irrigation will no longer be practiced.
(D) Ultrasonic cleaning is not recommended.
(E) Stain removal with air polishers is not possible.

139. Brent should plan to tell the mother that sealants are only necessary for children who do not receive fluoride treatments.

Brent should plan to tell the mother that sealants can seal pits found in occlusal surfaces.
(A) Both statements are true.
(B) Both statements are false.
(C) The first statement is true, the second is false.
(D) The first statement is false, the second is true.

140. Which of the following is a tooth abnormality that is specifically caused by the grinding of teeth?
(A) Bruxism
(B) Abrasion
(C) Erosion
(D) Attrition
(E) Occlusion

141. The amount of pressure needed for periodontal probing of the gingival sulcus is
(A) 10–20 grams of pressure.
(B) 20–30 grams of pressure.
(C) 30–40 grams of pressure.
(D) 40–50 grams of pressure.
(E) 50–60 grams of pressure.

142. When recording periodontal assessment factors, a blue X drawn over a tooth would indicate a(an)
    (A) missing tooth.
    (B) exudate.
    (C) frenum pull.
    (D) blunted papilla.
    (E) furcation involvement.

143. Which of the following is wear caused by chemical wear?
    (A) Erosion
    (B) Abrasion
    (C) Attrition
    (D) Anodontia
    (E) Taurodontism

144. Maintaining confidentiality is one of the ethical principles of the dental hygiene profession. Each of the following is a situation when this principle does not apply **EXCEPT** one. Which one is the **EXCEPTION**?
    (A) A patient is being abused.
    (B) A patient has tuberculosis.
    (C) A patient has an infected wound.
    (D) A patient is a type 2 diabetic.
    (E) A patient has a stab wound.

145. After a procedure, a dental hygiene professional plans to clean clinical contact surfaces such as door handles and countertops to help with the dental practice's overall infection-control efforts. The dental hygiene professional can use a low-level disinfectant for this task if it
    (A) can destroy vegetative bacteria.
    (B) is capable of killing HIV.
    (C) can kill tuberculosis bacteria.
    (D) is able to kill some fungi.
    (E) can destroy bacterial spores.

146. If a sealant fails, it is **MOST LIKELY** from
    (A) operator error.
    (B) patient movement.
    (C) chemical malfunction.
    (D) adhesive failure.
    (E) polymerization error.

147. The gingiva adjoins the oral mucosa at the
    (A) mucogingival junction.
    (B) periodontal ligament.
    (C) gingival sulcus.
    (D) papillae.
    (E) alveolar bone.

148. A pregnant patient is receiving dental care. Which of the following dental drugs is generally considered safe for pregnant women?
    (A) Metronidazole
    (B) Nitrous oxide
    (C) NSAIDs
    (D) Aspirin
    (E) Amoxicillin

149. Which of the following is the most common tissue used to replace diseased gingival tissue during a free soft-tissue graft?
    (A) Tongue tissue
    (B) Palate
    (C) Tissue of the upper lip
    (D) Uvula
    (E) Tissue of the lower lip

150. Each of the follow is a radiopaque landmark **EXCEPT** one. Which one is the **EXCEPTION**?
    (A) Genial tubercles
    (B) Maxillary sinus
    (C) Mandibular tori
    (D) Nasal septum
    (E) Maxillary tuberosity

151. A positive response to which of the following health history screening questions may indicate a current or past history of tuberculosis?
    (A) Do you have night sweats?
    (B) Are you frequently thirsty?
    (C) Do you bruise easily?
    (D) Have you ever had a blood transfusion?
    (E) Do you have to urinate more than six times a day?

152. A patient presenting with angular cheilitis, pallor or atrophy of the oral tissues, and a sore tongue would **MOST LIKELY** be diagnosed with
    (A) aplastic anemia.
    (B) thalassemia.
    (C) iron-deficiency anemia.
    (D) polycythemia.
    (E) pernicious anemia.

153. Which of the following endocrine glands is the first to form?
    (A) Pineal
    (B) Thymus
    (C) Thyroid
    (D) Adrenal
    (E) Pituitary

154. Which of the following **BEST** describes how anthracycline chemotherapeutic agents work?
   (A) They prevent cell division and slow tumor growth.
   (B) They form free radicals that inhibit DNA production.
   (C) They impact the cell cycle to impair DNA transcription.
   (D) They make tumors more recognizable to the immune system.
   (E) They inhibit the assembly of microtubules in cells.

155. Each of the following is a part of the digestive system **EXCEPT** one. Which one is the **EXCEPTION**?
   (A) Spleen
   (B) Pancreas
   (C) Rectum
   (D) Small intestine
   (E) Large intestine

156. Each of the following should be included on an informed refusal form **EXCEPT** one. Which one is the **EXCEPTION**?
   (A) A list of risks associated with non-treatment
   (B) An outline of the dental hygiene plan of treatment
   (C) The signatures of the client, dentist, and witness
   (D) A client statement explaining refusal of service
   (E) A list of refused procedures

157. A dental hygienist is speaking to an elementary class about the importance of flossing. The hygienist presents several charts showing the benefits of flossing and also shares some stories of what might happen in the future if students do not floss on a regular basis. If the principles of teleological ethics are applied, which of the following would be used to decide whether the actions of the hygienist were right or wrong?
   (A) The relationship between the hygienist and students
   (B) The students' emotional reactions to the stories
   (C) The characteristics of the individual students
   (D) The reasons why the hygienist told the stories
   (E) The number of students who started flossing

158. It is necessary to take an initial impression using a rocking motion when using which of the following impression materials?
   (A) Polysulfide
   (B) Alginate hydrocolloid
   (C) Zinc oxide and eugenol
   (D) Polyether
   (E) Silicone

159. While conducting individualized patient education, it is crucial for dental hygiene professionals to make all clients aware of
   (A) the link between oral health and mental health.
   (B) the connection between periodontal disease and diabetes.
   (C) the link between smoking and various oral cancers.
   (D) the connection between oral health and birth weight.
   (E) the link between oral health and general health.

160. In most cases, a small sample size is preferable to a large one **BECAUSE** it reduces the standard error of the sample mean.
   (A) Both the statement and the reason are correct and related.
   (B) Both the statement and the reason are correct but NOT related.
   (C) The statement is correct, but the reason is NOT.
   (D) The statement is NOT correct, but the reason is correct.
   (E) NEITHER the statement NOR the reason is correct.

161. Each of the following is a compound approved by the ADA as an anti-gingivitis agent **EXCEPT** one. Which one is the **EXCEPTION**?
   (A) Chlorhexidine gluconate
   (B) Listerine®
   (C) Phenolic compounds
   (D) Triclosan
   (E) Stannous fluoride

162. An autograft is a type of bone graft taken from the patient.

    An alloplast is a type of bone graft taken from another animal species.
    (A) Both statements are true.
    (B) Both statements are false.
    (C) The first statement is true, but the second statement is false.
    (D) The first statement is false, but the second statement is true.

163. For a dental health professional's education to be effective in terms of changing behavior, the patient must hold several beliefs. Each of the following makes it more likely that a client will accept a hygienist's health recommendations **EXCEPT** one. Which one is the **EXCEPTION**?
    (A) The patient must believe that a condition can be cured easily.
    (B) The patient must believe she is at risk of developing a condition.
    (C) The patient must believe a given condition will have marked adverse effects.
    (D) The patient must believe she could have a condition without showing symptoms.
    (E) The patient must believe a behavior change is capable of yielding positive results.

164. Sealants are a thin coating placed in the pits and grooves of teeth to act as a(n)
    (A) adhesive bond.
    (B) oxygen-inhibited layer.
    (C) enamel protector.
    (D) polymerizing filler.
    (E) physical barrier.

165. A patient in a dental office suffers from erosion of tooth enamel, xerostomia, and goose bumps. What is the **MOST LIKELY** diagnosis?
    (A) Vitamin toxicity
    (B) HIV or AIDS
    (C) Scurvy
    (D) Eating disorder
    (E) Dehydration

166. A dental hygienist who is sitting in a chair and wants to show a patient she is paying attention to what is being said should lean forward.

    Leaning backward in a chair puts a barrier between the dental hygienist and the patient.
    (A) Both statements are true.
    (B) Both statements are false.
    (C) The first statement is true, the second is false.
    (D) The first statement is false, the second is true.

167. A study that follows a selected group of participants over an extended period of time to identify some change or development within the group is referred to as
    (A) longitudinal.
    (B) prospective.
    (C) cross-sectional.
    (D) retrospective.
    (E) cohort.

168. Which of the following was the first city in the United States to fortify its public drinking water with fluoride in 1945?
    (A) Green Bay, Wisconsin
    (B) Grand Junction, Iowa
    (C) Grand Rapids, Michigan
    (D) Grove City, Ohio
    (E) Grandview, Missouri

169. When viewing a radiograph, which part of the anatomy is often mistaken for a periapical pathological condition?
    (A) Genial tubercles
    (B) Mental foramen
    (C) Submandibular fossa
    (D) Lateral pterygoid plate
    (E) Nasal fossae

170. A dental hygienist should use proper, technical terms when communicating with patients **BECAUSE** it will make them feel more confident in the abilities of the dental hygiene professional.
    (A) Both the statement and reason are correct and related.
    (B) Both the statement and reason are correct but NOT related.
    (C) The statement is correct, but the reason is NOT.
    (D) The statement is NOT correct, but the reason is correct.
    (E) NEITHER the statement NOR the reason is correct.

171. Clients who have undergone corrective surgery for cardiac or vascular disorders are susceptible to transient bacteremias.

    These clients must be given prophylactic antibiotic premedication for up to 9 months after surgery.
    (A) Both statements are true.
    (B) Both statements are false.
    (C) The first statement is true, the second is false.
    (D) The first statement is false, the second is true.

172. When providing health advice, a dental hygiene professional should use an authoritarian approach **BECAUSE** it is more effective than strategies that invite a client's participation.
    (A) Both the statement and reason are correct and related.
    (B) Both the statement and reason are correct but NOT related.
    (C) The statement is correct, but the reason is NOT.
    (D) The statement is NOT correct, but the reason is correct.
    (E) NEITHER the statement NOR the reason is correct.

173. Each of the following is a bone that articulates at an immovable joint called a suture **EXCEPT** one. Which one is the **EXCEPTION**?
    (A) Mandible
    (B) Maxilla
    (C) Condyle
    (D) Parietal bone
    (E) Sphenoid bone

174. A dental hygiene professional is shopping online for a new chair for clients that will help reduce the spread of infection. Each of the following is a characteristic the dental hygiene professional should look for in a chair that will help reduce the spread of infection **EXCEPT** one. Which one is the **EXCEPTION**?
    (A) The chair has few or no buttons.
    (B) The chair has a minimal number of seams.
    (C) The chair has a firm stuffing and feel.
    (D) The chair is upholstered with vinyl.
    (E) The chair is controlled with a foot pedal.

175. A dental practice is treating a patient who has diabetes. Which of the following should be administered to this patient with caution?
    (A) Thiazolidinediones
    (B) NSAIDs
    (C) Acetaminophen
    (D) Epinephrine
    (E) Biguanides

176. Administering a vasoconstrictor to a patient who is currently taking antidepressants may lead to
    (A) hypertensive crisis.
    (B) elevated blood pressure.
    (C) arrhythmia.
    (D) elevated heart rate.
    (E) hypotension.

177. Each of the following is a component that should be included in an instructional objective **EXCEPT** one. Which one is the **EXCEPTION**?
    (A) Criterion
    (B) Performance
    (C) Method
    (D) Conditions
    (E) Time

178. A rad is a unit of measurement of
    (A) absorbed radiation.
    (B) dose equivalents.
    (C) the cause of biological effects.
    (D) the energy absorbed per unit mass of tissue.
    (E) the psychological effects of medication.

179. Fibrous dysplasia is swelling of the bone that may result in physical deformities.

    Orally, fibrous dysplasia affects the maxilla more frequently than the mandible.
    (A) Both statements are true.
    (B) Both statements are false.
    (C) The first statement is true, the second is false.
    (D) The first statement is false, the second is true.

180. When performing an occlusal evaluation, you should be careful to note any wear-patterns, including tooth-to-tooth wear, which is known as
    (A) abrasion.
    (B) erosion.
    (C) attrition.
    (D) furcation.
    (E) abfraction.

181. What structure is responsible for removing waste from the blood?
    (A) Kidneys
    (B) Liver
    (C) Ureters
    (D) Nephrons
    (E) Bladder

182. An example of a high-potency antipsychotic is Thorazine.

    Dyskinesia, a side effect associated with antipsychotic use, is a dental concern.
    (A) Both statements are true.
    (B) Both statements are false.
    (C) The first statement is true, the second is false.
    (D) The first statement is false, the second is true.

183. Each of the following is a symptom of toxic shock syndrome **EXCEPT** one. Which one is the **EXCEPTION**?
    (A) Fever
    (B) Convulsion
    (C) Vomiting
    (D) Rash
    (E) Diarrhea

184. Each of the following is something a dental hygienist would make use of during a type 2 assessment examination **EXCEPT** one. Which one is the **EXCEPTION**?
    (A) Percussion
    (B) An explorer
    (C) Supplemental illumination
    (D) Radiography
    (E) A mouth mirror

185. A well-written article must always include both current and classic references.

    Such an article must also be based on an adequate and clearly stated hypothesis.
    (A) Both statements are true.
    (B) Both statements are false.
    (C) The first statement is true, the second is false.
    (D) The first statement is false, the second is true.

186. Oxygen may not flow easily to the brain **BECAUSE** bad news, unpleasant smells, or the sight of medical apparatuses can all cause stress.
    (A) Both the statement and reason are correct and related.
    (B) Both the statement and reason are correct but NOT related.
    (C) The statement is correct, but the reason is NOT.
    (D) The statement is NOT correct, but the reason is correct.
    (E) NEITHER the statement NOR the reason is correct.

187. Masks are a vital part of infection control in the practice of dental hygiene. Each of the following is a guideline for mask use that will maximize their effectiveness as an infection-control strategy **EXCEPT** one. Which one is the **EXCEPTION**?
    (A) The mask should be handled by the portion covering the face when removed.
    (B) The mask should be changed any time the hygienist notices that it is moist.
    (C) The mask should be swapped out for a new one before each new client arrives.
    (D) The mask should be positioned so that it fits snugly against the hygienist's face.
    (E) The mask should be disposed of properly and not left hanging around the neck.

188. The deductive reasoning approach to diagnosis yields specific information about the patient's oral condition based on generalizations regarding oral health.

    The inductive reasoning approach to diagnosis yields specific information about the patient's oral condition based on potential patterns identified through oral observations.
    (A) Both statements are true.
    (B) Both statements are false.
    (C) The first statement is true, but the second is false.
    (D) The first statement is false, but the second is true.

189. Antineoplastic agents only destroy malignant cells **BECAUSE** they affect cells with the slowest life cycles first.
    (A) Both the statement and reason are correct and related.
    (B) Both the statement and reason are correct but NOT related.
    (C) The statement is correct, but the reason is NOT.
    (D) The statement is NOT correct, but the reason is correct.
    (E) NEITHER the statement NOR the reason is correct.

190. Which of the following bacteria are responsible for causing syphilis?
    (A) *Treponemapallidum*
    (B) *Streptococcus pyogenes*
    (C) *Neisseria gonorrhoeae*
    (D) *Staphylococcus aureus*
    (E) *Trypanosomabrucei*

191. An inadequate amount of attached gingiva should be indicated on a periodontal assessment when the measurement of attached gingiva is equal to or less than
    (A) 0.5 mm.
    (B) 1 mm.
    (C) 1.5 mm.
    (D) 2 mm.
    (E) 2.5 mm.

192. A dental hygiene professional discussing halitosis prevention should instruct clients to concentrate on the front portion of the tongue when using a scraper.

    A dental hygiene professional discussing the prevention of halitosis should cover the benefits of interdental brushes.
    (A) Both statements are true.
    (B) Both statements are false.
    (C) The first statement is true, the second is false.
    (D) The first statement is false, the second is true.

193. Which inferential statistical technique is used to determine if a statistically significant difference exists between two related samples?
    (A) Variance analysis
    (B) Chi-square test
    (C) Paired t-test
    (D) Discriminant analysis
    (E) Student's t-test

194. Each of the following is true of the Bergonie-Tribondeau law of radiosensitivity **EXCEPT** one. Which one is the **EXCEPTION**?
    (A) The more mature the cell, the more resistant it is to radiation.
    (B) The younger the tissues and organs, the greater its radiosensitivity.
    (C) The higher the metabolic activity of the cell, the higher its radiosensitivity.
    (D) The higher the proliferation rate of the cell, the higher its radiosensitivity.
    (E) The more specialized in function the cell, the less resistant it is to the effects of radiation.

195. Affective treatment plan goals should be focused on altering the client's attitudes, beliefs, and values regarding his or her oral health.

    Cognitive treatment plan goals should be focused on the development of the client's deficient oral skill sets.
    (A) Both statements are true.
    (B) Both statements are false.
    (C) The first statement is true, but the second is false.
    (D) The first statement is false, but the second is true.

196. Each of the following conditions can be treated with nitrous oxide **EXCEPT** one. Which one is the **EXCEPTION**?
(A) Hypertension
(B) Cardiovascular disease
(C) Mental retardation
(D) Cerebral palsy
(E) Multiple sclerosis

197. Which of the following monosaccharides link to form the disaccharide sucrose?
(A) Galactose and dextrose
(B) Glucose and dextrose
(C) Dextrose and fructose
(D) Glucose and fructose
(E) Galactose and glucose

198. A dental hygiene professional is handling instruments that were just used to complete a filling. The dental hygienist knows they are contaminated with blood and saliva. To stop the spread of infection, which of the following types of gloves should the hygienist wear while cleaning the instruments?
(A) Ambidextrous gloves
(B) Sterile gloves
(C) Overgloves
(D) Utility gloves
(E) Nonsterile gloves

199. What is a problem associated with detecting occlusal caries radiographically?
(A) It is difficult to maneuver the X-ray machine into the proper position.
(B) It is difficult to detect the radiolucent shadows under the enamel.
(C) It is difficult to position the patient's chin upward to get the proper angle.
(D) They are only able to be seen once they have become very large.
(E) They are located on the biting surfaces of posterior teeth and are difficult to film.

200. Fluoride can prevent and even reverse tooth decay by advancing remineralization **BECAUSE** fluorides are present naturally in water and soil.
(A) Both the statement and the reason are correct and related.
(B) Both the statement and the reason are correct but NOT related.
(C) The statement is correct, but the reason is NOT.
(D) The statement is NOT correct, but the reason is correct.
(E) Neither the statement NOR the reason is correct.

COMPONENT B

Directions: Study the case components and answer questions 1–10.

SYNOPSIS OF PATIENT HISTORY

CASE *PT2-1*

Age __15__

Sex __Male__

Height __5'4"__

Weight __125__ lbs

__56.70__kgs

Vital Signs

Blood pressure __115/70__

Pulse rate __74__

Respiration rate __18__

---

1. Under Care of Physician
   Yes ☑ No ☐

   Condition: _____

2. Hospitalized within the last 5 years
   Yes ☐ No ☑

   Reason: _____
   _____

3. Has or had the following conditions:

   Attention deficit hyperactivity disorder (ADHD)
   _____

4. Current medications:

   Adderall
   _____
   _____

5. Smokes or uses tobacco products
   Yes ☑ No ☐

6. Is pregnant
   Yes ☐ No ☐ N/A ☑

MEDICAL HISTORY:
The patient was diagnosed with ADHD when he was 6 years old. He started taking Adderall a few months ago, but has lost weight and had trouble sleeping since doing so. He drinks about 4 to 5 cups of coffee per day with sugar, which he says helps him concentrate. He also says he has started smoking because this also calms him and helps him concentrate. His mother does not know about his smoking. He says that he smokes one or two cigarettes per day on school days.

DENTAL HISTORY:
The patient has a history of good, regular care. During his last visit, he had 4 dental caries. He now has 6.

SOCIAL HISTORY:
The patient is a good student who, despite being fidgety and restless, does well in school. His parents are divorced, and he lives with his mother and sister. He says he has several good friends in school and is happy most of the time.

CHIEF COMPLAINT:
Checkup and cleaning.

CLINICAL EXAMINATION

Case PT2-1

KEY

Clinically visible carious lesion

Clinically missing tooth

Furcation

"Through and through" furcation

Probe 1: initial probing depth

Probe 2: probing depth 1 month after scaling and root planing

SUPPLEMENTAL ORAL EXAMINATION FINDINGS

1. Current Oral Hygiene Status: Fair/Poor.
2. Moderate calculus deposits generally.
3. Visible dental decay.
4. Mild staining and discoloration.

1. This patient's dental appointments should be scheduled at what time of day?
   (A) Early morning
   (B) Early afternoon
   (C) Late afternoon
   (D) Early evening

2. You should expect all of the following behaviors from this patient **EXCEPT** one. Which one is the **EXCEPTION**?
   (A) Extreme nervousness
   (B) Restlessness
   (C) Frequently wanting to get up
   (D) Excessive talking

3. Which of the following **MOST LIKELY** contributed to this patient's increase in dental caries?
   (A) Drinking coffee
   (B) Poor oral hygiene
   (C) Medication
   (D) Both (A) and (B)

4. Which of the following is a side effect of your patient's medication?
   (A) Bruxism
   (B) Dysgeusia
   (C) Xerostomia
   (D) All of the above

5. You should do all of the following when treating a patient with ADHD **EXCEPT** one. Which one is the **EXCEPTION**?
   (A) Tell the patient what is expected of him during the visit.
   (B) Introduce new procedures using a "tell-show-do" approach.
   (C) Give the patient difficult instructions in writing.
   (D) Give the patient breaks as needed.

6. Which of the following is most important in improving this patient's overall health?
   (A) Quitting smoking
   (B) Limiting coffee
   (C) Brushing more frequently
   (D) Visiting the dentist regularly

7. This patient has a carious lesion on which of the following teeth?
   (A) #1
   (B) #5
   (C) #21
   (D) #28

8. This patient is missing which of the following teeth?
   (A) #5
   (B) #16
   (C) #18
   (D) #29

9. Which of the following is true of this patient's blood pressure?
   (A) The diastolic pressure is higher than normal.
   (B) The systolic pressure is lower than normal.
   (C) Both the systolic and diastolic pressure are higher than normal.
   (D) Both the systolic and diastolic pressure are normal for his age.

10. The stains on this patient's teeth are **MOST LIKELY** from which of the following?
    (A) Smoking
    (B) Taking medication
    (C) Drinking coffee
    (D) None of the above

Directions: Study the case components and answer questions 11–20.

SYNOPSIS OF PATIENT HISTORY

CASE *PT2-2*

Age ___25___

Sex *Male*

Height *5'8"*

Weight *160* lbs

72.57 kgs

Vital Signs

Blood pressure ___*120/78*___

Pulse rate ___*74*___

Respiration rate ___*18*___

1. Under Care of Physician
   Yes ☑ No ☐

   Condition: _____

2. Hospitalized within the last 5 years
   Yes ☐ No ☑

   Reason: _____
   _____

3. Has or had the following conditions:

   Patient is under care of a physician
   for stress and anxiety.

4. Current medications:

   Zoloft
   _____
   _____

5. Smokes or uses tobacco products
   Yes ☑ No ☐

6. Is pregnant
   Yes ☐ No ☐ N/A ☑

MEDICAL HISTORY:
The patient says he has suffered from problems with stress and anxiety throughout most of his life. He takes Zoloft. He smokes nearly a pack of cigarettes per day. Other than this, he is healthy.

DENTAL HISTORY:
The patient has not visited the dentist in several years and has never before visited this office.

SOCIAL HISTORY:
The patient is a high school teacher who is recently divorced. He now lives alone. He says he does not eat a balanced diet and practically lives on take-out food.

CHIEF COMPLAINT:
The patient complains of painful, swollen, bleeding gums. He said he has bad breath and a metal taste in his mouth.

ADULT CLINICAL EXAMINATION

Case PT2-2

	1	2	3	4	5	6	7	8	9	10	11	12	13	14	15	16
Probe 2 / 1		434	535	333	333	333	323	323	323	323	323	325	523	434	434	

facial

R

palatal

| Probe 1 / 2 | | 424 | 525 | 323 | 323 | 323 | 323 | 323 | 323 | 323 | 323 | 325 | 523 | 434 | 434 | |

| Probe 2 / 1 | | 524 | 335 | 334 | 424 | 434 | 434 | 434 | 434 | 434 | 435 | 333 | 425 | 535 | 535 | |

lingual

R

facial

| Probe 1 / 2 | | 525 | 535 | 333 | 434 | 434 | 434 | 434 | 434 | 434 | 435 | 434 | 434 | 525 | 535 | |

| 32 | 31 | 30 | 29 | 28 | 27 | 26 | 25 | 24 | 23 | 22 | 21 | 20 | 19 | 18 | 17 |

KEY

Clinically visible carious lesion

Clinically missing tooth

△ Furcation

▲ "Through and through" furcation

Probe 1: initial probing depth

Probe 2: probing depth 1 month after scaling and root planing

SUPPLEMENTAL ORAL EXAMINATION FINDINGS

1. Current Oral Hygiene Status: Poor.
2. Moderate halitosis.
3. Tissues visibly inflamed.
4. Cannot probe due to patient's extreme pain and discomfort.
5. Generalized moderate plaque and stain.
6. Gray film on gums.

11. Which of the following is **MOST LIKELY** the diagnosis for this patient's condition?
    (A) Chronic gingivitis
    (B) Aggressive periodontitis
    (C) Necrotizing ulcerative periodontitis (NUP)
    (D) Necrotizing ulcerative gingivitis (NUG)

12. You should ask this patient all of the following questions **EXCEPT** one. Which one is the **EXCEPTION**?
    (A) "How long have you had these symptoms?"
    (B) "Is your current personal situation causing you much stress?"
    (C) "Have you had these symptoms before?"
    (D) "How much do you smoke?"

13. Which of the following are factors that may have led to this patient's condition?
    (A) Poor nutrition
    (B) Poor oral hygiene
    (C) Infections of the mouth
    (D) All of the above

14. All of the following are symptoms of this patient's condition **EXCEPT**
    (A) sores on the gums.
    (B) swollen gums.
    (C) sore throat.
    (D) tooth discoloration.

15. You should recommend which of the following for self-care for this patient?
    (A) Refrain from tobacco and alcohol.
    (B) Rinse with warm salt water.
    (C) Use an antibacterial mouthwash.
    (D) All of the above.

16. Which of the following would **MOST LIKELY** be performed on the patient's second visit to the dental office?
    (A) Antibiotic therapy
    (B) Scaling and root planing
    (C) Radiographs
    (D) Removal of tartar

17. This patient's condition is caused by which of the following?
    (A) A virus
    (B) Bacteria
    (C) An injury
    (D) An allergy

18. All of the following are risk factors for this condition **EXCEPT** one. Which one is the **EXCEPTION**?
    (A) Poor diet
    (B) Poor oral hygiene
    (C) Excess of Vitamin A
    (D) Stress

19. All of the following are characteristic of this patient's condition **EXCEPT** one. Which one is the **EXCEPTION**?
    (A) Develops rapidly
    (B) Affects the surrounding bone
    (C) Is painful even when no pressure is on gums
    (D) Gum tissue between teeth appears flat

20. If your patient follows instructions from the dental team, about how long will it take to cure his condition?
    (A) About 2 days
    (B) About 2–3 weeks
    (C) About 4–6 weeks
    (D) About 2–6 months

Directions: Study the case components and answer questions 21–30.

SYNOPSIS OF PATIENT HISTORY

CASE *PT2-3*

Age _____*58*_____

Sex _____*Female*_____

Height *5'9"*_____

Weight *160* lbs

_____*72.57*kgs

Vital Signs

Blood pressure _____*150/90*_____

Pulse rate _____*65*_____

Respiration rate _____*14*_____

---

1. Under Care of Physician
   Yes ☑ No ☐

   Condition: _____

2. Hospitalized within the last 5 years
   Yes ☑ No ☐

   Reason: _____

3. Has or had the following conditions:
   Patient had breast cancer 6 months ago and had
   a mastectomy along with chemotherapy and radiation.
   She also suffers from occasional migraines.

4. Current medications:

   Imitrex as needed
   _____
   _____

5. Smokes or uses tobacco products
   Yes ☐ No ☑

6. Is pregnant
   Yes ☐ No ☑ N/A ☐

MEDICAL HISTORY:
The patient was diagnosed with breast cancer 6 months ago and underwent a mastectomy of the right breast along with chemotherapy and radiation. Her physician says her prognosis is good. She occasionally suffers from migraines.

DENTAL HISTORY:
The patient frequently visits this dental office for checkups and amalgam restorations; she frequently has dental caries.

SOCIAL HISTORY:
The patient is a happily married college professor with two grown children. Before being diagnosed with breast cancer, she exercised at least 3 times a week.

CHIEF COMPLAINT:
"My mouth is red inside and very sore. I also wish I would stop getting so many cavities."

ADULT CLINICAL EXAMINATION

Case PT2-3

KEY

Clinically visible carious lesion

Clinically missing tooth

Furcation

"Through and through" furcation

Probe 1: initial probing depth

Probe 2: probing depth 1 month after scaling and root planing

SUPPLEMENTAL ORAL EXAMINATION FINDINGS

1. Current Oral Hygiene Status: Good.
2. Amalgam restorations.

21. You determine that the redness in your patient's mouth is oral mucositis, a common complication of chemotherapy. She does not have ulcers in her mouth, so the mucositis assessment is grade
(A) 0.
(B) 1.
(C) 2.
(D) 3.

22. The American Heart Association (AHA) classifies this patient's blood pressure as which of the following?
(A) Normal
(B) Prehypertension
(C) Stage 1
(D) Stage 2

23. The Imitrex this patient takes is intended to treat which of the following?
(A) Breast cancer
(B) Migraines
(C) Mucositis
(D) Blood pressure

24. This patient has a carious lesion on which of the following teeth?
(A) #14
(B) #15
(C) #18
(D) #19

25. Which of the following is an oral side effect of chemotherapy?
(A) Tooth decay
(B) Oral pain
(C) Gingivitis
(D) All of the above

26. You should recommend all of the following for this patient's self-care **EXCEPT** one. Which one is the **EXCEPTION**?
    (A) Use an alcohol-based mouthwash.
    (B) Use a soft toothbrush.
    (C) Use toothpaste with fluoride.
    (D) Use dental floss gently.

27. All of the following are treatment options for oral mucositis **EXCEPT** one. Which one is the **EXCEPTION**?
    (A) Mucosal cell stimulants
    (B) Antiseptics
    (C) Topical anesthetics
    (D) Clonazepam

28. If you are examining this patient's mouth for oral cancers, these cancers occur most often on the
    (A) roof of the mouth.
    (B) cheeks.
    (C) floor of the mouth.
    (D) tongue.

29. Your patient tells you that her mouth has been very dry. Which of the following is **MOST LIKELY** the cause of her xerostomia?
    (A) Surgery
    (B) Dental caries
    (C) Chemotherapy
    (D) All of the above

30. You should recommend that this patient brush her teeth and gums
    (A) once a day.
    (B) in the morning and at night.
    (C) after each meal.
    (D) None of the above

Directions: Study the case components and answer questions 31–40.

SYNOPSIS OF PATIENT HISTORY   CASE *PT2-4*

Age _*62*_

Sex _*Female*_

Height _*5'5"*_

Weight _*210*_ lbs

_*95.25*_kgs

Vital Signs

Blood pressure _*195/100*_

Pulse rate _*70*_

Respiration rate _*18*_

---

1. Under Care of Physician
   Yes ☑   No ☐

   Condition: _____

2. Hospitalized within the last 5 years
   Yes ☑   No ☐

   Reason: _____
   _____

3. Has or had the following conditions:

   Hypertension, high cholesterol
   _____

4. Current medications:

   Avapro, Lipitor
   _____
   _____

5. Smokes or uses tobacco products
   Yes ☐   No ☑

6. Is pregnant
   Yes ☐   No ☑   N/A ☐

MEDICAL HISTORY:
The patient has suffered from high blood pressure and high cholesterol throughout most of her life. She was hospitalized for stroke-like symptoms 4 years ago. In addition to taking medication, her physician suggests that she improve her health through diet and exercise.

DENTAL HISTORY:
The patient's last dental visit was one year ago. She is missing several teeth from extraction.

SOCIAL HISTORY:
She is divorced and lives with her grown daughter. She is low income.

CHIEF COMPLAINT:
"Sometimes my gums bleed a little when I floss."

ADULT CLINICAL EXAMINATION

Case PT2-4

	1	2	3	4	5	6	7	8	9	10	11	12	13	14	15	16
Probe 2 / 1		435	534	333		333	333	333	333	333	444	334				

facial

R

palatal

| Probe 1 / 2 | | 435 | 534 | 333 | | 323 | 333 | 333 | 333 | 434 | 545 | 334 | | | | |

| Probe 2 / 1 | | | 544 | 333 | 333 | 333 | 333 | 333 | 323 | 324 | | 544 | 444 | | | |

lingual

R

facial

| Probe 1 / 2 | | | 534 | 333 | 333 | 333 | 333 | 333 | 324 | 324 | | 333 | 444 | | | |

| 32 | 31 | 30 | 29 | 28 | 27 | 26 | 25 | 24 | 23 | 22 | 21 | 20 | 19 | 18 | 17 |

KEY

(tooth)	Clinically visible carious lesion
(X)	Clinically missing tooth
△	Furcation
▲	"Through and through" furcation

Probe 1: initial probing depth

Probe 2: probing depth 1 month after scaling and root planing

SUPPLEMENTAL ORAL EXAMINATION FINDINGS

1. Current Oral Hygiene Status: Good.
2. Generalized 3–4 mm periodontal pockets.
3. Bleeding on probing.

---

31. Upon examination, you note that this patient has an increase in dental caries. This is **MOST LIKELY** caused by
(A) high-blood pressure medication
(B) poor oral hygiene
(C) high-cholesterol medication
(D) None of the above

32. The American Heart Association (AHA) classifies this patient's blood pressure as which of the following?
(A) Normal
(B) Prehypertension
(C) Stage I hypertension
(D) Stage II hypertension

33. Your patient has a visible dental lesion on which of the following teeth?
(A) #1
(B) #3
(C) #5
(D) #11

34. All of the following are considered risk factors for hypertension **EXCEPT** one. Which one is the **EXCEPTION**?
(A) Smoking
(B) Weight
(C) Age
(D) Oral hygiene

35. This patient is missing which of the following teeth?
    (A) #1, #5, #7, and #16
    (B) #1, #5, #16, #13, #14, #15, #17, #18, #19, #22, and #32
    (C) #1, #5, #7, #16, #13, #14, #15, #16, #17, #18, #19, and #22
    (D) #1, #2, #5, #16, #17, #18, #19, and #22

36. According to the American Association of Periodontology, this patient's periodontal classification is which of the following?
    (A) Type I
    (B) Type II
    (C) Type III
    (D) Type IV

37. If this patient does not get treatment for her gums, she is at risk for which of the following?
    (A) Abscess of the gingiva
    (B) Tooth loss
    (C) Severe periodontitis
    (D) All of the above

38. As a dental hygienist, you will look for signs of periodontitis in this patient using which of the following?
    (A) Periodontal probing
    (B) Radiographs
    (C) Both (A) and (B)
    (D) Neither (A) nor (B)

39. You should first refer this patient to which of the following?
    (A) Periodontist
    (B) Physician
    (C) Nutritionist
    (D) Oral surgeon

40. This patient's gums should be treated with which of the following?
    (A) Root planing
    (B) Scaling
    (C) Mouthwashes containing chlorhexidine
    (D) All of the above

Directions: Study the case components and answer questions 41–50.

SYNOPSIS OF PATIENT HISTORY

CASE *PT2-5*

Age   *10*

Sex   *Male*

Height *4'7"*

Weight *80* lbs

36.29 kgs

Vital Signs

Blood pressure   *99/63*

Pulse rate   *70*

Respiration rate   *20*

1. Under Care of Physician
   Yes ☑   No ☐
   Condition: _____

2. Hospitalized within the last 5 years
   Yes ☐   No ☑
   Reason: _____

3. Has or had the following conditions:
   Allergies and asthma

4. Current medications:
   Biweekly allergy injections; Albuterol

5. Smokes or uses tobacco products
   Yes ☐   No ☑

6. Is pregnant
   Yes ☐   No ☐   N/A ☑

MEDICAL HISTORY:
The patient has a history of allergies and asthma and is under the care of an allergist and a pediatrician.

DENTAL HISTORY:
The patient visits the dental regularly for checkups and restorations.

SOCIAL HISTORY:
He lives with his parents and three brothers. He enjoys school. In his spare time, he likes to read and play with his dog.

CHIEF COMPLAINT:
"I had a toothache last week, but it seems to have gone away."

ADULT CLINICAL EXAMINATION

Case PT2-5

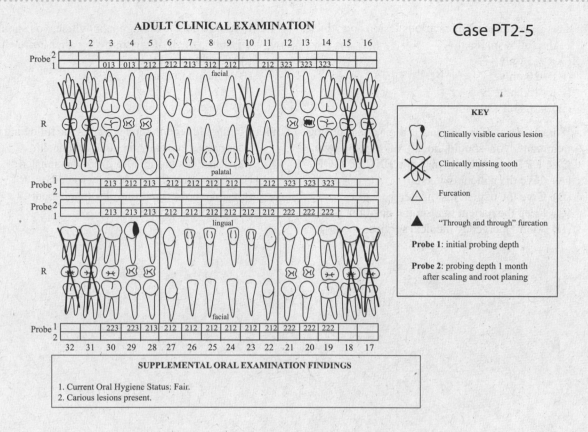

SUPPLEMENTAL ORAL EXAMINATION FINDINGS

1. Current Oral Hygiene Status: Fair.
2. Carious lesions present.

41. Before treating this patient, you should ask his mother which of the following?
(A) "How often does he have asthma attacks?"
(B) "What precipitates these attacks?"
(C) "How severe are these attacks?"
(D) All of the above

42. If this patient suffers an asthma attack during treatment, you should do all of the following **EXCEPT** one. Which one is the **EXCEPTION**?
(A) Immediately stop treatment.
(B) Give the patient a bronchodilator.
(C) Inject the patient with epinephrine.
(D) Allow the patient to position himself comfortably.

43. Which of the following dental materials might cause your patient to suffer an asthma attack?
(A) Tooth enamel dust
(B) Fissure sealants
(C) Dentifrices
(D) All of the above

44. Which of the following guidelines concerning rubber dams should you follow when treating this patient?
(A) Refrain from using rubber dams.
(B) Use rubber dams cautiously.
(C) Use rubber dams freely.
(D) Use rubber dams as quickly as possible.

45. If your patient's asthma is not severe, which of the following may be used to reduce his stress?
(A) Nitrous oxide
(B) Barbiturates
(C) Local anesthetic containing sodium metabisulfite
(D) None of the above

46. All of the following are side effects of Albuterol **EXCEPT** one. Which one is the **EXCEPTION**?
(A) Sore or dry throat
(B) Lethargy
(C) Nausea
(D) Dizziness

47. This patient has visible carious lesions on which of the following teeth?
    (A) #13 only
    (B) #20 only
    (C) #13 and #29
    (D) #20 and #29

48. If the patient suffers an acute asthma attack during treatment, you should do all of the following **EXCEPT** one. Which one is the **EXCEPTION**?
    (A) Give the patient oxygen.
    (B) Give the patient his inhaler.
    (C) Keep the patient in a supine position.
    (D) Alert emergency medical services.

49. If your patient is taking theophylline, you should give him which of the following after treatment?
    (A) Erythromycin
    (B) Phenobarbitals
    (C) Acetaminophen
    (D) None of the above

50. You should recommend which of the following to your patient to maintain good oral health?
    (A) Rinse his mouth after using his inhaler.
    (B) Brush and floss at least twice a day.
    (C) Take prescribed fluoride supplements.
    (D) All of the above

Directions: Study the case components and answer questions 51–60.

SYNOPSIS OF PATIENT HISTORY

CASE *PT2-6*

Age ___10___

Sex ___Male___

Height ___4'6"___

Weight ___105___ lbs

___47.63___kgs

Vital Signs

Blood pressure ___100/60___

Pulse rate ___80___

Respiration rate ___20___

1. Under Care of Physician
   Yes ☑   No ☐

   Condition: _____

2. Hospitalized within the last 5 years
   Yes ☐   No ☑

   Reason: _____
   _____

3. Has or had the following conditions:

   Patient has Down syndrome
   _____

4. Current medications:
   _____
   _____
   _____

5. Smokes or uses tobacco products
   Yes ☐   No ☑

6. Is pregnant
   Yes ☐   No ☐   N/A ☑

MEDICAL HISTORY:
The patient has Down syndrome; he just finished a course of antibiotics for an ear infection. He received surgery for a cardiac abnormality shortly after birth.

DENTAL HISTORY:
The patient visits the dental office regularly for checkups and restorations. He is a mouth breather and has xerostomia, and mild fissuring on the lips and tongue. He has had past dental caries.

SOCIAL HISTORY:
He is a lively, curious child who lives with his siblings and parents. He has adequate language and verbal development for effective communication.

CHIEF COMPLAINT:
Regular checkup. His mother says his breath stinks.

CLINICAL EXAMINATION

Case PT2-6

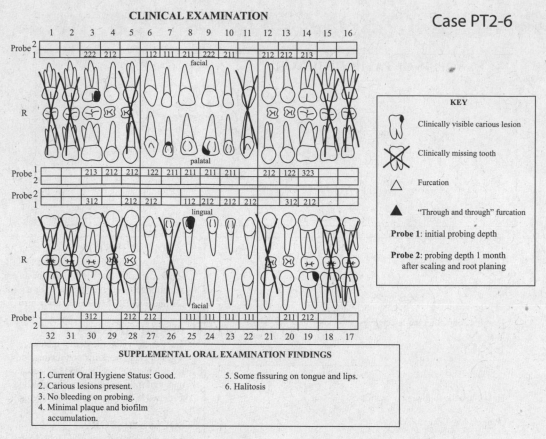

SUPPLEMENTAL ORAL EXAMINATION FINDINGS

1. Current Oral Hygiene Status: Good.
2. Carious lesions present.
3. No bleeding on probing.
4. Minimal plaque and biofilm accumulation.

5. Some fissuring on tongue and lips.
6. Halitosis

51. Patients with Down syndrome are at a high risk of developing which of the following dental disorders?
(A) Periodontal disease
(B) Recurrent aphthous ulcers
(C) Oral candidiasis
(D) Herpes simplex viral infections

52. This patient's appointment should be scheduled
(A) at noon.
(B) early in the morning.
(C) late in the morning.
(D) late in the afternoon.

53. All of the following conditions are common in patients with Down syndrome **EXCEPT** one. Which one is the **EXCEPTION**?
(A) Mouth breathing
(B) Missing permanent teeth
(C) Obesity
(D) Oversized teeth

54. When managing patients with Down syndrome, you should do all of the following **EXCEPT** one. Which one is the **EXCEPTION**?
(A) Limit distractions.
(B) Talk to caregivers about behavior techniques beforehand.
(C) Perform the first oral exam using only dental instruments.
(D) Involve the entire dental team in the patient's care.

55. Patients with Down syndrome are prone to all of the following **EXCEPT** one. Which one is the **EXCEPTION**?
(A) Low blood pressure
(B) Xerostomia
(C) Chronic respiratory infections
(D) Dental caries

56. Which of the following medical conditions is common in patients with Down syndrome?
    (A) Cardiac disorders
    (B) Hypotonia
    (C) Compromised immune system
    (D) All of the above

57. To determine whether this patient's missing teeth are congenital, you should take which of the following X-rays?
    (A) Bitewing X-rays
    (B) Periapical X-rays
    (C) Panoramic X-rays
    (D) All of the above

58. This patient's halitosis is **MOST LIKELY** caused by which of the following?
    (A) Xerostomia
    (B) Dental caries
    (C) Plaque accumulation
    (D) Poor oral hygiene

59. When instructing this patient's caregiver, you should do all of the following **EXCEPT** one. Which one is the **EXCEPTION**?
    (A) Recommend that the caregiver use a sweet food or drink as a reward.
    (B) Recommend the use of an antimicrobial agent such as chlorhexidine.
    (C) Demonstrate proper brushing and flossing techniques.
    (D) Recommend the caregiver use the same location and time for oral health care.

60. A Down syndrome patient's missing teeth may be caused by which of the following?
    (A) Periodontal disease
    (B) Genetics
    (C) Delayed eruption
    (D) All of the above

Directions: Study the case components and answer questions 61–70.

SYNOPSIS OF PATIENT HISTORY　　　CASE *PT2-7*

Age　　_30_

Sex　　_Female_

Height　_5'5"_

Weight　_135_ lbs

　　　　_61.4_ kgs

Vital Signs

Blood pressure　　_130/75_

Pulse rate　　　　_68_

Respiration rate　　_19_

---

1. Under Care of Physician
   Yes ☐　No ☑
   　　　　　Condition: _____

2. Hospitalized within the last 5 years
   Yes ☐　No ☑
   　　　　　Reason: _____
   　　　　　_____

3. Has or had the following conditions:

   Feeling run down lately
   _____

4. Current medications:

   _____
   _____
   _____

5. Smokes or uses tobacco products
   Yes ☑　No ☐

6. Is pregnant
   Yes ☐　No ☑　N/A ☐

MEDICAL HISTORY:
The patient had a history of good health but admits to feeling tired and run down the past six weeks, with headaches. She has not had a physical exam since she was in her mid 20s. "I'm always fine!"

DENTAL HISTORY:
Good care, a few restorations previously, from childhood.

SOCIAL HISTORY:
The patient is a single, working professional woman. She has many friends, is close to family, and is currently not dating anyone in particular. She has been experiencing high stress and pressure related to her work.

CHIEF COMPLAINT:
Need teeth cleaned. Teeth are sensitive, mouth "hurts," headaches.

ADULT CLINICAL EXAMINATION

Case PT2-7

	1	2	3	4	5	6	7	8	9	10	11	12	13	14	15	16
Probe 2 / 1			325	325	435	333	313	333	323	423	334	435	435	435		

facial

R

palatal

	1	2	3	4	5	6	7	8	9	10	11	12	13	14	15	16
Probe 1 / 2			335	335	325	323	313	333	323	323	334	335	335	335		

	32	31	30	29	28	27	26	25	24	23	22	21	20	19	18	17
Probe 2 / 1			345	345	323	323	324	324	324	333	323	323	335	335	335	

lingual

R

facial

	32	31	30	29	28	27	26	25	24	23	22	21	20	19	18	17
Probe 1 / 2			345	345	323	323	324	324	324	333	323	323	335	335	335	335

KEY

Clinically visible carious lesion

Clinically missing tooth

△ Furcation

▲ "Through and through" furcation

Probe 1: initial probing depth

Probe 2: probing depth 1 month after scaling and root planing

SUPPLEMENTAL ORAL EXAMINATION FINDINGS

1. Current Oral Hygiene Status: Fair/Good.
2. Light calculus and stain, especially lower anteriors.
3. Probes 1–3 mm.
4. FMX taken reveals widening of periodontal ligament in several areas, but no alveolar bone loss.
5. Teeth show evidence of bruxism.

61. The diagnosis for this patient's periodontal condition is which of the following?
    (A) Gingivitis
    (B) Localized chronic periodontitis
    (C) Health
    (D) Occlusal trauma

62. The American Academy of Periodontology (AAP) classification for this disease is which of the following?
    (A) Type IV
    (B) Type V
    (C) Type VI
    (D) Type VIII

63. What would be the appropriate technique to use to debride this patient's teeth at a maintenance visit?
    (A) Gross scaling
    (B) Deep scaling, two appointments
    (C) Light ultrasonic scaling, fine scaling as needed
    (D) Based on clinical findings, she does not need her teeth cleaned

64. If the patient is bruxing, what is the recommended treatment?
    (A) Refer her to a meditation center.
    (B) Each time she catches herself, make a point of stopping to break the habit.
    (C) Fabricate a night-guard appliance.
    (D) Provide an occlusal adjustment on the areas of concern.

65. A night guard can be all of the following **EXCEPT** one. Which one is the **EXCEPTION**?
    (A) Substituted for a sleep apnea appliance
    (B) A solution
    (C) Purchased over the counter
    (D) Customized and created in the laboratory

66. If the patient had a history of previous periodontal disease, her diagnosis would be which of the following?
    (A) Primary occlusal trauma
    (B) Secondary occlusal trauma
    (C) Tertiary occlusal trauma
    (D) Traumatic occlusion

67. Which of the following is **NOT** an alternative solution for this patient?
    (A) Stress reduction therapy
    (B) Referral to TMJ specialist
    (C) Braces
    (D) Wearing her night guard during day hours as well

68. Clinical indicators of occlusal trauma may include all of the following **EXCEPT** one. Which one is the **EXCEPTION**?
    (A) Progressive tooth mobility
    (B) Throbbing of the first molars
    (C) Fremitus of certain teeth
    (D) Thermal sensitivity on chewing or percussion

69. Radiographic indicators may include all of the following in cases of occlusal trauma **EXCEPT** one. Which one is the **EXCEPTION**?
    (A) Widened periodontal ligament space
    (B) Bone loss
    (C) Increasing areas of radiopacity at apices of traumatized teeth
    (D) Root resorption

70. If a tooth has experienced previous attachment or bone loss, all of the following may result from occlusal trauma **EXCEPT** one. Which one is the **EXCEPTION**?
    (A) Rapid bone loss
    (B) Pocket formation
    (C) Acute periapical abscess
    (D) Mobility

Directions: Study the case components and answer questions 71–80.

SYNOPSIS OF PATIENT HISTORY

CASE *PT2-8*

Age _____45_____

Sex _____Female_____

Height _5'1"_

Weight _115_ lbs

_52.3_ kgs

Vital Signs

Blood pressure _____125/78_____

Pulse rate _____70_____

Respiration rate _____15_____

1. Under Care of Physician
   Yes ☑ No ☐

   Condition: _Anxiety, depression, sinus infection_

2. Hospitalized within the last 5 years
   Yes ☐ No ☑

   Reason: _____

3. Has or had the following conditions:

   Anxiety, depression
   _____

4. Current medications:

   Antidepressant, she does not remember the name.
   _____
   _____

5. Smokes or uses tobacco products
   Yes ☑ No ☐

6. Is pregnant
   Yes ☐ No ☑ N/A ☐

MEDICAL HISTORY:
The patient has a history of fair health. She talks about quitting smoking, but says 1/4 pack a day is not significant in her mind. She recently had a long bout with a sinus infection. She did not take probiotics during her prescription, and is now suffering from a yeast infection.

DENTAL HISTORY:
Excellent care, comes in regularly, a few restorations previously, from childhood.

SOCIAL HISTORY:
Divorced, working as a waitress. Lives with her senior mother. Patient drinks a lot of coffee at home and at work.

CHIEF COMPLAINT:
In for her 4-month maintenance visit; worried she has bad breath.

ADULT CLINICAL EXAMINATION

Case PT2-8

	1	2	3	4	5	6	7	8	9	10	11	12	13	14	15	16

Probe 2 / 1: 333 433 333 323 323 322 313 223 313 223 233 233 334 334

facial

R

palatal

Probe 1 / 2: 333 433 333 323 323 322 313 223 313 223 233 233 334 334

Probe 2 / 1: 334 424 323 323 322 222 222 212 212 312 334 334 334 334

lingual

R

facial

Probe 1 / 2: 334 424 323 323 322 222 222 212 212 312 324 334 334 334

32 31 30 29 28 27 26 25 24 23 22 21 20 19 18 17

KEY

Clinically visible carious lesion

Clinically missing tooth

Furcation

"Through and through" furcation

Probe 1: initial probing depth

Probe 2: probing depth 1 month after scaling and root planing

SUPPLEMENTAL ORAL EXAMINATION FINDINGS

1. Current Oral Hygiene Status: Excellent.
2. Light calculus and stain, linguals of maxillary and mandibular anteriors.
3. Probes 1–3 mm. Tissues show signs of mild chronic inflammation.
4. 4 Horizontal BWs taken; unremarkable, no attachment loss.
5. Tongue is very coated.

---

71. The diagnosis for this patient's periodontal condition is which of the following?
    (A) Gingivitis
    (B) Generalized chronic periodontitis
    (C) Healthy
    (D) None of the above

72. What factors may be contributing to this patient's halitosis?
    (A) Smoking
    (B) Dry mouth from her medication
    (C) Excessive coffee consumption
    (D) All of the above

73. What would be the **BEST** technique to use to polish this patient's teeth at a maintenance visit?
    (A) Use a course pumice to get the stain off.
    (B) Use desensitizing toothpaste.
    (C) Use an air polisher.
    (D) There is no need to polish this patient's teeth.

74. Current research suggests that the **BEST** way for this patient to reduce her halitosis is which of the following?
    (A) Flossing twice a day
    (B) Brushing with an automatic toothbrush
    (C) Tongue scraping
    (D) Using a mouth rinse

75. What information should you provide to this patient regarding her antidepressant medication?
    (A) It causes xerostomia.
    (B) The antidepressant can cause staining.
    (C) Her cigarette smoking will increase the therapeutic effect of the medication.
    (D) Her coffee drinking will reduce the therapeutic effect of the medication.

76. Which of the following is an accurate description of oral malador?
    (A) The patient's periodontal status will not contribute to malador.
    (B) Oral malador is exacerbated by xerostomia.
    (C) Most cases of malador are due to systemic causes.
    (D) Organaleptic means are never used to diagnose malador.

77. All of the following should be recommended to this patient to help control her halitosis **EXCEPT** one. Which one is the **EXCEPTION**?
    (A) Use a humidifier.
    (B) Discontinue tobacco use.
    (C) Use candy mints to mask odor.
    (D) Use a tongue scraper.

78. Smoking is a primary risk factor for all of the following **EXCEPT** one. Which one is the **EXCEPTION**?
    (A) Periodontal disease
    (B) Diabetes
    (C) Chronic obstructive lung disease
    (D) Heart disease

79. Which of the following would **NOT** be an effective intervention for this patient's smoking habit?
    (A) Setting a quit date for her
    (B) Referring her to a quitline
    (C) Learning via questioning as to the patient's history of smoking
    (D) Recommending pharmacologic adjuncts to help her quit

80. All of the following are true regarding this patient's adhering to a preventive regiment **EXCEPT** one. Which one is the **EXCEPTION**?
    (A) Quality of communication between the hygienist and the patient is critical.
    (B) The patient needs to be encouraged to share responsibility for her own oral health.
    (C) An authoritarian message from the hygienist will probably be very effective, as it will encourage the patient to "get in line."
    (D) The hygienist must recognize that old behaviors are difficult to change, as they satisfy certain needs.

Directions: Study the case components and answer questions 81–90.

SYNOPSIS OF PATIENT HISTORY ·   CASE *PT2-9*

Age   *25*

Sex   *Male*

Height *5'11"*

Weight *175* lbs

79.5 kgs

Vital Signs

Blood pressure   *120/80*

Pulse rate   *66*

Respiration rate   *17*

---

1. Under Care of Physician
   Yes ☐   No ☑
           Condition: _____

2. Hospitalized within the last 5 years
   Yes ☐   No ☑
           Reason: _____
                   _____

3. Has or had the following conditions:
   _____
   _____

4. Current medications:
   _____
   _____
   _____

5. Smokes or uses tobacco products
   Yes ☐   No ☑

6. Is pregnant
   Yes ☐   No ☐   N/A ☑

MEDICAL HISTORY:
The patient has a history of excellent health. He takes no medications and has never been hospitalized.

DENTAL HISTORY:
He has never been to a dentist.

SOCIAL HISTORY:
Patient has recently moved here from South America. He is working as a laborer. He lives with other laborers on a farm. He speaks Spanish fluently and English fairly well. He is outgoing.

CHIEF COMPLAINT:
Need teeth cleaned. "I have never been to the dentist."

ADULT CLINICAL EXAMINATION   Case PT2-9

	1	2	3	4	5	6	7	8	9	10	11	12	13	14	15	16
Probe 2 / 1		434	535	333	333	333	323	323	323	323	323	325	523	434	434	

facial

R

palatal

	1	2	3	4	5	6	7	8	9	10	11	12	13	14	15	16
Probe 1 / 2		434	525	323	323	323	323	323	323	323	323	323	323	424	424	
Probe 2 / 1	535	424	335	334	424	434	434	434	434	434	435	333	425	535	535	535

lingual

R

facial

Probe 1 / 2	535	535	333	434	435	435	535	535	434	434	434	434	434	525	525	525
	32	31	30	29	28	27	26	25	24	23	22	21	20	19	18	17

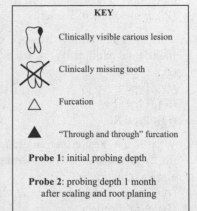

KEY

- Clinically visible carious lesion
- Clinically missing tooth
- △ Furcation
- ▲ "Through and through" furcation
- **Probe 1**: initial probing depth
- **Probe 2**: probing depth 1 month after scaling and root planing

SUPPLEMENTAL ORAL EXAMINATION FINDINGS

1. Current Oral Hygiene Status: Fair.
2. Calculus generally, with slight tissue inflammation.
3. Probes 1–3 mm, except #18 distal and #31 distal (5 mm); bleeding in numerous areas.
4. FMX taken shows no alveolar bone loss.
5. Four areas of clinical decay noted, on each first molar.
6. #32 and #17 are partially erupted and impacted.

81. The diagnosis for this patient's periodontal condition is which of the following?
   (A) Gingivitis
   (B) Generalized chronic periodontitis
   (C) Health
   (D) None of the above

82. The American Academy of Periodontology (AAP) classification for this disease is which of the following?
   (A) Type I
   (B) Type II
   (C) Type III
   (D) Type IV

83. Which of the following is the appropriate method for debriding this patient's teeth?
   (A) Gross scaling
   (B) Deep scaling with anesthesia, two appointments, ½ the mouth at each visit

(C) Ultrasonic scaling, fine scaling, dispersed over two appointments
(D) Based on clinical findings, he does not need his teeth cleaned.

84. The deep pocketing on the distal of the lower second molars is **MOST LIKELY**
   (A) an acute periodontal abscess.
   (B) loss of attachment with vertical bone loss.
   (C) pseudopocketing.
   (D) swelling that should disappear after debridement.

85. All of the following tooth brushing methods would be recommended for this patient when using a manual toothbrush **EXCEPT** one. Which one is the **EXCEPTION**?
   (A) Leonard method
   (B) Modified Bass
   (C) Modified Stillmans
   (D) Rolling

86. All of the following are desirable characteristics in a manual toothbrush **EXCEPT** one. Which one is the **EXCEPTION**?
    (A) Easily and efficiently manipulated
    (B) Flexible and medium
    (C) Impervious to moisture
    (D) End-rounded filaments

87. This patient's embrasures are occupied by the interdental papillae. What are they classified as?
    (A) Type 0
    (B) Type I
    (C) Type II
    (D) Type III

88. What is the most effective interdental device for the hygienist to give this patient given his general clinical conditions?
    (A) Interdental wedges
    (B) Pipe cleaners
    (C) Interdental brushes
    (D) Dental floss (Ideal for Type I embrasures)

89. Using which of the following would most help the patient to clean the distal areas of his lower second molars?
    (A) End tuft brush
    (B) Child-size brush
    (C) Power oral irrigation device
    (D) Dental tape

90. The patient heals well after debridement appointments. Which of the following is the **BEST** maintenance schedule?
    (A) 3 months
    (B) 4 months
    (C) 6 months
    (D) Annually

Directions: Study the case components and answer questions 91–100.

SYNOPSIS OF PATIENT HISTORY

CASE *PT2-10*

Age _51_

Sex _Male_

Height _6'0"_

Weight _217_ lbs

_98.43_ kgs

Vital Signs

Blood pressure _135/88_

Pulse rate _100_

Respiration rate _16_

---

1. Under Care of Physician
   Yes ☑ No ☐

   Condition: _____

2. Hospitalized within the last 5 years
   Yes ☐ No ☑

   Reason: _____
   _____

3. Has or had the following conditions:

   Diabetic since age 12
   _____

4. Current medications:

   Insulin by injection; has taken his insulin today;
   Advil in the past 24 hours for mouth pain.
   _____

5. Smokes or uses tobacco products
   Yes ☐ No ☑

6. Is pregnant
   Yes ☐ No ☐ N/A ☑

MEDICAL HISTORY:
Patient was diagnosed with diabetes when he was 12. Takes insulin by injection daily.

DENTAL HISTORY:
Last recall was three years ago. Wears removable partial denture with #20 and #28 as abutment teeth. No current radiographs available.

SOCIAL HISTORY:
Not married and lives by himself. Still works full-time as a banker.

CHIEF COMPLAINT:
Soreness and bleeding; slight odor when brushing. #28 d is very sensitive and bleeds. Knows he is overdue for a cleaning and was late to the appointment, but he would like something done today.

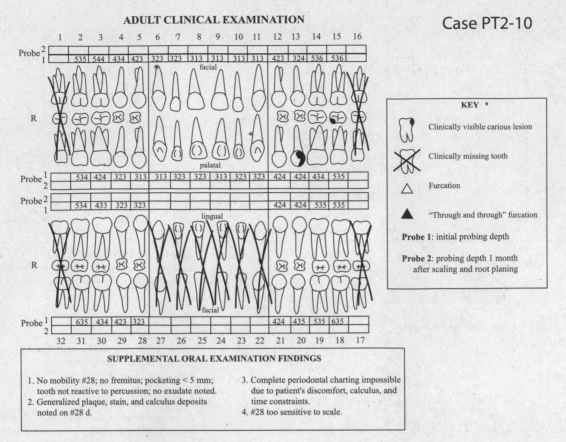

ADULT CLINICAL EXAMINATION

Case PT2-10

SUPPLEMENTAL ORAL EXAMINATION FINDINGS

1. No mobility #28; no fremitus; pocketing < 5 mm; tooth not reactive to percussion; no exudate noted.
2. Generalized plaque, stain, and calculus deposits noted on #28 d.
3. Complete periodontal charting impossible due to patient's discomfort, calculus, and time constraints.
4. #28 too sensitive to scale.

91. What is **MOST LIKELY** the diagnosis of this patient's periodontal condition?
(A) Chronic periodontitis
(B) Primary herpetic gingiva stomatitis
(C) Necrotizing ulcerative gingivitis
(D) Not enough data available for definitive provisional diagnosis

92. Which of the following is standard protocol for treating this patient's condition?
(A) Antibiotic therapy only
(B) Self-care regime only
(C) Root planning and scaling the entire mouth
(D) Debridement with localized pain management

93. You are concerned about a possible hypoglycemic episode and decide to forgo radiographs. All of the following are questions that should be asked of the patient **EXCEPT** one. Which one is the **EXCEPTION**?
(A) "Who is your emergency contact?"
(B) "When did you last eat, and what did you have?"

(C) "Who is your dental insurance carrier?"
(D) "When was the last time you had a hypo-glycemic episode?"

94. Consider your **BEST** plan for patient treatment. All of the following are likely **EXCEPT** one. Which one is the **EXCEPTION**?
(A) Explain to the patient that you want to do the best for his situation today.
(B) Start root planning as soon as possible since time is of the essence.
(C) Remove much of the deposit in the entire mouth, including the sensitive tooth.
(D) Explain that reevaluation and follow-up treatment will be needed.

95. When removing deposits from #28 distal, you should use
(A) a topical anesthetic only.
(B) a local, ester anesthetic agent.
(C) an amide local anesthetic agent.
(D) Mepivicaine (less vasodilation).

96. Since there are no radiographs or periodontal charting, which procedure is the **BEST** choice?
    (A) SRP four quads
    (B) Simple prophy
    (C) Debridement
    (D) No treatment

97. All of the following are part of the treatment for this patient's condition during the first appointment **EXCEPT** one. Which one is the **EXCEPTION**?
    (A) Subgingival instrumentation
    (B) Gentile supragivgival instrumentation with pain management #28
    (C) Patient self-care discussion for continued treatment
    (D) SRP and antibiotic therapy

98. Polishing agents should **NOT** be used during this visit because they contain a(an)
    (A) foaming agent.
    (B) abrasive agent.
    (C) thickening agent.
    (D) moisturizing agent.

99. The patient complains of sensitivity and says that he used a desensitizing agent 3 years ago which helped. What would you suggest for desensitizing #28 after treatment?
    (A) Placing a sealant on his tooth
    (B) Switching brands of sensitivity paste
    (C) Using mouthwash
    (D) Using the same desensitizing paste

100. What should be done to provide pain management for #28 distal?
    (A) An IANB, L should be given on the right side.
    (B) Infiltration anesthesia should be given only around #28.
    (C) 1:50,000 of lidocaine should be administered.
    (D) Bupivocaine should be administered.

Directions: Study the case components and answer questions 101–111.

SYNOPSIS OF PATIENT HISTORY   CASE *PT2-11*

Age   _7_

Sex   *Female*

Height *3'8"*

Weight _50_ lbs

   22.71 kgs

Vital Signs

Blood pressure   *93/56*

Pulse rate   *85*

Respiration rate   *25*

---

1. Under Care of Physician
   Yes ☐   No ☑

   Condition: _____

2. Hospitalized within the last 5 years
   Yes ☐   No ☑

   Reason: _____
   _____

3. Has or had the following conditions:

   Asthma _____
   _____

4. Current medications:

   Albuterol; inhaler and nebulizer _____
   _____
   _____

5. Smokes or uses tobacco products
   Yes ☐   No ☑

6. Is pregnant
   Yes ☐   No ☑   N/A ☐

MEDICAL HISTORY:
Patient is an active 7-year-old girl who has asthma. She uses an inhaler and a nebulizer.

DENTAL HISTORY:
Has lost teeth; no history of sealants.

SOCIAL HISTORY:
First grader at a local school who enjoys Barbies.

CHIEF COMPLAINT:
"She is hungry and one tooth bothers her a lot." Child came in crying; the mother says that her child is particularly cranky today and has attempted to bribe her with a new Barbie after the exam.

CLINICAL EXAMINATION

Case PT2-11

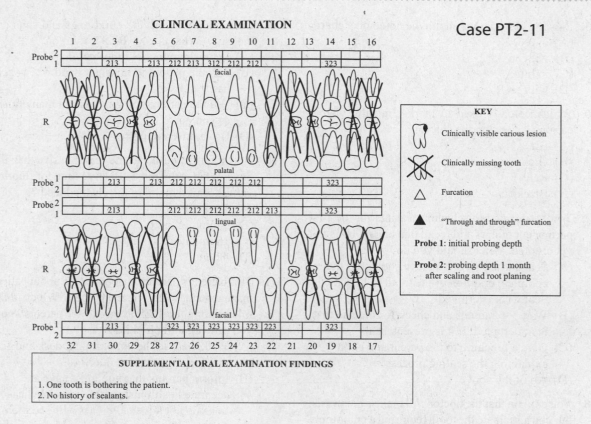

KEY

Clinically visible carious lesion

Clinically missing tooth

Furcation

"Through and through" furcation

Probe 1: initial probing depth

Probe 2: probing depth 1 month after scaling and root planing

SUPPLEMENTAL ORAL EXAMINATION FINDINGS

1. One tooth is bothering the patient.
2. No history of sealants.

---

101. All of the following are acceptable approaches for bringing the patient into the operatory **EXCEPT** one. Which one is the **EXCEPTION**?
(A) Let the parent come in, and interview her about medical history, health issues, dental problems, and parent concerns.
(B) Ask the parent to escort the child unless the child will come with you voluntarily.
(C) Tell the parent you do not approve of bribing the child with a Barbie and will see the child alone.
(D) Give the child a new toothbrush and tell her you are going to show her how to use it when she is seated in the chair.

102. You explain that a thorough medical history is important because sedation or other medications are often used if dental work needs to be done. About which of the following are you concerned?
(A) Episodic Asthma
(B) The anxiety displayed today
(C) The pain the child is in
(D) All of the above

103. While examining the patient, you note a dark area between the teeth with a smaller dark area on the opposite side, #S, mandibular right first deciduous molar. Which of the following do you do next?
(A) Advise the parent of your concerns, and recommend radiographs.
(B) Take bitewing radiographs and a periapical of the tooth causing discomfort.
(C) Place a lead shield with thyroid protection on the patient.
(D) All of the above

104. What marking should you use to note suspected caries for this patient?
(A) Mark findings in blue.
(B) Mark an X on the corresponding tooth in the chart.
(C) Mark findings in red.
(D) Mark findings in pencil.

105. Existing restorations should be noted on a chart
    (A) in red.
    (B) with an X.
    (C) in blue.
    (D) with an R.

106. Which color is used to mark clinically visible carious lesions on the chart?
    (A) Blue
    (B) Green
    (C) Red
    (D) Black

107. You've decided to schedule sealants for the first permanent molars and recall that one molar is not yet erupted. What should you do?
    (A) Sealants are most effective soon after the complete eruption of the tooth to be sealed. Seal what is erupted.
    (B) Wait 3–6 months and check for the one that is not erupted. If it is present, seal.
    (C) Give a brochure to the parent and child explaining the sealing process.
    (D) All of the above

108. You explain that the doctor will make a diagnosis, but you anticipate the tooth requiring a pulpotomy and crown. Which of the following statements will **BEST** explain a pulpotomy to the parent?
    (A) When a cavity gets really deep, close to the nerve of a tooth, or even into the pulp, the nerve tissue becomes irritated and inflamed.
    (B) This is usually the toothache you feel. If the inflammation and infection continues without treatment, the tooth will likely abscess eventually.
    (C) A pulpotomy is when the inflamed pulp chamber, usually on a baby molar, is removed, the area sterilized, and the chamber sealed.
    (D) All of the above

109. During a polishing, the child gags and spits out the paste. What is your **BEST** solution?
    (A) Let the patient hold the suction.
    (B) Ask the patient to raise her hand when she has to spit.
    (C) Tell the patient you will suction many times as you go.
    (D) Use a different paste.

110. New fluoride varnishes are less invasive than the trays. What is the most effective time for fluoride varnishes to remain on the cleaned teeth?
    (A) 1 minute
    (B) 5 minutes
    (C) 15 minutes
    (D) 4 hours

111. This patient's parents are concerned about patient management, sedation, and process. Which of the following is the **BEST** way to let parents know you care about their child's visit?
    (A) Walk them to the appointment desk and then out to the office door.
    (B) Inform parents that you must have an accurate health history to ensure medications do not adversely react with sedation.
    (C) Tell the parents that they should wait in the waiting room and you will come and get them if the child needs them.
    (D) Weigh the child yourself even if the parents are certain of their child's current weight.

Directions: Study the case components and answer questions 112–122.

SYNOPSIS OF PATIENT HISTORY

CASE *PT2-12*

Age   *43*

Sex   *Male*

Height *5'5"*

Weight *285* lbs

      129.27 kgs

Vital Signs

Blood pressure   *160/98*

Pulse rate   *100*

Respiration rate   *25*

1. Under Care of Physician
   Yes ☐   No ☑
         Condition: _____

2. Hospitalized within the last 5 years
   Yes ☐   No ☑
         Reason: _____
   _____

3. Has or had the following conditions:

   Depression _____
   _____

4. Current medications:

   4–6 aspirin daily for aches and pains;
   amitriptyline as an antidepressant
   _____

5. Smokes or uses tobacco products
   Yes ☐   No ☑

6. Is pregnant
   Yes ☐   No ☐   N/A ☑

MEDICAL HISTORY:
Patient demonstrates hypertension at rest but is not currently taking medication or seeing a doctor about the condition. Takes 4–6 aspirin a day for aches and pains. Takes amitriptyline, an antidepressant, daily.

DENTAL HISTORY:
Has come in today for a scaling and root planning procedure in the mandibular right quadrant.

SOCIAL HISTORY:
Leads a sedentary lifestyle. Is divorced and lives alone.

CHIEF COMPLAINT:
Has aches and pains. Not necessarily oral.

ADULT CLINICAL EXAMINATION

Case PT2-12

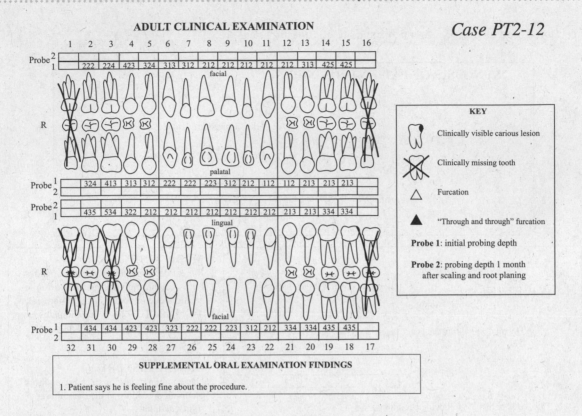

SUPPLEMENTAL ORAL EXAMINATION FINDINGS

1. Patient says he is feeling fine about the procedure.

112. What items should you have at arm's length to avoid paper shuffling and patient anxiety?
(A) FMX radiographs or computer images
(B) Treatment plan
(C) Periodontal charting
(D) Armamentarium set up

113. You will be administering local anesthesia and are concerned with all of the following **EXCEPT** one. Which one is the **EXCEPTION**?
(A) Hypertensive episode
(B) Adrenergic agent
(C) Daily aspirin intake
(D) Patient's body weight

114. Which of the following teeth has a visible carious lesion?
(A) #25
(B) #28
(C) #29
(D) #30

115. Based on radiographs and clinical examination, you notice an over-contoured crown on #30. You should do which of the following?
(A) Advise the patient that the crown may require eventual replacement.
(B) Continue your plan to scale and root plane the entire quadrant.
(C) Attempt to remove the crown before beginning treatment.
(D) (A) and (B) only

116. Root surface debridement remains the primary treatment modality for the professional management of chronic periodontitis.

The full-mouth debridement approach has proven to be the better method of nonsurgical treatment for chronic periodontitis.
(A) Both statements are true.
(B) Both statements are false.
(C) The first statement is true, the second is false.
(D) The first statement is false, the second is true.

117. Which of the following injections is **BEST** to reduce risk to the patient?
    (A) Infiltration only
    (B) Infraorbital nerve block
    (C) Mental nerve block
    (D) Inferior alveolar nerve block

118. What is the **BEST** choice of local anesthetic drugs to use?
    (A) Licocaine 1:100,000 or lidocaine 1:50,000
    (B) Marcaine
    (C) Mepivicaine 3 percent without vasoconstrictor
    (D) Procaine

119. All of the following are reasons why giving a mandibular block with long buccal minimizes patient risk **EXCEPT** one. Which one is the **EXCEPTION**?
    (A) You get pulpal anesthesia with fewer injection sites, causing anxiety from multiple sites.
    (B) You are definitely using less drug to achieve pulpal anesthesia.
    (C) You give the long buccal along with the IANB by reinsertion in the same general area for B.
    (D) Your working time will be longer because the medication will last longer.

120. You have anesthetized your patient, who is now comfortable. You check for changes in health. He reports he is fine, so you continue using your scaling and root planning skills
    (A) using both ultrasonic and hand-held instruments.
    (B) adapting to the root surfaces to remove toxins.
    (C) checking surfaces with an explorer for residual calculus deposit.
    (D) All of the above

121. You have planned some local delivery of antibiotics in one or two sites. Which of the following treatments should you use?
    (A) Atridox
    (B) Chlorhexadine irrigation
    (C) Arestin or minocycline beads
    (D) Hydrogen peroxide

122. All of the following are good post-operative recommendations to make **EXCEPT** one. Which one is the **EXCEPTION**?
    (A) Do not floss sites for a few days where local delivery was placed.
    (B) Do not floss any teeth for a week.
    (C) Do not rinse vigorously until tomorrow.
    (D) Reschedule for reevaluation or continued treatment.

Directions: Study the case components and answer questions 123–131.

SYNOPSIS OF PATIENT HISTORY

CASE *PT2-13*

Age _____67_____

Sex _____Female_____

Height _5'2"_

Weight _92_ lbs

_41.73_ kgs

Vital Signs

Blood pressure _____118/62_____

Pulse rate _____90_____

Respiration rate _____10_____

---

1. Under Care of Physician
    Yes ☐ No ☑
    Condition: _____

2. Hospitalized within the last 5 years
    Yes ☐ No ☑
    Reason: _____

3. Has or had the following conditions:
    _Strained knee_____
    _____

4. Current medications:
    _Advil for knee pain_____
    _____
    _____

5. Smokes or uses tobacco products
    Yes ☐ No ☑

6. Is pregnant
    Yes ☐ No ☑ N/A ☐

MEDICAL HISTORY:
Sees a physician only when needed. Has a strained knee and takes Advil for any associated pain.

DENTAL HISTORY:
First visit to the dentist was her initial examination a few weeks ago. Radiographs and periodontal charting were done during initial visit. Scheduled for scaling and root planing this visit.

SOCIAL HISTORY:
Married; does not have any children.

CHIEF COMPLAINT:
Is embarrassed that she has never before visited the dentist.

ADULT CLINICAL EXAMINATION

Case PT2-13

Probe 2/1

	1	2	3	4	5	6	7	8	9	10	11	12	13	14	15	16
Probe 2/1	223	323	212	212	212	212	212	212	212	212	212	212	212	224	433	433

facial

R

palatal

| Probe 1/2 | 213 | 212 | 212 | 211 | 211 | 212 | 212 | 212 | 212 | 212 | 212 | 323 | 322 | 323 | 333 | 333 |

| Probe 2/1 | 223 | 323 | 212 | 212 | 212 | 212 | 212 | 112 | 111 | 212 | 222 | 222 | 212 | 212 | 212 |

lingual

R

facial

| Probe 1/2 | 213 | 213 | 213 | 211 | 211 | 212 | 212 | 212 | 212 | 324 | 424 | 212 | 212 | 212 | 212 | 212 |

| 32 | 31 | 30 | 29 | 28 | 27 | 26 | 25 | 24 | 23 | 22 | 21 | 20 | 19 | 18 | 17 |

KEY

Clinically visible carious lesion

Clinically missing tooth

△ Furcation

▲ "Through and through" furcation

Probe 1: initial probing depth

Probe 2: probing depth 1 month after scaling and root planing

SUPPLEMENTAL ORAL EXAMINATION FINDINGS

1. Moderate marginal periodontitis.
2. Heavy subgingival calcified deposits.
3. Pocketing on #30 and #19.

4. Calculus on roots.
5. Full compliment of 32 teeth.

123. Your patient has never had a local anesthetic before. With which of the following are you most concerned?
(A) Which vasoconstrictor to use
(B) Duration of action of the drug
(C) Hypoglycemic episode
(D) Maximum dosage of the drug

124. Knowing that working time with soft-tissue anesthesia and pulpal anesthesia are important, you have decided to use two injections. Which of the following anesthetics should you choose?
(A) Lidocaine without vasoconstrictor
(B) Mepivicaine with vasoconstrictor
(C) Bupivicaine 1:200,000
(D) Prilocaine Citanest Plain

125. Upon examination of the patient, you discover deeper pockets on the mesial of #19 and #18 than were first indicated on the radiograph. Which of the following **BEST** describes your treatment plan change?
(A) You decide to include some subgingival irrigation.

(B) You decide to place site-specific local delivery.
(C) You decide to make changes on the periodontal charting.
(D) All of the above

126. Which injection type will give the patient pulpal anesthesia using the least amount of drug?
(A) Infiltration only
(B) Mental nerve block only
(C) Inferior alveolar nerve block
(D) Nasopalatine block

127. You have decided to use Mepivicaine because there is less vasodilation. Which of the following **BEST** describes why less vasodilation is preferred?
(A) Longer working time
(B) Less drug is used
(C) Decreased bleeding
(D) Increased pocket depth

128. The patient is anesthetized and comfortable. You continue procedures using your scaling and planning skills
(A) using only ultrasonic instruments.
(B) removing some stain, calculus, and debris.
(C) checking surfaces with curet for residual calculus deposits.
(D) adapting to root surfaces to remove toxins.

129. You plan to use local delivery of antibiotics in only two sites. Which of the following treatments should you use?
(A) Doxycycline Rx for a week
(B) Amoxicillin Rx for two weeks
(C) Atridox in all sites
(D) Arestin in specified sites locally

130. All of the following are good post-operative recommendations for this patient **EXCEPT** one. Which one is the **EXCEPTION**?
(A) Do not floss local delivery sites for 3 days.
(B) Do not floss any teeth for at least a week.
(C) Brush carefully tonight before going to bed.
(D) Schedule a reevaluation appointment before you leave.

131. Which of the following is the **BEST** exit strategy for this patient?
(A) Continue scaling and planing regime appointments.
(B) Schedule a recall in 6 weeks to reevaluate this quadrant.
(C) Schedule a recall in 3 months for periodontal maintenance and charting.
(D) All of the above should be implemented into an exit plan for this patient.

Directions: Study the case components and answer questions 132–142.

SYNOPSIS OF PATIENT HISTORY

CASE *PT2-14*

Age _____ *60* _____

Sex _____ *Male* _____

Height *5'8"*

Weight *160* lbs

72.57 kgs

Vital Signs

Blood pressure _____ *130/70* _____

Pulse rate _____ *95* _____

Respiration rate _____ *15* _____

---

1. Under Care of Physician
   Yes ☐   No ☑
   Condition: _____

2. Hospitalized within the last 5 years
   Yes ☐   No ☑
   Reason: _____
   _____

3. Has or had the following conditions:
   _____
   _____

4. Current medications:
   _____
   _____
   _____

5. Smokes or uses tobacco products
   Yes ☐   No ☑

6. Is pregnant
   Yes ☐   No ☐   N/A ☑

MEDICAL HISTORY:
Patient is in good health. Is a competitive runner who sees his doctor annually for routine checkups.

DENTAL HISTORY:
Patient is here today for periodontal maintenance appointment. Scaling and root planing have been performed in all four quadrants using local delivery antibiotics in select areas.

SOCIAL HISTORY:
Married with two children. Runs in approximately five races per year.

CHIEF COMPLAINT:
Slight bleeding near one tooth. Mouth is feeling better after scaling and root planing procedure.

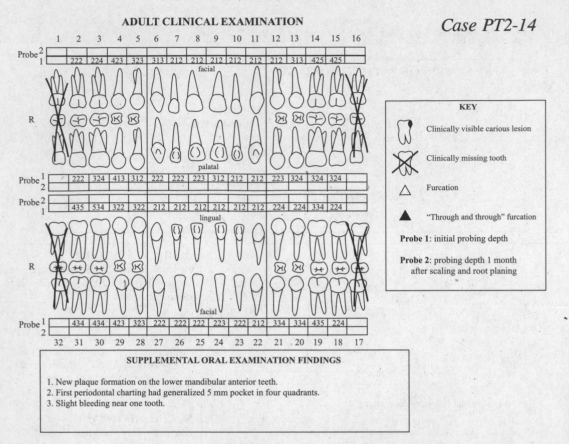

ADULT CLINICAL EXAMINATION   *Case PT2-14*

KEY

Clinically visible carious lesion

Clinically missing tooth

Furcation

"Through and through" furcation

Probe 1: initial probing depth

Probe 2: probing depth 1 month after scaling and root planing

SUPPLEMENTAL ORAL EXAMINATION FINDINGS

1. New plaque formation on the lower mandibular anterior teeth.
2. First periodontal charting had generalized 5 mm pocket in four quadrants.
3. Slight bleeding near one tooth.

132. All of the following are acceptable first steps in this periodontal maintenance appointment **EXCEPT** one. Which one is the **EXCEPTION**?
(A) Update medical and dental history.
(B) Complete a mucosal examination.
(C) Interpret the patient's radiographs.
(D) Asses the patient's oral hygiene regimen.

133. All of the following should be included in the periodontal and reevaluation examinations **EXCEPT** one. Which one is the **EXCEPTION**?
(A) Dental caries
(B) Gingival recession
(C) Furcation involvement
(D) Probing depths

134. The hygienist should continuously assess this patient's teeth and periodontum for
(A) mobility.
(B) areas that bleed.
(C) change in pocket depth.
(D) All of the above

135. All of the following are acceptable approaches for improving the patient's self-reported oral hygiene regimen **EXCEPT** one. Which one is the **EXCEPTION**?
(A) Recommend angling the brush at a 90-degree angle.
(B) Give the patient a soft brush and suggest he try it.
(C) Discuss the benefits he might realize by using an electric brush.
(D) Recommend using tarter-control toothpaste to control plaque.

136. Which of the following would you anticipate finding when performing a maintenance procedure to remove all new deposits on this patient?
(A) Leftover residual deposits
(B) Less calculus
(C) Less bleeding
(D) All of the above

137. All of the following are acceptable responses to finding one pocket that did not respond to the treatment **EXCEPT** one. Which one is the **EXCEPTION**?
    (A) Note the discrepancy on the periodontal charting.
    (B) Find an overhanging restoration in the increased area.
    (C) Deliver a local, site-specific agent again.
    (D) Advise the patient that he needs to increase his vitamin intake.

138. The patient asks, "If things are better, why must I come back so many times?" With which of the following do you respond?
    (A) "We need to monitor the need for more treatment and infections."
    (B) "Studies show scaling is beneficial over time."
    (C) "Local delivery of antimicrobial agents may need to be reapplied."
    (D) All of the above responses are acceptable as well as truthful.

139. All of the following are possible follow-up scenarios for this periodontal maintenance patient **EXCEPT** one. Which one is the **EXCEPTION**?
    (A) Advise the patient that an examination and radiographs are due at the next visit.
    (B) Each maintenance visit will involve some scaling, but should become easier with subsequent visits.
    (C) Put the patient on a recall schedule of once a month over the course of the next year.
    (D) Have the doctor evaluate the overhanging restoration, which may be contributing to pocket bleeding.

140. An example of supportive treatments and services includes the application of
    (A) desensitizing agents.
    (B) fluoride treatments during each recall visit.
    (C) tooth-whitening agents.
    (D) sealants to all teeth.

141. Radiographs must be taken during this patient's next visit **BECAUSE** it is important to look for improvements in areas of bone loss on current radiographs to make comparisons.
    (A) Both the statement and reason are correct and related.
    (B) Both the statement and reason are correct but NOT related.
    (C) The statement is correct, but the reason is correct.
    (D) The statement is NOT correct, but the reason is correct.

142. If a tooth is not responding, or a new pocket suddenly develops which is deeper, a bitewing X-ray should be taken.

    The origin of the problem may be endodontic rather than periodontic.
    (A) Both statements are true.
    (B) Both statements are false.
    (C) The first statement is true, the second is false.
    (D) The first statement is false, the second is true.

Directions: Study the case components and answer questions 143–150.

SYNOPSIS OF PATIENT HISTORY

CASE *PT2-15*

Age _____43_____

Sex _____Female_____

Height _5'4"_

Weight _155_ lbs

_70.31_ kgs

Vital Signs

Blood pressure _____140/90_____

Pulse rate _____60_____

Respiration rate _____15_____

---

1. Under Care of Physician
   Yes ☑ No ☐

   Condition: _____

2. Hospitalized within the last 5 years
   Yes ☑ No ☐

   Reason: *Patient had a complete hysterectomy three years ago*

3. Has or had the following conditions:

   Bipolar disorder, anxiety. Sees her primary care physician once a month and a psychologist once a week.

4. Current medications:

   Lithium, Ativan
   _____
   _____

5. Smokes or uses tobacco products
   Yes ☐ No ☑

6. Is pregnant
   Yes ☐ No ☑ N/A ☐

MEDICAL HISTORY:
Was diagnosed with bipolar disorder last year and currently takes Lithium and Ativan for her condition. Sees her primary care physician once a month and a psychologist once a week. Had a complete hysterectomy three years ago.

DENTAL HISTORY:
Last recall was five years ago.

SOCIAL HISTORY:
Single mother of a 13-year-old daughter and 16-year-old son. On disability for depression.

CHIEF COMPLAINT:
"Has a sore in her mouth for about two months. It hurts when she chews. Her lower left tooth hurts."

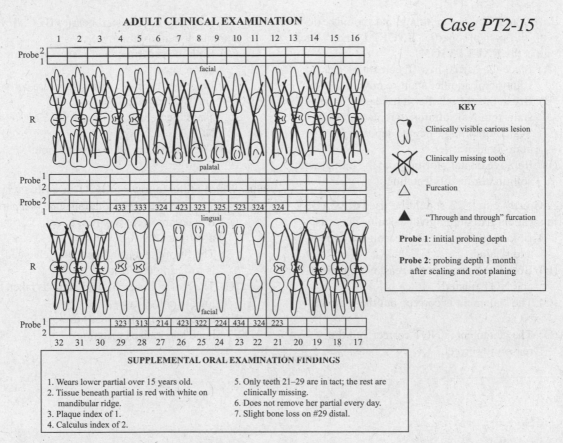

ADULT CLINICAL EXAMINATION

Case PT2-15

KEY

Clinically visible carious lesion

Clinically missing tooth

Furcation

"Through and through" furcation

Probe 1: initial probing depth

Probe 2: probing depth 1 month after scaling and root planing

SUPPLEMENTAL ORAL EXAMINATION FINDINGS

1. Wears lower partial over 15 years old.
2. Tissue beneath partial is red with white on mandibular ridge.
3. Plaque index of 1.
4. Calculus index of 2.
5. Only teeth 21–29 are in tact; the rest are clinically missing.
6. Does not remove her partial every day.
7. Slight bone loss on #29 distal.

143. You are talking with your patient about care of her partial denture. Which of the following do you suggest?

(A) She should take her partial out every night and place it in hot water.

(B) Use a denture brush every day to brush the tooth and base.

(C) Avoid the clasp when brushing with a dental brush and dentifrice.

(D) Soak nightly in a solution consisting of bleach, water softener, and water.

144. As you examine the patient, you notice a smooth, velvety, red, flat lesion. It is **MOST LIKELY**

(A) angular cheilitis.

(B) erythematous candidiasis.

(C) lichen planus.

(D) leukoplakia.

145. You took the patient's blood pressure at the beginning of the examination. Based on the results, your plan of action should be to

(A) recheck the patient's blood pressure in about 5 minutes.

(B) call the patient's primary care provider for guidance.

(C) explain to the patient that her blood pressure is too high, and you cannot continue the exam.

(D) ask the patient if she is on blood pressure medication, and if so, when she last took it.

146. The lesion under the partial is **MOST LIKELY**

(A) leukoplakia.

(B) nicotine stomatitis.

(C) hairy leukoplakia.

(D) hyperkeratosis.

147. All of the following are things that should be done with the patient's partial **EXCEPT** one. Which one is the **EXCEPTION**?

(A) Place the partial in a 10 percent bleach solution or another stain-removal solution.

(B) Brush the partial after it has been in the stain-removal solution to remove residues.

(C) Scale remaining calculus deposits using an abrasive dentifrice.

(D) Remove dental biofilm from the partial with solution or instrumentation.

148. A Gracey curet 1/2 should be used **BECAUSE** this patient has subgingival calculus deposits.

(A) Both the statement and reason are correct and related.

(B) Both the statement and reason are correct and NOT related.

(C) The statement is correct, but the reason is NOT.

(D) The statement is NOT correct, but the reason is correct.

149. This patient is not at risk for caries **BECAUSE** of infrequent denture removal.

(A) Both the statement and reason are correct and related.

(B) Both the statement and reason are correct and NOT related.

(C) The statement is correct, but the reason is NOT.

(D) The statement and reason are both incorrect.

150. Which of the following **BEST** describes why the patient is experiencing irritation under her partial?

(A) It is common for a partial to cause irritation after age 10.

(B) The fit of the partial may have changed, and is irritating the lesion.

(C) The partial never fit well and has taken this long to cause irritation.

(D) Osteoporosis often leads to bone loss, and bone loss causes irritation.

ANSWER KEY AND EXPLANATIONS

Component A

1. C	41. A	81. C	121. C	161. E
2. C	42. B	82. B	122. E	162. C
3. D	43. A	83. D	123. A	163. A
4. D	44. D	84. C	124. B	164. E
5. A	45. A	85. A	125. E	165. D
6. A	46. A	86. C	126. C	166. C
7. A	47. D	87. C	127. A	167. A
8. C	48. E	88. E	128. B	168. C
9. D	49. D	89. D	129. E	169. B
10. C	50. C	90. B	130. A	170. E
11. D	51. A	91. C	131. A	171. C
12. B	52. C	92. D	132. E	172. E
13. D	53. E	93. A	133. A	173. A
14. C	54. D	94. A	134. A	174. C
15. C	55. D	95. A	135. E	175. D
16. E	56. C	96. C	136. B	176. A
17. E	57. A	97. B	137. E	177. C
18. B	58. E	98. A	138. D	178. A
19. E	59. E	99. D	139. D	179. C
20. E	60. D	100. D	140. A	180. C
21. C	61. C	101. E	141. A	181. D
22. B	62. B	102. A	142. A	182. D
23. B	63. B	103. E	143. A	183. A
24. C	64. E	104. E	144. D	184. A
25. C	65. A	105. B	145. B	185. D
26. E	66. B	106. B	146. A	186. A
27. A	67. E	107. C	147. A	187. A
28. A	68. E	108. B	148. E	188. A
29. D	69. B	109. C	149. B	189. E
30. B	70. E	110. C	150. B	190. A
31. B	71. A	111. C	151. A	191. B
32. D	72. C	112. A	152. C	192. D
33. C	73. C	113. A	153. C	193. C
34. B	74. A	114. D	154. B	194. E
35. E	75. B	115. B	155. A	195. C
36. A	76. C	116. D	156. D	196. C
37. A	77. B	117. C	157. E	197. D
38. D	78. C	118. C	158. E	198. D
39. E	79. C	119. E	159. E	199. D
40. A	80. C	120. C	160. E	200. B

1. **The correct answer is (C).** Hepatitis D can only be contacted in the presence of hepatitis B. Both hepatitis B and D can be contacted through infected blood and are sometimes passed from an infected mother to her baby. Hepatitis D can cause liver failure in extreme cases.

2. **The correct answer is (C).** The first measurement of attached gingival is from the CEJ to the muco-gingival line, but the second measurement is from the CEJ to the base of the gingival pocket. Then you subtract the second measurement from the first to find the amount of attached gingiva.

3. **The correct answer is (D).** During the lag phase of bacterial replication, bacteria grow and mature, but they do not yet divide. After bacteria mature, they enter the log phase and begin to replicate at a high rate.

4. **The correct answer is (D).** Discovery learning uses an indirect format to guide the learner to use logic to come to the right conclusion. One possible disadvantage of using discovery learning as a dental health education method is that students must be guided towards the correct conclusions. Another disadvantage is that the learner's responses may be interpreted as guessing.

5. **The correct answer is (A).** Airway obstructions occur more easily in dental settings because patients are often in the supine position. Foreign bodies that may obstruct airways include cotton rolls, extracted teeth or fragments, restorative materials, and vomit. Several types of airway obstructions exist. A partial foreign body airway obstruction occurs when the airway is not completely blocked and the patient is able to cough forcibly and speak. A partial foreign body airway obstruction with air exchange occurs when the patient is unable to cough forcibly and wheezing occurs when the patient inhales. A complete foreign body airway obstruction blocks the airway completely and the patient can neither speak nor breathe.

6. **The correct answer is (A).** Treatments for gastroesophageal reflux disease, which include famotidine (Pepcid AC) and ranitidine (Zantac 75), work by blocking acids secreted by the stomach. These acids can cause pain and damage the esophagus. Choices (B), (C), (D), and (E) are generic and brand names of adrenocorticosteroids used to treat asthma.

7. **The correct answer is (A).** Tooth mobility is measured during the periodontal assessment because it is a risk factor for the progression of periodontal disease and the measurement of mobility is taken by bidigital palpitation only when the teeth are occluded. When the teeth are occluded, the measurement is taken by direct observation.

8. **The correct answer is (C).** Neutrophils are specialized mobile cells within the periodontal pocket that migrate to the area of invading microbes by sensing the chemicals given off by these microbes. This process is called chemotaxis. Neutrophils are also known as polymorphonuclear leukocytes (PMNs).

9. **The correct answer is (D).** Parasitic population would be considered an agent factor of a disease state, not an environmental factor. Parasites benefit from living on or within their hosts.

10. **The correct answer is (C).** Plaque biofilm is a nonmineralized biofilm made of microorganisms and food debris. A coccus is any number of bacteria that is sphere-shaped.

11. **The correct answer is (D).** Local anesthesia blocks the perception of pain by preventing sodium from entering neurons. If the neuron cannot take in sodium, it cannot transmit nerve impulses to the brain.

12. **The correct answer is (B).** The stratified sampling method is used to achieve a proportionate representation of subgroups in a sample when their existence in the population is established.

13. **The correct answer is (D).** Phase I therapy focuses on controlling risk factors responsible for disease, which includes self-care education, diet control, antimicrobial therapy, and dental caries management.

14. **The correct answer is (C).** The primary purpose of assessing a population as part of developing a community health program is to isolate a target group. This will help define the parameters of the program.

15. **The correct answer is (C).** Zinc oxide-eugenol (ZOE) is a mixture that can irritate connective tissues and has a pH between 7 and 8. The presence of clove oil in ZOE can cause an allergic reaction.

16. **The correct answer is (E).** The cell's flagellum is a filament connected to the cell wall that allows mobility. The jelly-like substance inside the cell is the cytoplasm. A microtubule is a cylinder that supports the cell's structure.

17. **The correct answer is (E).** The first-choice agents for absence, or petit mal, seizures are ethosuximide and valproate. First-choice agents for tonic-clonic, or grand mal, seizures are carbamazepine (Tegretol), phenytoin (Dilantin), and valproate.

18. **The correct answer is (B).** The adult human body has 206 bones. At birth, humans are born with 300 bones. As we grow, some of our bones fuse together to form fewer, larger bones.

19. **The correct answer is (E).** A blunted papilla would be indicated on a periodontal assessment by drawing a straight horizontal line.

20. **The correct answer is (E).** Candidiasis is a common oral symptom only among patients suffering from acute, rather than chronic, leukemia.

21. **The correct answer is (C).** The film size varies by number. Typically, a film speed of 0 is used on children. A speed of 2 is used for adult dentitions—both periapicals and bitewings. A speed of 1 is used on mixed dentition, a number 3 on long bitewings, and a number 4 on occlusal films.

22. **The correct answer is (B).** Steroids can reduce the inflammation associated with conditions such as asthma and arthritis. This class of drugs can be used to treat arthritic TMJ disease. It will often be injected directly into the joint to provide symptom relief.

23. **The correct answer is (B).** An injury to the buccinator muscle could cause food to get trapped in the cheek, and the buccinator muscle does aid in whistling; however, these statements are unrelated. An injury to the buccinator muscle could cause food to get trapped in the check because this muscle pulls the cheek in to keep food over the surface area of the teeth.

24. **The correct answer is (C).** Calcium channel blockers reduce the movement of calcium that muscles need for contraction. Channel blockers also contribute to the contraction of gingival hyperplasia. Because research has proven that a connection between periodontal disease and coronary artery disease exists, a dental hygienist must build a rapport with patients with either coronary artery disease or periodontal disease because good oral hygiene will promote good coronary health.

25. **The correct answer is (C).** The object of a health education plan plays a vital role in dynamic teaching for students and teachers alike because it provides teachers with an organized approach for presenting given subjects and concepts in order to achieve a stated objective.

26. **The correct answer is (E).** Bimanual palpitation involves the simultaneous use of the index finger of one hand and the fingers and thumb of the other hand to move or compress the tissue of the floor of the client's mouth.

27. **The correct answer is (A).** The movements of every part of the body (gestures, expressions, etc.) and even the way people carry themselves (posture) are all part of body language. Paralanguage is how people convey meaning through the way they speak (volume, tone, placing emphasis on certain words, etc.).

28. **The correct answer is (A).** Intraoral radiographs are used to interpret and diagnose any dental conditions or diseases. The periapical and bitewing views are included in the full-mouth series. The occlusal view is not.

29. **The correct answer is (D).** The increased exposure to fluoride, through fluoridated water, fluoride supplements, fluoride dentifrices, and dental sealants, is believed to be the primary reason for the noted decrease in dental caries over the last few decades.

30. **The correct answer is (B).** Patients who are hesitant to make eye contact may have some anxieties or concerns, and may interpret a dental hygienist's hesitancy to make eye contact as a sign that he is holding something back from the patient. In general conversation, people will maintain eye contact about 25 percent of the time.

31. **The correct answer is (B).** Slander is a type of oral defamation in which untrue information about somebody is shared with a third party. Libel is also a type of defamation, but involves making untrue and potentially harmful statements about another person in writing.

32. **The correct answer is (D).** One type of intentional tort that is considered an invasion of privacy is publicity of private life, which is the legal violation the hygienist in this example committed. A dental hygienist is generally not permitted to reveal patient information without written consent, even to the patient's spouse, family, or friends.

33. **The correct answer is (C).** In certain instances, patient information can be disclosed to individuals and agencies without the patient's consent. Workers' Compensation is permitted to request and access information without requesting permission if an individual files a claim.

34. **The correct answer is (B).** To be considered competent to give consent, individuals must be of legal age and must be considered mentally competent. Oral consent is sufficient in emergency situations, but in this case the hygienist should have gotten the child's parent or guardian to sign the consent form.

35. **The correct answer is (E).** Patients with a phosphorus deficiency may have dental caries and weak bones. Phosphorus helps create and maintain bone in the body. If a patient has a phosphorus deficiency, the teeth may weaken, making dental caries more likely.

36. **The correct answer is (A).** Ethical duties dental hygienists have to clients include avoiding discriminatory actions (or ones that may be perceived as such), keeping client relationships confidential, and looking out for the welfare of clients. Choices (B), (C), and (D) are ethical duties dental hygienists have to colleagues, while choice (E) is an ethical obligation dental hygienists have to society.

37. **The correct answer is (A).** It is true that a multi-therapeutic approach to administering fluoride effectively includes topical (toothpaste), systemic (fluoridated water), and professional (gels, foams or varnishes) methods of fluoride to protect teeth against decay.

38. **The correct answer is (D).** Osseous surgery is a type of surgical modification that corrects bone defects caused by periodontitis. It involves resculpting the alveolar bone to attain a more physiologic form.

39. **The correct answer is (E).** Soft-tissue implants are not a type of dental implant since all of the metal implants used must osseointegrate into bone. Soft tissue would be used to replace diseased gingival tissue, but not bone.

40. **The correct answer is (A).** During polishing, it is best to keep the circulation motion consistent and hold the polishing instrument at a 90-degree angle when working on the occlusal tooth surfaces.

41. **The correct answer is (A).** The final state or condition the student can demonstrate following an instructional event is referred to as the terminal product. The terminal product is one of the instructional objectives important to successful instruction and learning.

42. **The correct answer is (B).** Dental hygienists have an ethical duty to the dental hygiene profession to spend time promoting the profession, working to advance the profession, and making efforts to develop a positive image of the profession (among other duties). Dental hygienists have an ethical duty to themselves as individuals to maintain a healthy lifestyle, get advice on ethical matters, and recognize their own limits (among others).

43. **The correct answer is (A).** Hyperdontia is the condition of having supernumerary teeth. These teeth are usually underdeveloped. This abnormality occurs during the initiation stage of development.

44. **The correct answer is (D).** The scaler has rigid shanks that reduce tactile sensitivity. Other reasons the scaler should not be used subgingivally are because it is so large, it may damage the gingival tissue, and its pointed tip will not adapt to the curvature of the tooth surface.

45. **The correct answer is (A).** Common dental abnormalities that occur during the cap stage include dens in dente, germination, tubercles, and fusion. Enamel pearls, a term that describes a condition in which enamel is found somewhere unusual (such as the surface of the root), usually occur during the bell stage.

46. **The correct answer is (A).** Patients with thiamin (vitamin B1) deficiencies should eat more whole grains, legumes, nuts, fish, pork, and brown rice. These foods are naturally rich in thiamin and will help the patients increase their thiamin levels.

47. **The correct answer is (D).** Psittacosis is a bacterial infection that can infect humans when they inhale dust covered in the excretions of infected birds. Psittacosis can often cause cold-like symptoms in infected humans.

48. **The correct answer is (E).** A radicular, or root-end cyst, can be treated with root canal therapy. The cysts in choices (A), (B), (C), and (D) would require surgical intervention.

49. **The correct answer is (D).** Responsibility for oral health relates to the presence of plaque and calculus, as well as inadequate parental supervision of oral health care and inadequate frequency of dental examinations.

50. **The correct answer is (C).** In time-temperature processing, optimal results will occur when the temperature is 68 degrees Fahrenheit, and the time the film should stay in the developer is 4.5 minutes.

51. **The correct answer is (A).** Discrete data can be measured using the nominal and ordinal scales.

52. **The correct answer is (C).** A root resection involves the removal of one root on a multirooted tooth while leaving the crown still intact. In both a root resection and root hemisection, in which the crown is removed, further endodontic treatment is required.

53. **The correct answer is (E).** Optimally, tooth extractions should be done between day 23 and day 28 of a woman's oral contraceptive cycle. Performing extractions during this time period minimizes the chances that the patient will develop a dry socket after the procedure.

54. **The correct answer is (D).** The pulp cavity is part of the inner tooth and is not considered part of the periodontium. The periodontium comprises the specialized tissues that surround and support the teeth.

55. **The correct answer is (D).** Photopolymerizing refers to using visible light to help cure the resin compound of a sealant to provide a smooth, colorless, and transparent surface on the tooth.

56. **The correct answer is (C).** Laws emphasize behaviors that benefit a society, while ethics emphasize moral behaviors that benefit individuals who are part of a society. Laws are related to the actual actions of individuals, while ethics are related to why individuals act the way they do.

57. **The correct answer is (A).** Both of these statements about dentin are true. Dentin makes up the majority of the tooth structure and it continues forming throughout a person's life.

58. **The correct answer is (E).** All of the substances listed are commonly found in dentifrices such as toothpaste and tooth powder. The detergents in these products assist with plaque removal because they use a foaming action to help reduce surface tension, which loosens plaque and makes it easier to remove.

59. **The correct answer is (E).** The range of vibrations per second for most ultrasonic debridement tools is usually 30,000–50,000. These vibrations are acoustical vibrations that cannot be heard by the human ear.

60. **The correct answer is (D).** During the extraoral examination, the client's thyroid gland can be assessed for symmetry and enlargement through a combination of bidigital palpation and circular compression. In addition, the patient, ideally in an upright seat position, should be asked to swallow.

61. **The correct answer is (C).** The three fingers used in the Modified Pen Grasp are the thumb, index, and middle finger. The ring finger acts as the fulcrum and rests on the tooth next to the one being examined and should be used to balance the hand.

62. **The correct answer is (B).** Periapical cemento-osseous dysplasia is most often diagnosed in patients in their mid-thirties. This diagnosis is also particularly common among females and African Americans.

63. **The correct answer is (B).** The mucobuccal fold mesial to the canine eminence is the correct penetration site to use to anesthetize the anterior superior alveolar nerve and to reduce the pain caused by needle insertion.

64. **The correct answer is (E).** Primary and secondary sources can both be useful when assessing populations and defining objectives for a community oral health program. Primary data is information that is collected through firsthand observation and experience (indices, interviews, questionnaires, etc.), while secondary data is collected by other parties (organizations that create public policies, federal agencies, etc.).

65. **The correct answer is (A).** Good objectives are specific, measurable, appropriate, realistic, and time bound. Choice (A) has a deadline (the end of the program), is measurable since a specific percentage is included, is realistic, is specific and clearly stated, and is appropriate since it is relevant to the target population's needs.

66. **The correct answer is (B).** Those responsible for designing and presenting programs should keep the principles of teaching in mind. In this case, Kim failed to remember that the audience level must be considered when choosing activities. Showing the cartoon described might be a good way to educate children about the oral health problems associated with smoking but will probably not be effective with an audience of grown men.

67. **The correct answer is (E).** Evaluation can help determine the overall success of a community program and should take place at all stages of learning. Issuing multiple-choice tests after each unit would help the oral health professionals evaluate and, if necessary, tweak their approach. Evaluation should focus on the outcomes of a program and whether it is successfully meeting the original goals. In this case, the oral health professionals would want to assess how well their program promotes awareness of smoking-related oral diseases.

68. **The correct answer is (E).** Patients with cystic fibrosis often exhibit an unusually low rate of caries and a plaque accumulation with increased calculus deposits. It is believed that this phenomenon may be related to changes in the saliva from long-term antibiotic use.

69. **The correct answer is (B).** The statement and the reason are both true but unrelated. An article that appears in a journal published by a professional society would be preferred over one appearing in a journal published by a commercial firm because of the likelihood of bias on the part of the commercial firm.

70. **The correct answer is (E).** The bacteria *Staphylococcus aureus* arrange into clumps or clusters. *Streptococcus mutans* and *Streptococcus pneumoniae* arrange themselves into chains. *Neisseria gonorrhoeae* and *Moraxella catarrhalis* arrange themselves into pairs.

71. **The correct answer is (A).** A microorganism feeding off decaying plant matter is an example of syntrophism. Syntrophism occurs when two seemingly unrelated organisms can benefit from one another.

72. **The correct answer is (C).** When the body's immune system causes inflammation, it causes redness, swelling, heat, and pain. The redness of inflammation is caused by increased blood flow at the sight of the infection or injury.

73. **The correct answer is (C).** Diuretics help rid the body of excess fluids and also act as vasodilators, which make them a useful treatment for hypertension or high blood pressure. Hypokalemia, hyperglycemia, and hyperuricemia are possible adverse reactions to diuretics.

74. **The correct answer is (A).** The bisecting technique uses geometry to determine the angle the film should be set at to the capture the correct image. In this technique, an imaginary line is drawn down the axis of the tooth with another imaginary line bisecting the imaginary line of the tooth and the angle of the film. The X-ray beam is directed perpendicular to the imaginary bisecting line.

75. **The correct answer is (B).** The cancellous bone fills in bone tissue between the cortical bone and the alveolar bone. It provides support for the bone tissue surrounding the root of the teeth.

76. **The correct answer is (C).** Dyspnea is a term used to describe an unusual respiration rate when breathing is difficult or labored. Tachycardia describes a heart rate that is greater than 100 BPM. Bradycardia describes a heart rate that is less than 60 BPM. Pulsus alternans describes heart beats that alternate between weak and strong, and premature

ventricular contractions (PVCs) is a name given to a longer than normal pause or a skip between heart beats.

77. **The correct answer is (B).** Milk or a calcium solution should be given if a large amount of fluoride is ingested. This will slow the absorption rate of the fluoride into the body until medical care can be obtained.

78. **The correct answer is (C).** Acidulated phosphate fluoride is used to strengthen tooth enamel and prevent tooth decay and caries. Ideally, it should be applied once every 6 months during a routine dental checkup.

79. **The correct answer is (C).** The dental hygiene profession is governed by several core values. Aside from the responsibility to protect clients and minimize harm (nonmaleficence), other core values include justice and fairness (choice (A)), veracity (choice (B)), confidentiality (choice (D)), and individual autonomy and respect for human beings (choice (E)).

80. **The correct answer is (C).** A vitamin K deficiency can cause bleeding disorders in some patients because vitamin K helps clot blood. People with too little vitamin K can bleed too much, so vitamin K deficiencies should be treated appropriately.

81. **The correct answer is (C).** Lines or stripes of Retzius indicate a gradual change in enamel. Retzius are incremental lines that may have a brown appearance. They are striations on the enamel rods that develop over time.

82. **The correct answer is (B).** The first statement describes an epidemic, whereas the second statement describes an endemic.

83. **The correct answer is (D).** The vessel that has the greatest pressure is the aorta. The pressure within vessels lessens as they become smaller and as they move farther away from the heart. The aorta is connected directly to the heart and has the highest pressure.

84. **The correct answer is (C).** The genioglossus muscle protrudes and depresses the tongue. This muscle runs from the chin to the tongue.

85. **The correct answer is (A).** Both of these statements are true. The glands of the head and neck aid in digestion through the production of saliva and strengthen the immune system by protecting the body from invading pathogens.

86. **The correct answer is (C).** The frontal sinuses drain through the middle nasal meatus. It is located between the middle and inferior conchae.

87. **The correct answer is (C).** The mandibular second premolars are the **MOST LIKELY** to have abnormalities. The third molars are also prone to abnormalities, such as anodontia.

88. **The correct answer is (E).** The presence of an excess number of roots is a characteristic of supernumerary roots. The most common teeth affected by this condition include the mandibular canines, premolars, and molars.

89. **The correct answer is (D).** The medulla oblongata is part of the central nervous system, not the peripheral nervous system. The medulla oblongata does regulate the respiratory system and circulatory system.

90. **The correct answer is (B).** Gout can be treated with a low-protein diet, along with medications. High-protein diets increase potassium in the body, but this does not have any impact on gout. A low-protein diet is effective because it decreases the amount of uric acid in the body, which in excess can cause gout.

91. **The correct answer is (C).** The status quo refers to the existing state of affairs within a population. The best way to gauge the status quo is through a written questionnaire. This method allows the researcher to reach a large number of people in a relatively short amount of time.

92. **The correct answer is (D).** A basic emergency kit must include injectable and noninjectable drugs as well as oxygen. Noninjectable drugs that must be included in a basic emergency kit include nitroglycerin for angina attacks, a bronchodilator, which is an asthma inhaler, a glucose source such as oral glucose gel, and aspirin, which prevents additional platelet activation and helps during cardiac events. Injectable drugs that must be included in a basic

emergency kit include epinephrine, also known as an EpiPen, and diphenhydramine, which is also known as Benadryl. Oxygen with positive pressure administration capabilities must also be present in a basic emergency kit.

93. **The correct answer is (A).** Gram staining is affected by the chemical and physical properties of bacteria's cell walls. The staining method divides cells into two large groups—Gram-positive and Gram-negative cells.

94. **The correct answer is (A).** Cheilitis is the swelling of the lips. This condition is usually accompanied by redness and by fissures or cracks in the lips or the angles of the mouth.

95. **The correct answer is (A).** Rett syndrome is a neurological condition caused by a genetic mutation and is not an autosomal dominant disorder. Autosomal dominant disorders, such as Huntington disease, are often passed from parents to children and people of both sexes are equally likely to be affected.

96. **The correct answer is (C).** A full-mouth debridement is a procedure that is used to remove hard and soft deposits on tooth structure. This is typically the first step in addressing periodontitis. Occlusal equilibrations and bacterial cultures are part of the first step in managing the disease only if the condition is chronic or aggressive. Scaling and root planing and prescribing antibiotics are done during subsequent visits.

97. **The correct answer is (B).** A type of graph that is used to depict interval- or ratio-scaled variables that are continuous in nature is called a histogram.

98. **The correct answer is (A).** Couples who are predisposed to genetic disorders should be referred to genetic counseling because genetic counseling involves determining genetic risks in future offspring. Genetic counseling is also important because it can confirm, diagnose, or rule out certain genetic disorders. Furthermore, it can provide psychological support.

99. **The correct answer is (D).** Concrescence is a dental defect in which a fusion takes place after root formation has been completed. This condition can also occur after a trauma or in the case of crowding.

100. **The correct answer is (D).** The hygienist's report indicates that the patient has excellent oral hygiene and no other signs or symptoms of periodontal disease. Therefore, his swollen gums are **MOST LIKELY** caused by the medication he recently started taking for his hypertension, as indicated in his medical history. Certain medications, such as the calcium channel blockers sometimes prescribed for hypertension, can cause gingival hyperplasia, or swollen gums.

101. **The correct answer is (E).** A PSR (periodontal screening and reporting) score of 0 indicates that no deposits were found. A higher PSR score indicates that plaque, calculus, or both are present and serves as evidence of periodontal disease.

102. **The correct answer is (A).** The plaque index (PI) is used to assess how much plaque a patient has on his or her teeth and is a good indicator of how well the patient cares for his or her teeth at home. A PI score of 0 is considered "Excellent." The calculus index (CI-S) is used to assess the amount of calculus a patient has. A score of 0.0 to 0.6 is considered "Good," the highest rating on this scale.

103. **The correct answer is (E).** A normal pulse rate, or heart rate, for an adult is 60–100. While a heart rate of 108 is considered normal for toddlers and school-age children, it's above average for an adult. A heart rate of 108 for an infant is considered low.

104. **The correct answer is (E).** Examining the hard and soft palate should be completed during the oral evaluation, not during the examination of the head and neck.

105. **The correct answer is (B).** Freedom from respiratory difficulties is not one of the eight human needs related to oral health and disease. The other needs not listed here include freedom from anxiety and stress, freedom from head and neck pain, responsibility for oral health, and conceptualization and understanding.

106. **The correct answer is (B).** The safelight bulb used to light a darkroom should be 15 watts or less with a red filter. The safelight should be at least 4 feet from the film. It is important to have the right amount of light in the correct position in the room in order to not damage the film.

107. The correct answer is (C). Patients with Parkinson's disease may encounter problems with dental prosthesis retention because of the side effects from medications used to treat conditions such as dry mouth, or xerostomia, not because of reduced oral motor functions and personal hygiene skills.

108. The correct answer is (B). When the patient's chin is tilted upward, the radiograph will produce a "frown" that will obscure the maxillary anterior teeth and make them difficult to view.

109. The correct answer is (C). Fluoride treatments are an integral part of a dental caries prevention strategy, and neutral fluoride is a suitable option for people with veneers and crowns, people undergoing chemotherapy, and people who have xerostomia. Stannous fluoride is available in gel or rinse form and can cause gingival sloughing following treatment.

110. The correct answer is (C). The greater the dispersion of the scores around the mean of the distribution, the greater the standard deviation and variance will be.

111. The correct answer is (C). To floss effectively, individuals should wrap floss around each interproximal tooth surface so that the floss has a "C" shape. Floss should gently be pushed into the embrasure and below the gingival margin. An up-and-down motion should be used to clean interproximal surfaces, and the type of floss a patient decides to use is largely a matter of personal preference.

112. The correct answer is (A). Accumulated radiation in the body accelerates the normal aging process.

113. The correct answer is (A). Chewing gum may help prevent dental caries because it increases the production of saliva, which can lower the acidity of the oral cavity. High acidity in the oral cavity is linked to caries formation. Xylitol is a sugar-free sweetener that can also play a role in preventing dental caries.

114. The correct answer is (D). Macrophages are cells that perform phagocytosis to ingest or engulf microbes. They are also attracted to the site of microbe infection by chemotaxis.

115. The correct answer is (B). Ultrasonic debridement tools are generally 0.3–0.6 mm wide, rather than 0.75–1.0 mm wide. Handheld tools, such as curettes, are larger and measure about 0.75–1.0 mm wide.

116. The correct answer is (D). The treatment for syncope, or fainting, is to place a patient in the Trendelenburg position. The Trendelenburg position requires the patient to lie down, usually in a dental chair, with her feet elevated higher than her head. Pregnant patients should lie on either side before their feet are elevated.

117. The correct answer is (C). Acidulated phosphate fluoride (APF) gels strengthen tooth enamel. APF gels demineralize acids on the outer layer of enamel and accelerate remineralization to prevent caries.

118. The correct answer is (C). The first statement is true and the second statement is false. While amalgam dental filling is a mixture of metal powders triturated with mercury and does give off a miniscule amount of mercury vapor, it has not been proven as a health risk to most patients. It can be harmful, however, to patients with a mercury allergy.

119. The correct answer is (E). Neither the statement nor the reason is correct. Ultrasonic cleaning should not be performed on a dental implant because this procedure may result in severe scratching of the implant. Scratches on an implant's surface can harbor bacteria.

120. The correct answer is (C). Certain universal moral principles can be applied to almost every situation to make ethical decisions, and veracity is one of them. The principle states that both the patient and health-care provider must be truthful with each other, and the hygienist is violating it by incorrectly stating that general anesthesia has no risks.

121. The correct answer is (C). The density and the kVp remain the same, so they are not a factor here. The formula is:

$$\frac{\text{old mA} \times \text{old impulse}}{\text{new mA}} = \text{new impulse}$$

$$\frac{18 \times 8}{12} = 24 \text{ impulses}$$

122. The correct answer is (E). A dental hygienist should avoid speaking too loudly when interacting with patients on an individual basis because it can seem like they are lecturing the patient. Hygienists can help patients understand their message by clearly explaining technical terms and not presenting the client with too much information at once.

123. The correct answer is (A). Hepatitis A commonly occurs in children and young adults and is often transmitted through contaminated water and food. Rarely, hepatitis A is transmitted through blood. Hepatitis B and Hepatitis D (choices (B) and (D)) are spread in a number of ways, including through blood and other body fluids.

124. The correct answer is (B). Primary strategies are preventive in nature, and may include applying dental sealants or removing biofilm. Secondary strategies such as performing oral cancer screenings are designed to spot diseases and begin treatment early, while tertiary strategies (such as fillings) are designed to halt the destruction of tissues and possibly restore function.

125. The correct answer is (E). When researchers examine a disease based on the number of new cases of the disease that occur within a particular population over a certain period of time, they are studying the disease in terms of its incidence. An incidence is typically expressed as a portion or ratio.

126. The correct answer is (C). The epithelial proliferations give rise to the salivary glands, which produce saliva and secrete enzymes.

127. The correct answer is (A). Patients who have too much vitamin A in their bodies often exhibit symptoms such as cracking and bleeding lips and bone hypertrophy. Patients with vitamin A toxicity can be treated by significantly decreasing their intake of vitamin A.

128. The correct answer is (B). Informed consent is an important ethical principle in the dental hygiene profession, and obtaining it involves providing information regarding the diagnosis, prognosis if left untreated, other possible courses of treatment, and the benefits and risks of a specific treatment. The patient should also be asked to sign a consent form written using non-technical language.

129. The correct answer is (E). When working with hemihydrates, the highest-strength stone requires the least amount of water. Too much water prolongs setting time and creates a weaker cast. Too little water results in increased expansion. The ideal amount of water is between 19–24 mL/100 g powder.

130. The correct answer is (A). Too much fluoride can lead to a condition known as dental fluorosis. Dental fluorosis is characterized by white streaks or specks on the enamel of the teeth, and it is caused by excessive amounts of fluoride over an extended period of time.

131. The correct answer is (A). Both statements are true. The first periodontal ligaments to be lost in periodontal disease are alveolar crest fibers, which connect cementum to alveolar crest bone. The interradicular fibers connect cementum to another cementum in instances of multirooted teeth.

132. The correct answer is (E). If the source-to-film distance becomes closer, the central ray becomes smaller and more powerful. Because of this, a decrease in exposure time is needed to produce a clearer image.

133. The correct answer is (A). Anticoagulants reduce the clotting ability of blood and are used to treat a variety of conditions associated with excessive clotting, including myocardial infarction, thrombophlebitis, atrial fibrillation, and embolisms. Von Willebrand disease reduces the clotting ability of blood, so an anticoagulant would not be a beneficial treatment for this condition.

134. The correct answer is (A). Chronic inflammatory diseases often to lead to fibrosis and scar tissue because the harmful stimuli are never removed and persistent tissue damage occurs.

135. The correct answer is (E). Infective endocarditis is an infection that is usually caused by microbes already present in the body, and any injuries to the heart make it more susceptible to infection. Drug abuse, heart-valve surgery, clogged arteries, and scarring on the heart valves are all factors that predispose patients to infective endocarditis. Arrhythmia, however, is not a risk factor for infective endocarditis because it is not an injury of the heart.

136. **The correct answer is (B).** Tongue piercings can lead to infections that can result in Ludwig angina, which causes the floor of the mouth to become infected. Other serious oral risks associated with tongue piercings include fractured teeth and nerve damage.

137. **The correct answer is (E).** Interdental brushes that are coated with plastic can be used on open embrasures, which are a common consequence of orthodontic treatment. Implant prostheses can be maintained using yarn, tufted floss, and floss threaders, and patients can employ the Bass method with a manual or rotary toothbrush.

138. **The correct answer is (D).** One of the main drawbacks of dental implants is that they can be scratched quite easily, and these compromised areas will serve as breeding grounds for bacteria. Ultrasonic cleaning is not used on those with dental implants because it can cause serious scratching, so air polishers are typically used for the purposes of stain removal.

139. **The correct answer is (D).** Sealants are not a replacement for fluoride treatments, but they can complement them by protecting tooth surfaces that fluoride cannot. Sealants are used to seal the pits and grooves that characterize the occlusal surfaces of the teeth, something that can help reduce the risk of carious lesions.

140. **The correct answer is (A).** Bruxism is a tooth abnormality that is specifically caused by the grinding of teeth. It is a form of attrition.

141. **The correct answer is (A).** In order to complete an adequate periodontal assessment, 10–20 grams of pressure is needed during probing of the gingival sulcus.

142. **The correct answer is (A).** When recording periodontal assessment factors, a blue X drawn over a tooth would indicate a missing tooth.

143. **The correct answer is (A).** Erosion is wear caused by chemical wear. There are a number of common foods and beverages, including fruits and soft drinks, that can cause erosion of the enamel.

144. **The correct answer is (D).** Situations in which a dental hygienist must violate the ethical principle of confidentiality and disclose information about patients do exist. Communicable diseases (TB is an example, diabetes is not), knife and gunshot wounds, suspected abuse of children or senior citizens, threats of self-harm, and threats of inflicting harm on others must all be reported to the authorities.

145. **The correct answer is (B).** Low-level disinfectants are able to kill vegetative bacteria as well as select viruses and fungi. The Centers for Disease Control and Prevention permit the use of low-level disinfectants to clean clinical contact surfaces if they can kill HIV and the hepatitis B virus, and are hospital disinfectants registered with the Environmental Protection Agency.

146. **The correct answer is (A).** Operator error is **MOST LIKELY** the reason if a sealant fails. Oil, debris, or moisture contamination in addition to not following manufacturer's instructions can all lead to a sealant not being applied properly by a dentist or dental hygienist.

147. **The correct answer is (A).** The gingiva adjoins the oral mucosa at the muscogingival junction, the definitive line that alters the texture of the tissue into a more relaxed mucosa.

148. **The correct answer is (E).** Many dental drugs are safe for pregnant women, including amoxicillin, lidocaine, penicillin, and epinephrine in limited amounts. Drugs such as metronidazole, nitrous oxide, NSAIDs, and aspirin should be avoided when treating expectant mothers.

149. **The correct answer is (B).** Tissue from the palate within the mouth is the tissue that most resembles gingival tissue. Therefore it is used frequently as a donor site to support free soft-tissue grafts of diseased gingival tissue.

150. **The correct answer is (B).** The maxillary sinus is a radiolucent landmark. In a radiograph, the maxillary sinus appears as a dark area on the film. Genial tubercles, mandibular tori, nasal septum, and maxillary tuberosity are radiopaque landmarks because they appear as light areas on radiographs.

151. **The correct answer is (A).** If a client answers yes when asked if he or she has night sweats, this response may be an indication that he or she may have a current or past history of tuberculosis.

152. **The correct answer is (C).** A patient who presents with angular cheilitis, pallor or atrophy of the oral tissues, and a sore tongue is exhibiting the classic oral signs of iron-deficiency anemia. Anemia is a condition in which the blood has an abnormally small amount of healthy red blood cells.

153. **The correct answer is (C).** The thyroid is the first endocrine gland to develop. The thyroid develops in the fourth week of gestation. It begins in the foramen cecum of the tongue and moves downward during the fifth week of development.

154. **The correct answer is (B).** Anthracyclines work by forming free radicals that inhibit DNA production and function. Examples of anthracyclines include Daunorubicin and Doxorubicin.

155. **The correct answer is (A).** The spleen is part of the lymphatic system. The spleen works to filter the blood and fight off infection. All of the other organs are part of the digestive system.

156. **The correct answer is (D).** When a patient refuses treatment, he or she must fill out an informed refusal form. An informed refusal form should include all of the above, except for a client statement explaining refusal of service.

157. **The correct answer is (E).** Teleological ethics focuses on the outcomes or consequences of actions and whether they are beneficial for a large number of individuals. If the hygienist's actions convinced a large number of students to start flossing (a positive outcome), those actions would be considered ethical according to the principles of teleological ethics.

158. **The correct answer is (E).** It is necessary to make an initial impression using a rocking motion when using silicone as the impression material. When you rock the initial impression as you position it into place, you create an open space around the tooth for wash material to be applied along with the final impression.

159. **The correct answer is (E).** A healthy oral cavity can help an individual maintain good overall health, while poor oral health can contribute to problems such as diabetes, heart disease, and low birth weight in infants. The dental hygiene professional should stress this connection to all clients.

160. **The correct answer is (E).** A large sample size is preferable to a small one because a large sample size reduces the standard error of the sample mean.

161. **The correct answer is (E).** Stannous fluoride has been approved by the ADA for its ability to deliver fluoride for the protection of teeth against cavities. However, it is not an accepted method by the ADA to reduce bacteria and gingivitis-reducing properties.

162. **The correct answer is (C).** The first statement is true. An autograft is a bone graft used to stimulate regeneration of bone when the bone is taken from the patient itself. The second statement is false. An alloplast is when synthetic bone is made and used to repair diseased bone. A xenograft is when bone from another animal species is used to replace degenerated human bone.

163. **The correct answer is (A).** Four components of the health belief model can help predict whether patients will act on dental health advice: susceptibility (the patient is at risk), severity (the outcomes are serious), the asymptomatic nature of disease (disease can be present without the patient knowing it), and the belief that changing the behavior will directly benefit the patient. The belief that a condition can be cured easily would not likely prompt patients to take a dental hygienist's health advice.

164. **The correct answer is (E).** Sealants act as a physical barrier to bacteria and debris in the mouth. Because back teeth are characterized by pits and grooves, they do not benefit from fluoride as smooth surfaces do. Sealants are a way to protect the teeth from settlement of bacteria to prevent dental caries.

165. **The correct answer is (D).** Common symptoms of eating disorders are erosion of tooth enamel, xerostomia (dry mouth), and goose bumps. Patients with eating disorders should generally be treated for their conditions by a psychologist or a physician.

166. **The correct answer is (C).** Body posture is an essential part of effective communication for those in the dental hygiene profession. Leaning forward while seated conveys attentiveness, leaning backward conveys a lack of empathy, and crossing the arms places a barrier between the hygienist and the patient.

167. **The correct answer is (A).** A study that follows a selected group of participants over an extended period of time to identify some change or development within the group is referred to as longitudinal. Longitudinal studies can be more than thirty years.

168. **The correct answer is (C).** Grand Rapids, Michigan, adjusted the fluoride level of its water supply to 1.0 parts per million and became the first city to administer community water fluoridation.

169. **The correct answer is (B).** On a radiograph, a periapical pathological condition may often be mistaken for the mental foramen, which is located inferior to mandibular premolar apices.

170. **The correct answer is (E).** A dental hygiene professional should avoid using technical jargon when communicating with patients because it can make them feel insecure and confused. Instead, the dental hygiene professional should clearly explain complex medical terms and use simpler words in place of more complex ones whenever possible.

171. **The correct answer is (C).** While clients who have undergone cardiac or vascular corrective surgery are susceptible to transient bacteremias, these clients must be given prophylactic antibiotic premedication for only up to 6 months after surgery.

172. **The correct answer is (E).** When dental hygiene professionals provide health advice, they should avoid both verbal messages and nonverbal cues that are authoritarian in nature. Instead, they should encourage the patient's involvement and encourage them to take responsibility for their own oral health.

173. **The correct answer is (A).** The mandible is the only bone in the skull with a moveable joint. The other bones in the skull are held together at immovable joints.

174. **The correct answer is (C).** A chair that has a firm stuffing and feel would not help prevent the spread of infection. The design of a dental office and the equipment it contains can help with infection-control efforts. Aside from the guidelines for choosing a chair mentioned in choices (A), (B), (D), and (E), dental offices should also look for items that do not contain knobs and hooks; look for sink faucets that can be operated with a foot pedal or electronically; and choose cabinets and counters made out of plastic laminate.

175. **The correct answer is (D).** Certain agents, including epinephrine, steroids, and analgesics, contain opioids that can reduce the amount of insulin released by the body or increase the body's insulin requirements. Caution should be used when administering these agents to patients with diabetes.

176. **The correct answer is (A).** Administering a vasoconstrictor, which contracts the smooth muscle in blood vessels, to a patient who is currently taking antidepressants may lead to a hypertensive crisis. A hypertensive crisis is a severe increase in blood pressure and can lead to stroke.

177. **The correct answer is (C).** A good instructional objective should include performance, conditions, criterion, and time components. These factors tell you what the learner is expected to be able to do (performance), describe the conditions under which the performance will occur (conditions), explain the conditions for an acceptable performance (criterion), and outline a time frame in which the learner is expected to perform adequately (time). Method describes the techniques that instructors use to impart information to the learner, and it is not a part of an instructional objective.

178. **The correct answer is (A).** The effects of radiation can be measured in a variety of ways. One way is to measure the amount of radiation absorbed in rads, which stands for radiation absorbed dose. Other units used to measure radiation include the Roentgen and rems (roentgen-equivalent-man).

179. **The correct answer is (C).** Fibrous dysplasia, which is a condition that presents with a swelling of the bone, occurs more frequently in the mandible than in the maxilla in oral cases.

180. **The correct answer is (C).** Tooth-to-tooth wear observed during an occlusal evaluation is known as attrition.

181. **The correct answer is (D).** Although the kidneys do remove waste from the blood, the nephrons are the tiny units inside the kidney that are actually responsible for removing waste. Each kidney has about a million nephrons.

182. **The correct answer is (D).** Thorazine is a low-potency antipsychotic; an example of a high-potency antipsychotic is Haldol. Dyskinesia is a side effect of antipsychotics in which individuals experience uncontrolled movement of the tongue and face. It is a dental concern because it could prevent individuals from performing proper dental care at home.

183. **The correct answer is (A).** Toxic shock syndrome, which is an infection caused by the bacteria *Staphylococcus aureus*, is characterized by violent nausea with vomiting and diarrhea, a rash, and convulsions. This infection does not, however, cause a fever.

184. **The correct answer is (A).** A dental hygienist performing a type 2 assessment examination would make use of all of these except percussion. Percussion would only be used in a type 1 assessment examination.

185. **The correct answer is (D).** While a well-written article must be based on an adequate and clearly stated hypothesis, it need not necessarily utilize both current and classic references. Current references are a must, but classic references are generally optional.

186. **The correct answer is (A).** Syncope, which is also known as fainting, is the most common emergency that occurs in dental offices. Syncope is most commonly caused by a lack of consciousness. A loss of consciousness is most often related to the lack of oxygen reaching the brain. A major cause for decreased oxygen to the brain is stress, which can be brought on by bad news, unpleasant smells, and the sight of blood, needles, or other apparatuses used in a dental office.

187. **The correct answer is (A).** When removing a mask, the dental hygiene professional should grasp the strings or elastic on the mask as opposed to the portion that actually covers the face. Guidelines for mask use other than the ones mentioned in choices (B) through (E) include changing the mask every 20 to 30 minutes, refraining from touching the mask during a procedure, and leaving the mask on after a procedure to help minimize the risk of inhaling aerosols.

188. **The correct answer is (A).** The deductive and inductive reasoning approaches to diagnosis both yield specific information about the patient's oral condition, but each does so differently. Using deductive reason, a dental hygienist would make a determination about the patient's condition based on common generalizations associated with oral health. Using inductive reasoning, the dental hygienist would make such a determination based on possible patterns that may emerge during oral observations.

189. **The correct answer is (E).** Antineoplastic agents are drugs used to combat the development of cancer cells. They destroy both malignant and normal cells and they affect cells with the fastest life cycles.

190. **The correct answer is (A).** Syphilis is caused by the bacteria *Treponemapallidum*. This disease has four distinct phases: primary, secondary, latent, and tertiary.

191. **The correct answer is (B).** An inadequate amount of attached gingiva should be indicated on a periodontal assessment when the measurement of attached gingiva is equal to or less than 1 mm.

192. **The correct answer is (D).** Tongue scrapers are an effective way to remove bacteria and prevent or manage halitosis, but the patient should be instructed to concentrate on the posterior (back) portion of the tongue surface. Interdental brushes, toothbrushes, and tooth scrapers should all be discussed during an educational session focusing on strategies to prevent halitosis.

193. **The correct answer is (C).** The paired t-test is the inferential statistical technique used to determine if a statistically significant difference exists between two related samples.

194. **The correct answer is (E).** Choice (E) is false because the more specialized in function a cell is, the more resistant it is to the biologic effects of radiation.

195. **The correct answer is (C).** Cognitive treatment plan goals should be focused on increasing the client's level of knowledge about oral health.

196. **The correct answer is (C).** Patients with multiple sclerosis should not be treated with nitrous oxide because nitrous oxide acts as a dilator and lowers blood pressure, which can lead to the loss of nerve function.

197. **The correct answer is (D).** A monosaccharide is the simplest form of sugar and cannot be broken down into a simpler sugar. A disaccharide is a sugar made up of two monosaccharides. The disaccharide sucrose is formed when the monosaccharide glucose and fructose link together.

198. **The correct answer is (D).** Utility gloves are tough, reusable gloves that are suitable to use when dealing with contaminated instruments and preparing chemicals. Nonsterile and ambidextrous gloves can be used for protection during most routine procedures; sterile gloves are used for surgical procedures; and overgloves are placed over regular gloves to avoid cross contamination of surfaces.

199. **The correct answer is (D).** Occlusal caries are able to be seen and diagnosed best through clinical examination because they do not appear on radiographs until they are large.

200. **The correct answer is (B).** It is true that fluoride can prevent and even reverse tooth decay, but it is not because fluorides are present naturally in water and soil. It is because fluorides obtained through systemic and topical methods are a preventive tool against caries and further decay.

Component B

1. A	31. A	61. D	91. D	121. C
2. A	32. D	62. D	92. D	122. B
3. D	33. B	63. C	93. C	123. D
4. D	34. D	64. C	94. B	124. B
5. C	35. B	65. A	95. D	125. D
6. A	36. B	66. B	96. C	126. C
7. C	37. D	67. C	97. D	127. C
8. B	38. C	68. B	98. B	128. D
9. D	39. B	69. C	99. D	129. D
10. C	40. D	70. C	100. B	130. B
11. D	41. D	71. C	101. C	131. D
12. B	42. C	72. D	102. D	132. C
13. D	43. D	73. C	103. D	133. A
14. D	44. B	74. C	104. C	134. D
15. D	45. A	75. A	105. C	135. A
16. B	46. B	76. B	106. C	136. D
17. B	47. C	77. C	107. D	137. D
18. C	48. C	78. B	108. D	138. D
19. B	49. C	79. A	109. C	139. C
20. B	50. D	80. C	110. D	140. A
21. D	51. A	81. A	111. B	141. A
22. C	52. B	82. A	112. D	142. D
23. B	53. D	83. C	113. D	143. B
24. D	54. C	84. C	114. D	144. B
25. D	55. A	85. A	115. D	145. A
26. A	56. D	86. B	116. C	146. D
27. D	57. C	87. B	117. D	147. C
28. C	58. A	88. D	118. C	148. A
29. C	59. A	89. C	119. D	149. D
30. C	60. D	90. B	120. D	150. B

1. **The correct answer is (A).** This patient is likely to be the least fatigued early in the morning. He will be most comfortable sitting in the dental chair during this time.

2. **The correct answer is (A).** ADHD patients are no more nervous than other patients. Their nervousness depends on their personality. Restlessness, frequently wanting to get up, and excessive talking are characteristic of patients with ADHD.

3. **The correct answer is (D).** This patient drinks coffee with sugar and does not practice good oral hygiene. These behaviors are **MOST LIKELY** responsible for his increase in dental caries.

4. **The correct answer is (D).** Bruxism, the grinding of teeth, and dysgeusia, a distorted sense of taste, and xerostomia, a dry mouth, are all side effects of stimulants such as Adderall.

5. **The correct answer is (C).** You should only give this patient brief instructions, and you should give these instructions one at a time.

6. **The correct answer is (A).** ADHD patients are known to become easily addicted to smoking;

therefore, quitting smoking is the most important action to improve this patient's health.

7. **The correct answer is (C).** According to this patient's dental chart, he has a carious lesion on tooth #5.

8. **The correct answer is (B).** According to this patient's dental chart, he is missing tooth #16.

9. **The correct answer is (D).** A teen between the ages of 13 and 15 usually has blood pressure of about 120/70, so this patient's blood pressure is normal.

10. **The correct answer is (C).** While the stains on his teeth could be from drinking coffee and smoking, this patient doesn't smoke often, and he drinks a lot of coffee. Therefore, the stains are **MOST LIKELY** from drinking coffee.

11. **The correct answer is (D).** The patient's symptoms and examination indicate that he has necrotizing ulcerative gingivitis (NUG), which affects only the gums. Necrotizing ulcerative periodontitis (NUP) affects both the gums and surrounding bone.

12. **The correct answer is (B).** You should not inquire into the patient's personal life. Your questions should relate to his condition only.

13. **The correct answer is (D).** The patient has necrotizing ulcerative gingivitis (NUG). Factors leading to this condition include poor nutrition, poor oral hygiene, infections of the mouth, and stress.

14. **The correct answer is (D).** Tooth discoloration is not a symptom of necrotizing ulcerative gingivitis (NUG). Symptoms other than those listed in the answer options include bad breath, gums that bleed easily, a gray film on the gums, and swollen glands.

15. **The correct answer is (D).** The patient should be instructed to keep his mouth clean, refrain from smoking or drinking alcohol, rinse with warm salt water, and use a prescription antibacterial mouthwash containing chlorhexidine. The patient may also be prescribed antibiotics.

16. **The correct answer is (B).** Scaling and root planing are usually performed on a second visit, when some of the patient's symptoms have begun to subside.

17. **The correct answer is (B).** Necrotizing ulcerative gingivitis (NUG) is caused by a bacterial infection.

18. **The correct answer is (C).** While a vitamin deficiency is a risk factor for necrotizing ulcerative gingivitis (NUG), there is no indication that an excess of vitamin A may put someone at risk.

19. **The correct answer is (B).** Necrotizing ulcerative gingivitis (NUG) affects only the gums and not the surrounding bone.

20. **The correct answer is (B).** If your patient follows instructions, his condition should be cured in about 2 to 3 weeks.

21. **The correct answer is (D).** Your patient has a sore mouth, but no ulcers. According to the World Health Organization, this is a grade 1 mucositis assessment.

22. **The correct answer is (C).** The American Heart Association (AHA) classifies this patient's blood pressure as Stage 1, which has a systolic range of 140–159 and a diastolic range of 90–99.

23. **The correct answer is (B).** Patients take Imitrex to reduce the symptoms of migraines.

24. **The correct answer is (D).** According to the dental chart, the patient has a dental lesion on tooth #19.

25. **The correct answer is (D).** Tooth decay, oral pain, and gingivitis are all side effects of chemotherapy. Other side effects include oral mucositis, and infections in the mouth or mouth lining.

26. **The correct answer is (A).** Patients undergoing chemotherapy should use an alcohol-free mouthwash.

27. **The correct answer is (D).** Clonazepam is used to treat anxiety and is not a treatment for oral mucositis.

28. **The correct answer is (C).** Oral cancers occur most often on the floor of the mouth.

29. **The correct answer is (C).** Chemotherapy causes xerostomia because it reduces the amount of saliva in the mouth. This, in turn, causes dental caries.

30. **The correct answer is (C).** Because patients who have undergone chemotherapy have a higher-than-average risk of tooth decay, you should recommend that your patient brush her teeth after each meal.

31. **The correct answer is (A).** Some high blood pressure mediation can cause xerostomia, or dry mouth. A lack of saliva increases a patient's risk of developing dental caries.

32. **The correct answer is (D).** This patient has Stage 2 hypertension, which means systolic blood pressure is 160 or higher, and her diastolic pressure is 100 or higher.

33. **The correct answer is (B).** According to this patient's dental chart, she has a visible carious lesion on tooth #3.

34. **The correct answer is (D).** A patient's oral hygiene does not put her at risk of hypertension.

35. **The correct answer is (B).** According to this patient's dental chart, she is missing the following teeth: #1, #5, #16, #17, #18, #19, #22, and #32.

36. **The correct answer is (B).** This patient's condition falls under the classification of Type II: Moderate chronic periodontitis. Her pocket depths are 3–4 mm.

37. **The correct answer is (D).** This patient is at risk for abscess of the gingival or the jaw bones, tooth loss, severe periodontitis, as well as ulceration of the gums.

38. **The correct answer is (C).** You would use both periodontal probing and radiographs to look for signs of periodontitis in this patient.

39. **The correct answer is (B).** This patient's blood pressure is dangerously high. She should first be referred to her physician.

40. **The correct answer is (D).** This patient's gums should be treated with root planing, scaling, mouthwashes containing chlorhexidine as well as flossing and interdental brushing.

41. **The correct answer is (D).** You should ask your patient's mother each question in the answer options. You should also inquire how to best manage an attack, should your patient have one.

42. **The correct answer is (C).** You should only inject the patient with epinephrine if his bronchodilator is not working.

43. **The correct answer is (D).** Tooth enamel dust, fissure sealants, and dentifrices may cause your patient to suffer an asthma attack. In addition, methyl methacrylate and fluoride trays and cotton rolls might also exacerbate your patient's asthma.

44. **The correct answer is (B).** Rubber dams might irritate your patient's airway. You can use them, but you should use them cautiously.

45. **The correct answer is (A).** As long as your patient's asthma is not severe, nitrous oxide may be used to relax him.

46. **The correct answer is (B).** Lethargy is not a side effect of Albuterol. Side effects other than those in the answer options include nervousness, sinus inflammation, and vomiting.

47. **The correct answer is (C).** According to this patient's dental chart, he has visible carious lesions on teeth #13 and #29.

48. **The correct answer is (C).** The patient should be allowed to position himself comfortably and should only be in a supine position for a short time.

49. **The correct answer is (C).** Acetaminophen is recommended for asthmatic patients after treatment. Patients taking theophylline should not be given erythromycin or phenobarbitals.

50. **The correct answer is (D).** You should recommend all of the above for your patient to maintain good oral health and avoid additional dental caries.

51. **The correct answer is (A).** Patients with Down syndrome have a higher-than-average risk of developing both periodontal disease and dental caries.

52. **The correct answer is (B).** Patients with Down syndrome should be scheduled early in the morning. They will be more alert and attentive at this time, and this will reduce their waiting time.

53. **The correct answer is (D).** Individuals with Down syndrome usually have smaller-than-average teeth with wide spaces between them.

54. **The correct answer is (C).** You should begin by first seating the patient in the dental chair. If the patient is comfortable, perform the first exam using only your fingers. If the patient is also comfortable with this, move on to dental instruments and then prophylaxis.

55. **The correct answer is (A).** Patients with Down syndrome are not prone to having low blood pressure. They are prone to developing chronic respiratory infections. They are often mouth breathers, which causes them to have xerostomia (dry mouth) and contributes to the development of dental caries.

56. **The correct answer is (D).** Cardiac disorders, hypotonia, and a compromised immune system are all common in persons with Down syndrome.

57. **The correct answer is (C).** A Down syndrome patient usually finds panoramic X-rays less threatening, and these X-rays will clearly show missing teeth.

58. **The correct answer is (A).** Xerostomia, or dry mouth, frequently causes halitosis.

59. **The correct answer is (A).** Sweet foods increase the risk of dental caries, so they should be avoided. Other types of rewards, such as stickers, may be used.

60. **The correct answer is (D).** Patients with Down syndrome frequently have congenitally missing teeth, teeth that have not erupted, and tooth loss due to periodontal disease.

61. **The correct answer is (D).** Based on the patient's symptoms and the observations you make during her examination, the **MOST LIKELY** diagnosis would be occlusal trauma.

62. **The correct answer is (D).** The AAP classification for this disease is Type VIII, which includes developmental or acquired deformities and conditions.

63. **The correct answer is (C).** The most appropriate technique to use to debride this patient's teeth at a maintenance visit would be light ultrasonic scaling and fine scaling as needed. This approach would be in compliance with normal debridement protocol.

64. **The correct answer is (C).** If the patient is bruxing, the recommended treatment would be to fabricate a night-guard appliance, as this would help to keep the patient's teeth apart and relax her muscles while she sleeps.

65. **The correct answer is (A).** A night guard cannot be substituted for a sleep apnea appliance, as these devices are designed to serve two different purposes and are not interchangeable.

66. **The correct answer is (B).** If the patient had a history of previous periodontal disease, her diagnosis would be secondary occlusal trauma, which occurs when there is a traumatic occlusion in a patient who has already had periodontal breakdown.

67. **The correct answer is (C).** Braces would not be an alternative solution for this patient because there is not enough information provided to indicate the patient requires referral to an orthodontist.

68. **The correct answer is (B).** Throbbing of the first molars is not necessarily a clinical indicator of occlusal trauma. Though patients with occlusal trauma may present with throbbing of the first molars, this symptom may alternatively be a sign of a different condition.

69. **The correct answer is (C).** Increasing areas of radiopacity at apices of traumatized teeth would not be a radiographic indicator of occlusal trauma.

70. **The correct answer is (C).** Acute periapical abscess would not be a likely result of occlusal trauma.

71. **The correct answer is (C).** Based on clinical and radiographic findings, this patient's periodontal condition would be diagnosed as healthy.

72. **The correct answer is (D).** All of the given factors may be contributing to the patient's halitosis. Smoking, drinking coffee, and taking certain medications can all exacerbate xerostomia, which is associated with halitosis.

73. **The correct answer is (C).** The best technique to use to polish this patient's teeth at a maintenance visit would be to use an air polisher, as this approach is the most effective for stain removal.

74. **The correct answer is (C).** According to current research, the best way for this patient to reduce her halitosis is tongue scraping. Though the other choices would be helpful, scraping the tongue helps to remove the majority of the microorganisms that cause halitosis.

75. **The correct answer is (A).** When discussing the patient's antidepressant medication, you should be sure to mention that it causes xerostomia, which is a contributing factor to halitosis.

76. **The correct answer is (B).** It has been documented in research that oral malador is exacerbated by xerostomia.

77. **The correct answer is (C).** Although you may suggest the use of candy mints to mask the odor of the patient's halitosis, you should always specifically recommend sugar-free mints.

78. **The correct answer is (B).** Diabetes is a disease that involves the body's ability to manage glucose. Smoking is not directly linked to diabetes.

79. **The correct answer is (A).** Setting a quit date for the patient would not be an effective intervention because it is her decision as to when she will be ready to quit.

80. **The correct answer is (C).** An authoritarian message from the hygienist would not be an effective means of ensuring the patient's adherence to a preventive regiment, because the patient needs to assume responsibility for herself and is more apt to do so if the hygienist allows her to be involved in the decision-making process.

81. **The correct answer is (A).** The diagnosis for this patient's periodontal condition would be gingivitis, as he presents with inflammation and bleeding with no sign of bone loss.

82. **The correct answer is (A).** The AAP classification for this disease is Type I, which is the gingival disease category.

83. **The correct answer is (C).** The appropriate method for debriding this patient's teeth would be ultrasonic scaling and fine scaling, dispersed over two appointments. This would reflect the prescribed protocol for debridement as based on the patient's clinical conditions and periodontal diagnosis.

84. **The correct answer is (C).** The deep pocketing on the distal of the lower second molars is **MOST LIKELY** pseudopocketing, which would be due to the partially impacted lower third molars.

85. **The correct answer is (A).** The Leonard method would not be recommended for this patient because vertical tooth brushing would not be advisable for his condition.

86. **The correct answer is (B).** Although flexibility is desirable, soft toothbrushes are preferable to medium toothbrushes because they are more effective and less traumatic.

87. **The correct answer is (B).** Embrasures that are occupied by the interdental papillae would be classified as Type I.

88. **The correct answer is (D).** Dental floss would be the most effective interdental device for the hygienist to give this patient because it is ideal for Type I embrasures.

89. **The correct answer is (C).** A power oral irrigation device would most help the patient to clean the distal areas of his lower second molars, given the presence of the partially erupted and impacted third molars.

90. **The correct answer is (B).** Based on the patient's level of healing, a maintenance schedule set at 4-month intervals would be recommended due to the presence of the partially impacted lower third molars and their effect on the health of #18 distal and #31 distal.

91. **The correct answer is (D).** Radiographs are not available for this patient and complete periodontal charting is impossible due to the patient's discomfort, calculus, and time constraints. Therefore, it is impossible to make a diagnosis.

92. **The correct answer is (D).** Debridement and localized pain management is the best treatment protocol, since the patient has pain in one area and wants treatment today. Without radiographs or periodontal charting, scaling and root planning cannot be done.

93. **The correct answer is (C).** Although a dental hygienist should be familiar with payment and insurance options, payment issues are handled normally by the office financial manager. In this case in particular, the hygienist should only be concerned with the patient's care and well-being.

94. **The correct answer is (B).** Root planning cannot be done without a diagnosis. In order to make a diagnosis, periodontal charting and radiographs of the entire mouth are required. A recall appointment will have to be scheduled for these procedures.

95. **The correct answer is (D).** Mepivicaine (Carbocaine with or without vasocontrictor) is the best choice because very few patients are allergic

to it. A topical will not give pulpal anesthesia. Esters are not a valid choice, because they have been replaced by amides.

96. **The correct answer is (C).** Debridement offers the best treatment for the patient today to eliminate some discomfort under the time constraints created due to his late arrival.

97. **The correct answer is (D).** Scaling and root planning are not an option during this initial visit because there are no radiographs and no periodontal charting. Due to the time constraints, it will be impossible to gather these necessary components during this visit, and the other options should be examined.

98. **The correct answer is (B).** Polishing agents are abrasive. They are not recommended to be used during this patient visit because of open tissue and sensitivity on #28 distal. There are other treatment options available to this patient, which will yield more desirable results.

99. **The correct answer is (D).** Even though it's been three years, the patient should try the same desensitizing paste again, since he had positive results before. If it doesn't work as well this time, then try a different desensitizing paste.

100. **The correct answer is (B).** Since one tooth is involved, infiltration should provide enough anesthesia to complete treatment on that tooth. Mepivicaine, with or without vasoconstrictor, is recommended because few allergies result from its use and it does not last long. It has less of a vasodilator than lidocaine.

101. **The correct answer is (C).** As a dental hygienist, you need to gain the child's and parent's cooperation using the most professional attitude. Many parents prefer to be in the operatory when their child is being seen. This is allowed as long as the parent does not interfere with treatment.

102. **The correct answer is (D).** Asthma is a concern when giving sedation, nitrous oxide, and local anesthetics. The child is in pain right now, so that is a concern, too. It is important to determine which tooth is bothering the patient and consider it during the radiographic assessment.

103. **The correct answer is (D).** For many children, the first radiographs can be scary. Even though this patient has had them before, it has been awhile. Let the child know that the film has to go in a certain place. Also, tell the patient that you must use the shield by law and that it protects them.

104. **The correct answer is (C).** All new findings for today's visit should be marked in red. Pencil is normally not an acceptable medium to use when marking a chart because it is not permanent.

105. **The correct answer is (C).** All existing restorations should be noted on the chart in blue.

106. **The correct answer is (C).** All current findings are marked in red. Since these were noted today during the examination, they should be marked in red. Blue is used to mark existing findings.

107. **The correct answer is (D).** Explain the process to the parent and the importance of sealing soon after the tooth has completely erupted. Then explain that, for this reason, you would like to seal the teeth that are fully in, and check on the unerupted tooth in 3–6 months.

108. **The correct answer is (D).** Parents worry about invasive procedures. The more you can prepare them, the better it will be for the parent and the patient. Some parents do not understand the importance of restoring baby teeth, because they know eventually they will fall out.

109. **The correct answer is (C).** Children like it if you take things in small steps and talk them through it. Suctioning a little at a time makes them feel in control. Time is of the essence with children since their attention spans are short.

110. **The correct answer is (D).** The new fluoride varnishes are designed to stay on teeth for up to 4 hours. They are sticky, like varnish. Directions say only soft foods should be consumed, no brushing or hot drinks during the 4 hours following treatment.

111. **The correct answer is (B).** Hygienists have a special responsibility to parents of small children to make both patient and parents comfortable. By explaining why you need information and the reason for taking the steps you are taking, you will earn the trust of parents and young patients.

112. **The correct answer is (D).** It is important to be prepared especially when dealing with a patient who is anxious and at risk for problems during the procedure. This patient's blood pressure is elevated while at rest and he takes antidepressant medication. It is important to reduce his anxiety as much as possible.

113. **The correct answer is (D).** Body weight is a consideration for administering local anesthetic drugs. However, in this case, the patient's body weight is not a consideration for overdose of the drug. Only one quadrant is being anesthetized. Therefore, the limited dosage is not a problem.

114. **The correct answer is (D).** There is a visible white marking on #30 d on the radiograph. This indicates a visible carious lesion and should be marked on the patient's dental chart as such. A recall plan will also need to be made to have the lesion taken care of.

115. **The correct answer is (D).** Never attempt to remove a crown. That decision is up to the doctor and beyond your scope of practice. Your treatment may improve the patient's condition, and he will be able to retain the tooth as is. Do instrument the tooth surfaces to the best of your ability to enhance the best postoperative evaluation.

116. **The correct answer is (C).** The only thing that has been proven is that mechanical debridement is an important component of treatment for chronic periodontitis. Even though both the traditional quadrant approach and the newer full-mouth debridement approach are both equally effective, most professionals continue to use the quadrant method of debridement.

117. **The correct answer is (D).** The IANB, L gives anesthesia with fewer site injections, less anxiety, and less drug needed to achieve pulpal anesthesia. The entire quadrant can be free from pain with two injections, not multiple infiltrations.

118. **The correct answer is (C).** Mepivicaine and carbocaine come with or without vasoconstrictor. While this drug has less vasodilation than lidocaine, it is still recommended without any vasoconstriction for this patient who has risk.

119. **The correct answer is (D).** A vasoconstrictor lengthens your working time. It has been determined that no vasoconstrictor is being used, so working time is much shorter. IANB will reduce patient risk by using less drug with fewer injection sites resulting in reduced anxiety.

120. **The correct answer is (D).** It is important to use both ultrasonic and hand-held instruments to achieve optimum results. It is also important to adapt to the root surfaces to remove toxins, and check surfaces with an explorer for residual calculus deposits. It is also important to remove stain, calculus, and debris.

121. **The correct answer is (C).** One or two sites requires Arestin placement. Atridox is used for many sites and you will be delivering the antibiotic to one or two sites. Chlorhexadine rinses or irrigation is not an antibiotic, nor is hydrogen peroxide.

122. **The correct answer is (B).** The patient may resume flossing all teeth other than sites that have been treated. Flossing facilitates the healing process. However, it is recommended that the local delivery site not be flossed for a few days so as not to disturb the site.

123. **The correct answer is (D).** The patient's body weight is low. Therefore, your only concern is the maximum dosage of the drug. Consult maximum dosage charts that match dosage in mg/lb to body weight.

124. **The correct answer is (B).** Mepivicaine gives 20-40 minutes of pulpal working time without vasoconstrictor. This is longer than lidocaine. Mepivicaine gives 60 minutes of pulpal working time with vasoconstrictor, and 3–5 hours of soft-tissue anesthesia.

125. **The correct answer is (D).** Subgingival irrigation, though not used much, helps sites not receiving local delivery antibiotics. Local delivery antibiotics are used in pockets 5 mm or deeper.

126. **The correct answer is (C).** IANB, L will give anesthesia using the least amount of drug and the fewest needle sticks. The entire quadrant will be free of pain with two injections. The other options will not have so profound an effect because the patient has pocketing in the molars and deep, tenacious calculus.

127. **The correct answer is (C).** Vasodilation is preferred because there will be less bleeding during

the procedure. Since this is the patient's first time having any dental procedure, ease is important.

128. **The correct answer is (D).** Good scaling and planing skills require using both ultrasonic and hand-held instruments; removing all stain, calculus, and debris; checking surfaces with an explorer for residual calculus deposits; and adapting to root surfaces to remove toxins. The only accurate answer is adapting to root surfaces to remove toxins.

129. **The correct answer is (D).** Arestin is made for local site delivery in up to two sites. It would be the best choice for this procedure. Although Atridox is used in multiple sites, it is costly if used in only two.

130. **The correct answer is (B).** The patient may immediately floss the teeth that were not affected by today's treatment. In fact, flossing facilitates the healing process. The patient can resume flossing local delivery sites in a few days.

131. **The correct answer is (D).** This patient needs to continue scaling and planing procedures and should schedule the appointments for this. The quadrant that was worked on today also needs to be reevaluated and monitored in approximately 6 weeks. In 3 months, further charting and periodontal maintenance are also required.

132. **The correct answer is (C).** Radiographs were taken before the initial therapy and were available for previous diagnosis. The purpose of today's visit is for reevaluation, and the patient is not due for new radiographs.

133. **The correct answer is (A).** Assessment of dental caries is part of the dental examination with restorative and prosthetic evaluation. All other choices are part of a periodontal charting examination.

134. **The correct answer is (D).** Hygienists should constantly monitor every patient's progress by marking their findings. From there, the hygienist can assess and retreat the patient if necessary.

135. **The correct answer is (A).** Brushing at a 45-degree angle will ensure optimum results when combined with the other suggested options. When making suggestions to patients, hygienists must first address any problems in self-reported oral hygiene regimens.

136. **The correct answer is (D).** The patient has reported that he has been following your oral hygiene regime instructions and the numbers have improved. The patient will still be monitored, however, every 3 months for the next year.

137. **The correct answer is (D).** Vitamins are helpful in maintaining good overall health and dental health. However, the site that is bleeding is **MOST LIKELY** not from a vitamin deficiency.

138. **The correct answer is (D).** All of the responses are acceptable and truthful. Although the patient is feeling better, and the scaling and planing procedure was successful, monitoring for at least a year is necessary to treat any further infections.

139. **The correct answer is (C).** The patient should be seen every 3 months for the first year, not every month. All of the other scenarios are acceptable based on this patient's presentation.

140. **The correct answer is (A).** Applying desensitizing agents will alleviate some of the patient's discomfort after the scaling and planing procedure. It is always good to tell the patient to call with any problems regarding sensitivity, discomfort, and excessive bleeding.

141. **The correct answer is (A).** Both the statement and reason are correct and related. Radiographs are important tools for determining whether treatment has been successful and whether or not any other follow-up treatments will be necessary. Radiographs taken prior to the procedure will be helpful when comparing the level of improvement.

142. **The correct answer is (D).** If a tooth is not responding, or a new pocket suddenly develops which is deeper, a periapical X-ray should be taken to determine the cause of this sudden increase. Regardless of whether the problem is endodontic or periodontic, it is necessary to consider the sudden increase to determine the appropriate intervention.

143. **The correct answer is (B).** Dentures should be brushed after each meal, and at the very least, every day. This includes the clasp. Dentures should be placed in warm water when taken out, not hot water. Hot water will distort the base.

144. **The correct answer is (B).** Based on the patient's dentures, the flat, red lesion is **MOST LIKELY**

erythematous candidiasis, which is a fungus typically found under dentures or on the mucous membranes of the tongue.

145. **The correct answer is (A).** Normal protocol recommends you retake the patient's blood pressure in 5 minutes. Based on her medical background, she presents with anxiety, which could be elevating her blood pressure. Her blood pressure reading is within the guidelines to be taken again.

146. **The correct answer is (D).** Hyperkeratosis is a localized chronic irritation that is whitish or paler than normal anywhere in the oral cavity. The patient stated that her tooth hurt, and upon examination you noticed beneath the partial was red with white on the mandibular ridge.

147. **The correct answer is (C).** Calculus should be removed from the denture. However, an abrasive dentifrice should not be used. Extreme care should be taken to not scratch a prosthetic because scratches house bacteria and may lead to gingival disease.

148. **The correct answer is (A).** There are several different sizes of Gracey curets. The 1/2 is used to remove subgingival calculus while the 7/8 curet is used for the facial and lingual surfaces of posterior teeth. The 11/12 curet is used for the mesial aspect of posterior teeth.

149. **The correct answer is (D).** This patient is not at a risk for caries because she does not have any natural teeth in tact. Normally, infrequent denture removal places a patient at a high risk for caries.

150. **The correct answer is (B).** The patient's partial is 15 years old. The irritation may be due to the age of the partial because the fit may have changed, and the partial may be interfering with the lesion. Osteoporosis was not mentioned in the patient's medical history, so it cannot be assumed that the patient has this condition simply because of her age.

APPENDIXES

Other Careers in Dentistry

In addition to dental hygienists, the dental industry is composed of many professionals dedicated to promoting oral health. There are many career opportunities within the field of dentistry. Some careers require more schooling than others. The following provides an overview of the most common careers in dentistry.

DENTISTS

Dentists are trained to recognize and treat a number of oral diseases and conditions. These highly trained professionals also work to promote good oral hygiene practices among their patients. Most dentists obtain a bachelor's degree before attending dental school. After completing a four-year program, dentists must pass an examination to receive a license to practice in a particular state. Some state boards require dentists to complete a minimum number of hours of continuing education before they can renew their licenses. Dentists who focus on special areas of expertise may require additional training and continuing education courses.

ORTHODONTISTS

Orthodontists are dental professionals who specialize in the recognition and correction of malocclusions, or improper bites. In addition to diagnosing malocclusions, orthodontists often design and create special appliances, such as braces or retainers, which help correct the alignment of the teeth. Many orthodontists receive a bachelor's degree before enrolling in dental school. After completing their four years of dental training, orthodontists usually spend two to three years enrolled in a full-time orthodontics program. To become licensed orthodontists, candidates must submit an application, pass a written examination, and pass a clinical examination.

PROSTHODONTISTS

Prosthodontists specialize in the restoration or replacement of teeth. Replacement of teeth may involve the use of permanent fixtures, such as crowns and dental implants, or removable fixtures, such as dentures. After graduating from dental school, prosthodontists receive additional training at hospitals or universities with programs accredited by the American Dental Association. Prosthodontists are also trained to treat traumatic injuries to the mouth, congenital abnormalities of the teeth or support structures, and sleep disorders, such as snoring.

ORAL AND MAXILLOFACIAL SURGEONS

Oral and maxillofacial surgeons are trained to perform surgery on the mouth, jaw, head, and neck structures to extract teeth, remove tumors, and correct abnormalities of these structures. Following dental school, candidates must complete a four- to six-year surgical residency that focuses on the maxillofacial region. Candidates also receive training in anesthesia, internal medicine, and emergency medicine. All candidates must pass a certifying examination to receive a license to practice.

EXPANDED FUNCTION DENTAL AUXILIARY/ASSISTANTS (EFDA)

An expanded function dental auxiliary/assistant (EFDA) is a dental assistant who can perform additional duties, such as placing restorations (fillings) after the dentist has prepped a tooth. Candidates must complete a specialized course to receive certification as an EFDA. Not all states allow dental assistants to receive certification as EFDAs. Check with your state board to see if it recognizes EFDAs.

DENTAL ASSISTANTS AND CERTIFIED DENTAL ASSISTANTS (CDA)

Dental assistants should not be confused with dental hygienists as they perform a different yet important set of clinical tasks. Most dental assistants are responsible for sterilizing and disinfecting instruments, preparing materials to treat patients, and obtaining and updating patient dental records. Dental assistants also help during dental procedures by handing the dentist instruments and suctioning the patient's mouth to keep it dry and clear. In some states, no formal training is required for entry-level dental assistants. Other states require dental assistants to complete licensing programs to receive certification. Certified dental assistants (CDAs) must complete an accredited dental assisting program before taking the certified dental assistant examination administered by the Dental Assisting National Board.

DENTAL LAB TECHNICIANS

Dental lab technicians work behind the scenes to create crowns, bridges, and dentures from impressions taken in the dentist's office. The dental lab technician then uses these impressions to create a model of the patient's mouth. This model helps the technician create the needed apparatus. Training requirements vary, but most dental lab technicians have completed high school and a one-year certification program. Some states require dental lab technicians to take continuing education courses.

Accredited Dental Education Programs by State

ALASKA

University of Alaska Anchorage
UAA Dental Hygiene Program
3211 Providence Drive
Allied Health Sciences, Room 160
Anchorage, AK 99508
Phone: 907-786-6925
Fax: 907-786-6938
www.uaa.alaska.edu

ARIZONA

Northern Arizona University
Department of Dental Hygiene
Health Professions Building, Room 202
P.O. Box 15065
Flagstaff, AZ 86011-5065
Phone: 520-523-5122
http://home.nau.edu

CALIFORNIA

Loma Linda University
School of Dentistry
Dental Hygiene Department
11092 Anderson Street
Loma Linda, CA 92354
Phone: 909-558-4631
www.llu.edu/dentistry/dentalhygiene/index.page

University of Southern California, Los Angeles
School of Dentistry
925 West 34th Street, Room 4313
Los Angeles, CA 90089
Phone: 213-740-1089
Fax: 213-740-1094
www.usc.edu

CONNECTICUT

University of Bridgeport
Fones School of Dental Hygiene
Division of Health Sciences
60 Lafayette Street
Bridgeport, CT 06604
Phone: 203-576-4138
Fax: 203-576-4220
www.bridgeport.edu/academics/fonesschool

University of New Haven
College of Arts and Sciences
Dental Hygiene Program
419 Boston Post Road
West Haven, CT 06516-1916
Phone: 203-931-6005
Fax: 203-931-6083
www.newhaven.edu

FLORIDA

Nova Southeastern University
College of Allied Health and Nursing
Bachelor of Health Science Program
3200 North University Drive
Ft. Lauderdale, FL 33314-7796
Phone: 954-288-9695
Fax: 954-262-1181
www.nova.edu/bhs

St. Petersburg College
College of Health Sciences
Dental Hygiene Program
7200 66th Street North
Pinellas Park, FL 33781
Phone: 727-341-4150
Fax: 727-341-4152
www.spcollege.edu/bachelors/dental

GEORGIA

Armstrong Atlantic State University
College of Health Professions
Dental Hygiene
11935 Abercorn Street
Savannah, GA 31419-1997
Phone: 912-344-2585
www.armstrong.edu

Clayton State University
College of Health
Dental Hygiene
2000 Clayton State Boulevard
Morrow, GA 30260-0285
Phone: 678-466-4905
http://healthsci.clayton.edu/DH/default.htm

Medical College of Georgia
School of Allied Health Sciences
Department of Dental Hygiene
1120 15th Street, AD 3103
Augusta, GA 30912-0200
Phone: 706-721-2938
Fax: 706-721-8857
www.georgiahealth.edu/

ILLINOIS

Southern Illinois University Carbondale
Dental Hygiene
School of Allied Health
College of Applied Sciences and Arts
Mail Code 6615
Carbondale, IL 62901-6615
Phone: 618-453-8869
www.sah.siuc.edu/DH/home.htm

INDIANA

Indiana University School of Dentistry
Periodontics and Allied Dental Programs
Dental Hygiene Programs
1121 West Michigan Street
Indianapolis, IN 46202
Phone: 317-274-7801
www.iusd.iupui.edu

Indiana University South Bend
College of Health Sciences
Dental Hygiene Program
1700 Mishawaka Avenue
P.O. Box 7111
South Bend, IN 46634-7111
Phone: 574-520-4405
www.iusb.edu/~sbdental/

University of Southern Indiana
College of Nursing and Health Professions
Dental Hygiene Program
8600 University Boulevard
Evansville, IN 47712-3596
Phone: 812-464-1702
Fax: 812-465-7092
www.usi.edu/health/acadprog/dhy/default.asp

IOWA

Iowa Western CC/Creighton University
School of Dentistry
Dental Hygiene
2700 College Road
Council Bluffs, IA 51503
Phone: 712-325-3200
www.iwcc.edu

KANSAS

Wichita State University
College of Health Professions
Dental Hygiene Department
1845 Fairmount
Wichita, KS 67260
Phone: 316-978-3456
www.wichita.edu/dh

KENTUCKY

Western Kentucky University
Allied Health and Human Services
Dental Hygiene Program
1906 College Heights Boulevard
Bowling Green, KY 42101
Phone: 270-745-3827
www.wku.edu

LOUISIANA

University of Louisiana at Monroe
College of Health Sciences
Department of Dental Hygiene
700 University Avenue
Monroe, LA 71209-0420
Phone: 318-342-1621
www.ulm.edu/dentalhygiene/

MAINE

University of Maine at Augusta
College of Mathematics and Professional Studies
Dental Hygiene Program
1 University Drive
Bangor, ME 04401-4331
Phone: 207-262-7876
Fax: 207-262-7871
www.uma.maine.edu

University of New England
College of Health Professions
Dental Hygiene Program
716 Stevens Avenue
Portland, ME 04103-2670
Phone: 207-221-4314
www.une.edu

MARYLAND

University of Maryland, Baltimore
Dental School
Dental Hygiene Program
650 West Baltimore Street
Baltimore, MD 21201
Phone: 410-706-7773
www.dental.umaryland.edu

MASSACHUSETTS

Massachusetts College of Pharmacy & Health Sciences
Forsyth School of Dental Hygiene
Master of Science in Dental Health
179 Longwood Avenue
Boston, MA 02115-5896
Phone: 617-879-5987
www.mcphs.edu/academics/programs/dental_hygiene

MICHIGAN

Ferris State University
Allied Health Sciences
200 Ferris Drive, VFS 210
Big Rapids, MI 49307
Phone: 231-591-2270
www.ferris.edu/

University of Detroit Mercy
School of Dentistry
Dental Hygiene Program
2700 Martin Luther King Jr. Boulevard
Detroit, MI 48208-2576
Phone: 313-494-6611
http://dental.udmercy.edu/

University of Michigan
School of Dentistry
Dental Hygiene Program
1011 North University Avenue, Room 3066
Ann Arbor, MI 48109-1078
Phone: 734-763-3392
Fax: 734-763-5503
www.dent.umich.edu/

MINNESOTA

Metropolitan State University
College of Nursing and Health Sciences
Dental Hygiene Program
700 East Seventh Street
St. Paul, MN 55106-5000
Phone: 651-793-1375
Fax: 651-793-1382
www.metrostate.edu/cnhs

Minnesota State University, Mankato
Department of Dental Hygiene
3 Morris Hall
Mankato, MN 56001
Phone: 507-389-1313
Fax: 507-389-5850
ahn.mnsu.edu/dental/

University of Minnesota, Twin Cities
School of Dentistry
Moos Health Sciences Tower
515 Delaware Street SE
Minneapolis, MN 55455-0213
Phone: 612-625-7477
http://www.dentistry.umn.edu/

MISSOURI

University of Missouri-Kansas City
School of Dentistry
Dental Hygiene Program
650 East 25th Street
Kansas City, MO 64108
Phone: 816-235-2100
http://dentistry.umkc.edu

NEVADA

College of Southern Nevada
School of Health Sciences
Dental Hygiene Program—W1a
6375 West Charleston Boulevard
Las Vegas, NV 89146
Phone: 702-651-5853
Fax: 702-651-7401
http://sites.csn.edu/health/dental/dental-hygiene(bs)
.html

NEW JERSEY

University of Medicine & Dentistry of New Jersey
School of Health Related Professions
Baccalaureate Program—SHRP
65 Bergen Street
Newark, NJ 07107
Phone: 973-972-8512
http://shrp.umdnj.edu/

NEW MEXICO

University of New Mexico
Health Sciences Center
Division of Dental Hygiene
Novitski Hall
MSC09 5020
1 University of New Mexico
Albuquerque, NM 87131-2039
Phone: 505-272-4513
www.unm.edu/

NEW YORK

Farmingdale State College of New York
School of Health Sciences
Department of Dental Hygiene
2350 Broadhollow Road
Farmingdale, NY 11735-1021
Phone: 631-420-2000
www.farmingdale.edu/

New York University
College of Dentistry
Dental Hygiene Program
345 East 24th Street
New York, NY 10010
Phone: 212-992-9800
www.nyu.edu/dental

SUNY at Canton
Dental Hygiene Program
34 Cornell Drive
Canton, NY 13617
Phone: 315-386-7011
www.canton.edu/sci_health/dhyg/

NORTH CAROLINA

**The University of North Carolina
School of Dentistry**
Dental Hygiene Program
3220 Old Dental Building
Chapel Hill, NC 27599-7450
Phone: 919-966-2800
www.dentistry.unc.edu/

OHIO

Ohio State University
College of Dentistry
Division of Dental Hygiene
305 West 12th Avenue
Columbus, OH 43210
Phone: 614-292–2401
www.dent.osu.edu/dhy

Youngstown State University
Bitonte College of Health and Human Services
Health Professions Bachelor's in Applied Science
One University Plaza
Youngstown, OH 44555-0001
Phone: 330-941-2000
www.ysu.edu

OREGON

Pacific University
School of Dental Health Science
Degree Completion Program
190 Southeast 8th Avenue, Suite 181
Hillsboro, OR 97123
Phone: 503-352-2900
www.pacificu.edu/dentalhealth

PENNSYLVANIA

Pennsylvania College of Technology
School of Health Sciences
Dental Hygiene Program
One College Avenue
Williamsport, PA 17701-5778
Phone: 570-320-8007
www.pct.edu

University of Pittsburgh
School of Dental Medicine
Salk Hall
3501 Terrace Street
Pittsburgh, PA 15261
Phone: 412-648-8432
www.dental.pitt.edu

TENNESSEE

East Tennessee State University
College of Clinical and Rehabilitative Health Sciences
Department of Allied Health Sciences
P.O. Box 70690
Johnson City, TN 37614-0690
www.etsu.edu/crhs/alliedhealth/bsdh

Tennessee State University
College of Health Sciences
Department of Dental Hygiene
3500 John A. Merritt Boulevard
Nashville, TN 37209-1561
Phone: 615-963-5000
www.tnstate.edu

University of Tennessee Health Science Center
College of Allied Health Sciences
Department of Dental Hygiene
930 Madison Avenue, Suite 600
Memphis, TN 38163
Phone: 901-448-6230
www.uthsc.edu/allied/dh/

TEXAS

Baylor College of Dentistry
Caruth School of Dental Hygiene
Texas A&M Health Science Center
3302 Gaston Avenue
Dallas, TX 75246
Phone: 214-828-8100
www.bcd.tamhsc.edu

Texas Woman's University
College of Health Sciences
Dental Hygiene Program
P.O. Box 425796
Denton, TX 76204-5796
Phone: 940-898-2870
www.twu.edu/hs/dh

University of Texas Health Science Center at Houston
Dental Branch
School of Dental Hygiene
6516 M. D. Anderson Boulevard, Suite 155
Houston, TX 77030
Phone: 713-500-4151
Fax: 713-500-4425
www.db.uth.tmc.edu

University of Texas Health Science Center at San Antonio
School of Health Professions
Department of Dental Hygiene
7703 Floyd Curl Drive
San Antonio, TX 78229-3900
Phone: 210-567-8820
Fax: 210-567-8843
www.uthscsa.edu/shp/dh/bachelor-completion.asp

UTAH

Dixie State College of Utah
Division of Nursing and Allied Health
Dental Hygiene Program
225 South 700 East
St. George, UT 84770-3876
Phone: 435-652-7500
www.dixie.edu

Weber State University
College of Health Professions
Dental Hygiene
Marriott Health Building, Room 475
Ogden, UT 84408-3920
Phone: 801-626-6130
Fax: 801-626-7304
www.weber.edu/dentalhyg

VERMONT

Vermont Technical College
School of Nursing and Allied Health
Dental Hygiene Department
301 Lawrence Place
Williston, VT 05495
Phone: 802-879-5632
www.vtc.edu

VIRGINIA

Old Dominion University
Gene W. Hirschfield School of Dental Hygiene
College of Health Sciences
4608 Hampton Boulevard
Health Science Building, Room 2011
Norfolk, VA 23529
Phone: 757-683-5235
http://hs.odu.edu/dental

WASHINGTON

Clark College/Eastern Washington University
Dental Hygiene Department
310 North Riverpoint Boulevard, Suite 160
Spokane, WA 99202
Phone: 509-828-1300
Fax: 509-828-1283
www.ewu.edu

University of Washington (South Campus)
Dental Hygiene
1959 Northeast Pacific Street
Health Sciences Building B-509
Seattle, WA 98195-7475
Phone: 206-543-5820
Fax: 206-685-4258
http://depts.washington.edu/dhyg/

WEST VIRGINIA

West Liberty University
School of Science/Health Sciences Department
Dental Hygiene Program
P.O. Box 295
West Liberty, WV 26074
Phone: 304-336-8030
www.westliberty.edu

West Virginia University
School of Dentistry
Division of Dental Hygiene
P.O. Box 9400
Morgantown, WV 26506-9400
Phone: 304-293-3417
www.hsc.wvu.edu/sod

DENTAL SPECIALTY CERTIFYING BOARDS

American Board of Dental Public Health
3085 Stevenson Drive, Suite 200
Springfield, IL 62703
Phone: 217-529-6941
Fax: 217-529-9120
www.aaphd.org/

American Board of Endodontists
211 East Chicago Avenue, Suite 1100
Chicago, IL 60611-2691
Phone: 800-872-3636
www.aae.org

American Board of Oral and Maxillofacial Pathology
P.O. Box 25915
Tampa, FL 33622-5915
Phone: 813-286-2444, Ext. 230
Fax: 813-289-5279

American Board of Oral and Maxillofacial Radiology
P.O. Box 231422
New York, NY 10023
www.aaomr.org/

American Board of Oral and Maxillofacial Surgery
625 North Michigan Avenue, Suite 1820
Chicago, IL 60611
Phone: 312-642-0070
Fax: 312-642-8584
www.aboms.org/

The American Board of Orthodontics
401 North Lindbergh Boulevard, Suite 300
St Louis, MO 63141-7839
Phone: 314-432-6130
Fax: 314-432-8170
www.americanboardortho.com/

American Board of Pediatric Dentistry
325 East Washington Street, Suite 208
Iowa City, IA 52240-3959
Phone: 319-341-8488
Fax: 319-341-9499
www.abpd.org/

American Board of Periodontology
4157 Mountain Road, PBN 249
Pasadena, MD 21122
Phone: 410-437-3749
Fax: 410-437-4021
www.abperio.org/

American Board of Prosthodontics
P.O. Box 271894
West Hartford, CT 06127-1894
Phone: 860-679-2649
Fax: 860-206-1169
www.prosthodontics.org/abp/

SPECIAL ADVERTISING SECTION

University of Medicine & Dentistry of New Jersey
Thomas Jefferson University School of Population Health
Saint Louis University John Cook School of Business
St. Mary's University Bill Greehey School of Business
The Winston Preparatory Schools

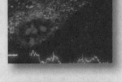
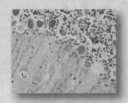
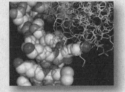
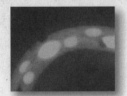
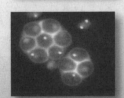
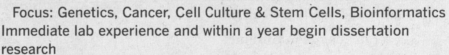
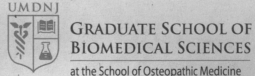
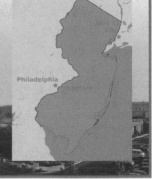

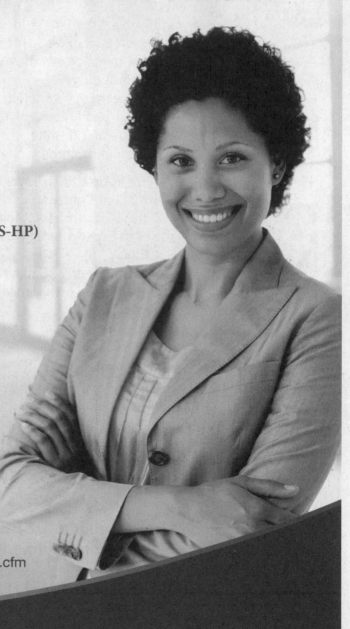
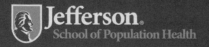

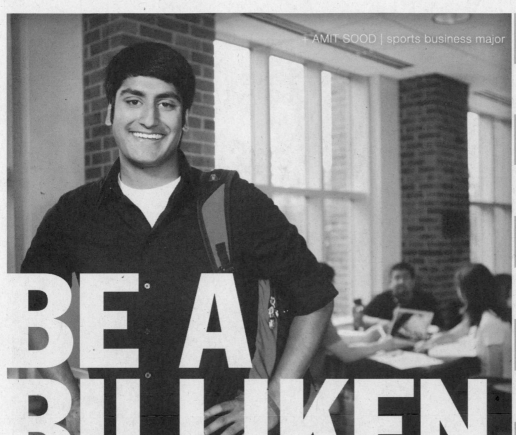

+ AMIT SOOD | sports business major

BE A BILLIKEN

Find out how the breadth and depth of the fully accredited undergraduate and graduate programs at Saint Louis University's **JOHN COOK SCHOOL OF BUSINESS** will give you the knowledge and tools necessary for success in today's global and highly technical business world.

— + Visit **BeABilliken.com** for more information on our undergraduate business programs and to see what life is like as a Billiken.

To learn about our graduate business programs, attend an open house or visit **gradbiz.slu.edu.** + —————

SAINT LOUIS UNIVERSITY

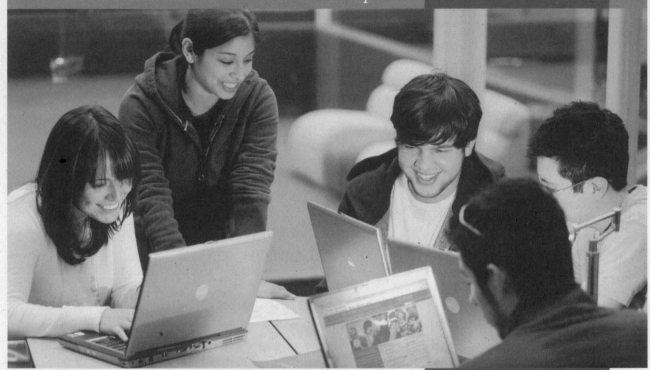

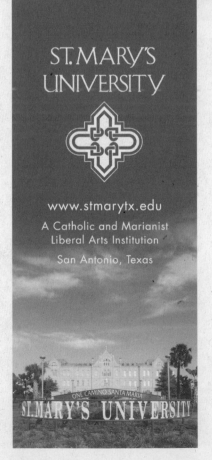

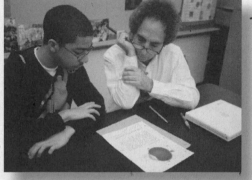
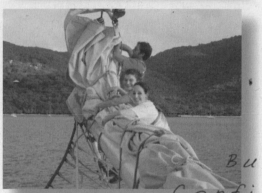
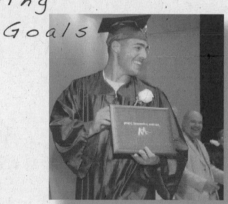
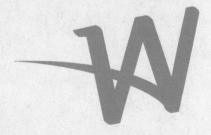

NOTES